# The Profit Motive and Patient Care

*A Twentieth Century Fund Report*

The Twentieth Century Fund is a research foundation undertaking timely analyses of economic, political, and social issues. Not-for-profit and nonpartisan, the Fund was founded in 1919 and endowed by Edward A. Filene.

# The Profit Motive and Patient Care

## The Changing Accountability of Doctors and Hospitals

BRADFORD H. GRAY

*A Twentieth Century Fund Report*
Harvard University Press
Cambridge, Massachusetts
London, England
1991

Copyright © 1991 by the Twentieth Century Fund, Inc.
All rights reserved
Printed in the United States of America
10 9 8 7 6 5 4 3 2 1

This book is printed on acid-free paper, and its binding materials have been chosen for strength and durability.

*Library of Congress Cataloging-in-Publication Data*

Gray, Bradford H., 1942–
    The profit motive and patient care : the changing accountability of doctors and hospitals / Bradford H. Gray.
        p.   cm.
    "A Twentieth Century Fund report."
    Includes index.
    ISBN 0-674-71337-0 (alk. paper)
    1. Medical economics–United States. 2. Hospitals–United States–Business management. 3. Medical care—United States. I. Title.
    [DNLM: 1. Delivery of Health Care—trends—United States. 2. Economics, Hospital—trends—United States. 3. Economics, Medical—trends—United States. 4. Financial Management—trends—United States. 5. Hospitals—trends—United States.
                                                                                    WX 157
G778p]
RA410.53.G73   1991
338.4'73621'0973—dc20
DNLM/DLC
for Library of Congress
                                                                            90-5119
                                                                               CIP

*To Helen*

# Contents

# Foreword

Americans pay more for health care than any other people in the world. Yet the cost is continuing to increase at a rate in excess of the growth of the economy and the rate of inflation. Not surprisingly, at a time when belief in market forces has achieved near religious status, many have seen changing the structure of health care services as a route to cost containment. Perhaps even more troubling is the fact that all this spending does not buy better health care. Why, for example, is our infant mortality rate so embarrassingly high? And what, if anything, can be done about the uninsured and underinsured? These are the sorts of questions that dominate the national dialogue, but are they, in fact, too broad?

Perhaps some of the answers to the high cost and the qualitative deficiencies of the U.S. health system lie in the conditions under which medical decisions are made on a day-to-day basis, particularly as they affect profitability. The health care field today includes a large group of new players—entrepreneurs large and small whose health care companies have brought about a transformation in the American health care system. In the past, those who provided health care were presumed to be governed by their belief in a set of ethical and social responsibilities that took precedence over economic concerns. Whether or not they all lived up to that ideal, it is clear that today, physicians are being pushed to take into consideration not only patients' needs but also the financial ramifications of treatment. Today, some hospital administrators are accountable to profit-oriented headquarters rather than local, community-oriented boards; state regulators are no longer monitoring purely local institutions but multi-institutional chains that span many different communities in different states; and third-party payers are trying to impose limits and conditions on levels of expenditures based on criteria other than altruism, professionalism, and an orientation toward service on the part of health care providers.

As a result, the mechanisms of accountability that were appropriate to an industry comprised largely of medical professionals and nonprofit institutions have been augmented by mechanisms appropriate to the corporate world. The system thus has to be modified to take account of the imperatives of corporate management, shareholders, and the investment community. The new, evolving accountability is complex, involving formal structures and regulations. The question is whether the new accountability systems being pieced together can ensure that public as well as private and professional interests will be served.

Put another way, what happens to the ideals of community service, trust, and professionalism that have long been associated with those who provide our health care in a world in which financial performance is being increasingly demanded of health care institutions by those who provide capital and those third-party payers, both private and governmental, who pick up much of the costs of service?

In an attempt to answer these complex and difficult questions, Bradford Gray, currently professor of public health at the Yale School of Medicine and director of the Yale Program on Non-Profit Organizations, who directed several studies over a decade at the Institute of Medicine and served as a special consultant to the President's Commission for the Study of Ethical Problems in Medicine and Biomedical and Behavioral Research, has provided us with this insightful analysis of the critical issue of how we as a nation should handle questions of accountability in health care.

It is the first of a series of studies on health issues that the Fund is sponsoring for publication, and we are grateful to him for it.

*Richard C. Leone, Director*
*The Twentieth Century Fund*

# Preface

This book is an analysis of the American health care system during a period of rapid change. In many different ways the profit motive—on the part of organizational providers of health care, suppliers of their capital, physicians, employers who provide health benefits for employees, and organizations that administer health benefit plans and monitor the performance of health care providers—has come to shape the behavior of all parties. An ethos that emphasizes trust, community service, professional autonomy, and devotion to the interests of individual patients is being replaced by undisguised self-interest, commercialization, competition, and the management of care by third parties. For the remainder of the century, these shifts will shape how providers and purchasers of services respond to the two great accountability problems that characterize health care: the vulnerability of the person who needs services and the absence of the payer at the point of service.

Although the roots of these changes go back many years, my main focus is on the 1980s. The decade began symbolically with the publication of Arnold Relman's article "The New Medical Industrial Complex" in the *New England Journal of Medicine* (October 23, 1980), which called alarmed attention to the growing presence of for-profit organizations among hospitals and other providers of health care. The decade closed with the passage of legislation funding a major research effort to assess the outcomes of the treatments being provided for common medical conditions and with the creation of an organization to develop standards and an accreditation process for utilization management programs, in which third-party payers or their agents become involved in physicians' patient care decisions. The decade began with signs of disquiet about the role of for-profit organizations as providers of medical services and, ironically, ended with skepticism about the legitimacy of nonprofit hospitals (particularly their tax exemptions), with rampant evidence of distrust of physicians, and with attempts to manage the health care system by third-party payers.

With health care costs in the United States now approaching $700 billion annually—about 12 percent of our gross national product—it is not surprising that money is central to the changes that have swept health care. Financial performance is demanded of health care institutions by the providers of their capital, and third-party payers (both governmental and private) have used their control over the flow of dollars to implement ever more specific mechanisms of formal accountability. Notwithstanding my attention to the role of the profit motive in shaping the health care system, however, this book is rooted more in the field of sociology than economics. My concern throughout is how social arrangements, including economic incentives, are affecting the behavior and mutual perceptions of the different parties.

For much of the past decade, I worked on these issues as the director of the Institute of Medicine's (IOM) studies on for-profit health care and on utilization management by third parties. The first draft of this book was written between these two projects. I owe major intellectual debts to the members of the two committees with whom I worked on those studies, particularly Walter McNerney, who chaired the Committee on For-Profit Enterprise in Health Care, and Richard Egdahl, who chaired the Committee on Utilization Management by Third Parties through much of its life, but also Jerry Grossman, Alex Capron, Bob Derzon, Eliot Freidson, Jack Moxley, Uwe Reinhardt, Arnold Relman, Steve Schroeder, Steve Shortell, Rosemary Stevens, Jim Todd, and Dan Wikler from the for-profit study committee, and Bob Berenson, John Burns, John Eisenberg, Paul Gertman, Alice Gosfield, Nat Hershey, Arnie Milstein, Alan Nelson, and Bob Patricelli from the utilization management study. That list, it should be noted, includes practicing physicians, health care administrators, practicing attorneys, and corporate executives, as well as scholars in law, economics, philosophy, history, sociology, and health services research. All of those perspectives have influenced this book; I hope I have done them reasonable justice.

My tenure at the Institute of Medicine was bracketed by the presidencies of David A. Hamburg and Samuel O. Thier, two remarkable men who moved from distinguished careers in academic medicine to become, through the force of their intellect, energy, and character, major national and international leaders in the field of health care. One learns from such people in ways that are both obvious and subtle.

I also owe many debts to colleagues and coworkers on the IOM staff, particularly Karl Yordy, director of the Division of Health Care Services, Eileen Connor, Marilyn Field, Kathy Lohr, Dick Rettig, Susan Sherman, and Jessica Townsend. Don Tiller brought great skill to the preparation and revision of the manuscript and patiently taught me an unfamiliar word processing program, consulting with me on its perplexities after I moved to New Haven.

I also want to express appreciation to many busy people who took my calls, shared their knowledge, located materials, and sometimes even did research to help me. This occurred over many years, so the list will inevitably be incomplete, but I particularly want to thank Peter Kralovek, Ross Mullner, and Paul Rettig of the American Hospital Association, James Todd and Lynn Jensen of the American Medical Association, Steve Long of the Congressional Budget Office, Janet Kline and Michael O'Grady of the Congressional Research Service, Samuel Mitchell of the Federation of American Healthcare Systems, Marsha Gold of the Group Health Association of America, Richard Merritt of the Intergovernmental Health Policy Project at George Washington University, Judy Miller Jones of the National Health Policy Forum, Bruce Steinwald of the Prospective Payment Assessment Commission, and James A. Simpson of the Western Center for the Health Professions, Inc.

I would also like to thank the ten hospitals that welcomed the site visit teams during the IOM study of for-profit health care, the twelve utilization management organizations that hosted site visits during the IOM study on that topic, and the committee and staff members who accompanied me on those extraordinarily educational visits; Thomas Frist, Jr., and Merlin K. DuVal for their role in making the IOM study of for-profit health care possible; Richard Sharpe of the John A. Hartford Foundation for intellectual and financial support at crucial stages of both the for-profit and utilization management studies at the IOM; David A. Jones for his time and the time of senior executives of Humana, Inc., during my 1987 visit to that company's corporate offices; Richard Edgahl for including me in two of the fine conferences that he and Diana Walsh conducted for corporate health benefits managers in 1988; Paul DiMaggio and Charles Perrow for welcoming my participation in their ongoing complex organizations seminar at Yale; and Richard F. Larson, the late A. B. Hollingshead, Bernard Barber, and John A. Simon for providing me with models of professional and scholarly responsibility.

Janet Hinson Shope provided superb research assistance during the first year of this project. Then a doctoral student in sociology at George Washington University, she went to original sources to compile much of the information on fraud and abuse, political contributions, and legal activity in Chapters 6 and 7.

Mark Schlesinger of the Harvard School of Public Health, who has done much pathbreaking empirical work on the topic of for-profit health care, provided detailed comments and useful suggestions about virtually every chapter of a late draft of the manuscript. David Mechanic of Rutgers University, who has been very generous with help and advice over many years, also made many helpful suggestions. I also took some good advice from several anonymous reviewers at both the Twentieth Century Fund and Harvard University Press, and I am grateful to them all.

This book could not have been written without the support of the Twentieth Century Fund, which made it possible for me to take a leave of absence from the Institute of Medicine to write the first draft. In addition to financial support from the Fund, I received many valuable comments and suggestions at different stages from Gary Nickerson, who originally approached me about the project, Beverly Goldberg, who saw the manuscript through its final steps, and, especially, Marcia Bystryn, whose detailed review and critique of one draft was an absolute model of clarity and helpfulness.

The National Academy of Sciences also provided a portion of my salary while on leave, and I thank Frank Press and Phil Smith for that investment in the professional development of staff. I also thank Fred Robbins and Karl Yordy of the Institute of Medicine for quietly allowing me to continue working in my office during that time.

The last two rounds of revision were done after I moved to Yale University to direct its Program on Non-Profit Organizations and teach in the Department of Epidemiology and Public Health at the Yale School of Medicine. The general support grants that the Ford Foundation, the Rockefeller Brothers Fund, and the William and Flora Hewlett Foundation made to the Program on Non-Profit Organizations provided a portion of my support during that period, and I am most appreciative.

Finally, I want to express my deep gratitude to my wife, Helen Darling. Having been exposed over my years at the Institute of Medicine to a Who's Who of American health policy, I can say with authority that she is one of the nation's smartest and most knowledgeable people in this area. I could not hope to enumerate her many intellectual contributions to this book. Beyond those, the moral support she provided went far beyond anything that could reasonably be expected. Dedicating the book to her is the least that I can do in return.

# The Changing Accountability
## of American Health Care

To whom and for what are our hospitals and physicians responsible? The answer to this question today is very different from what it was two decades ago. Significant changes have occurred in the control of organizations that provide medical care, in the conditions of physicians' work, in the ways in which medical care is paid for, and in the ethos of the health care system. This book documents and assesses these changes.

The American health care system is a complex mixture of public and private sector activities. The government's part in actually delivering health services is quite limited—either in specialized circumstances (for example, military and Veterans Administration hospitals; state psychiatric hospitals) or in a residual role (such as county or municipal public hospitals). The governmental systems are seldom viewed as models, and have been declining as a share of total hospital beds. Most individuals and organizations that provide medical services are in the private, nongovernmental sector. This sector includes, for example, about 95 percent of all doctors, about 75 percent of hospitals,[1] most nursing homes, ambulatory care centers, and home health care agencies, and all health maintenance organizations (HMOs). More than 60 percent of personal health services is privately financed, either through employment-based health benefits or direct payment by the patient.[2] In addition, most medical research is carried out in private hospitals, medical schools, and corporations.

Nevertheless, health care is heavily imbued with the notion of public interest. Many private hospitals were built with government funds (through the federal Hill-Burton program, as well as local funding), and subsidies via tax-exempt bond financing continue. Employment-based health benefits are subsidized (not being taxed as income to employees), and the biggest single financier of medical services and biomedical research is the federal government, most prominently through the Medicare and Medicaid programs and the extramural research programs of the National Institutes of Health.[3] Health care is subject to extensive governmental regulation by way of licensure requirements, reimbursement rules, and the various conditions of participation that apply to organizations that wish to seek or maintain eligibility for governmental funding.

In short, although the United States has never embraced any of the kinds of national health financing or delivery systems that characterize almost all other industrialized countries, neither has it left health care to the private market. Medicine is one of those areas of service for which communities seek to make provision, either through governmental processes or the work of community leaders. As they do with schools and post offices, small communities have gone to great lengths to establish and maintain a capacity for providing health services—by aggressively recruiting physicians in some instances and by building and struggling to maintain small hospitals even when expert opinion might judge them to be too small for efficiency or consistently high quality.[4]

The extensive governmental presence in health care notwithstanding, provision has not been made for the financing of medical services for the entire population.[5] The estimate of 37 million uninsured Americans is a well-known, melancholy characteristic of the present structure of financing health care, a flaw that the largely private system for providing services has somehow been expected to correct. The provision of charity care has had an important place in the history of both hospitals and the medical profession.[6] Nevertheless, the predominantly private character of the health care system has meant that providers of health services are not held accountable for failures to meet societal or community needs in the same way that they can be held accountable for failing to meet the needs of particular patients.

The glaring problem of the uninsured does not detract from the basic point that there is a sizable component of public interest in health care. The health care system and the elements therein can fairly be evaluated in terms of their contribution to the well-being of patients, individually and collectively. This involves issues not only of equity but also of how well scarce dollars are being spent.

## The Changing Health Care System

Until recent years the U.S. health care system could be fairly described in terms of independent nonprofit and small proprietary institutions and of independent physicians practicing alone or in very small groups. The few hospitals that were not independent were either government owned or were owned and operated by religious organizations. Third-party payers (both private and public) played their financing role passively, reluctant to interfere with medical decision making and the doctor-patient relationship. They paid for medical care by reimbursing for costs incurred or charges billed by health care providers and did little to control which services were provided or how much they cost.

For at least half a century nonprofit hospitals and the medical profession promoted the idea that in the largely private U.S. health care system medical care was nevertheless a community service that was provided in benevolent institutions by dedicated professionals who acted out of higher motivations than the pursuit of the dollar. Public acceptance of this idealistic image helps account for the fact that the United States does not have a more publicly accountable health care system.[7]

This book is concerned with the fact that the key elements lending plausibility to the idealistic image of hospitals and doctors have all changed since the late 1960s. Local control declined as large numbers of independent hospitals became part of multi-institutional systems (both for-profit and nonprofit). Ownership of institutions by publicly traded, investor-owned companies began and grew rapidly. Various kinds of new, mostly for-profit health care organizations—ranging from ambulatory care centers to HMOs—emerged without the traditional voluntary ethos. Some of the diagnostic, treatment, and rehabilitation centers are locally owned by entrepreneurs (often physicians) or hospitals. But there is also representation by investor-owned companies operating multiple facilities.

Changes in the organizations that provide medical care have not been limited to the for-profit sector. Because debt in private capital markets has become the primary source of capital for nonprofit as well as investor-owned hospitals, nonprofits now face a compelling pressure to perform well economically. Local control has declined as large numbers of independent nonprofit hospitals have joined multi-institutional systems and become subject to some control by central or regional offices located elsewhere. Large numbers of nonprofit hospitals are also now part of hybrid organizations that include both for-profit and nonprofit elements. These developments, along with increased marketing and a variety of other strategies used by nonprofit hospitals to maintain or increase market share, have led some observers to question how much today's nonprofit hospitals really differ from their for-profit counterparts.

Conditions of medical professionalism have also undergone significant changes. Officially, the medical profession retains a strong ethical orientation that obliges physicians to put the patient's interest before personal economic concerns. This orientation long rested implicitly on the fact that physicians were independent practitioners who depended on their patients for income and were obligated only to the patient. With physicians and procedural options both in relatively short supply, as they were through much of the century, adherence to high ethical standards did not necessarily require a sacrifice of income. During the past twenty years, however, dramatic increases in the number of physicians have led to rising competition and commercialism. Physicians are finding new ways to supplement their income by investing in equipment that they can use on their own patients or in facilities to which they can make referrals. Observers perceive new conflicts of interest.

Faced with declining patient loads, physicians are increasingly entering into arrangements with organizations—HMOs, hospitals, ambulatory care centers—that can offer access to large numbers of patients and, therefore, to income. As a result, physicians have become increasingly accountable to organizations that have their own agendas and economic interests and to which the physicians' income is tied. This has the potential to correct significant shortcomings in the traditional solo, fee-for-service system. As physicians become dependent on organizations for access to patients, however, new conflicts can arise with the physician's responsibility to act first and foremost on the behalf of the patient. Old concerns about the fee-for-service physician's obvious economic stake in doing and charging for additional, perhaps unnecessary, tests and procedures are now supplemented by concerns about new incentive arrangements that, under some circumstances, reward the physician (and the hospital) for performing fewer tests and procedures, perhaps even encouraging them not to provide all the services that may be in the patient's interest.

Finally, increasingly competitive conditions and growing pressures from purchasers of health care are forcing providers to find ways to control costs. Third-party purchasers have become more interested in keeping costs down than in respecting the physician's autonomy in making decisions about patient care. Purchasers are now willing to intervene directly in the patient care process through "utilization management" programs designed to minimize the provision of services deemed inappropriate or unnecessary. This may have real benefits—on costs, on the extraordinary variations in how different physicians respond to similar cases, and on quality of care—but pressure to eliminate "unnecessary" services could also inadvertently diminish the quality of care.

More broadly, and following ideologies that exalt competitive forces as a solution to the problems of the health care system, the health policy process has been dominated by efforts to create competitive conditions and the right set of economic incentives.

In sum, a continuing transformation—some would say revolution—is taking place in the economics, organization, and control of health care in the United States. Although charitable institutions and selfless professionals have not disappeared, health care has become an increasingly commercialized and competitive set. of activities that make up the fastest-growing element in the service sector of the nation's economy. The behavior of both providers of health care and third-party purchasers is driven more and more by the dollar. The question can be raised whether a role remains for idealism, for altruism, for looking to the needs of the patient and the community before attending to the bottom line.

No single concept adequately captures all of the changes that have occurred. Many descriptive terms have been used: commercialization, monetarization, corporatization, privatization, the proletarianization of the physician, the rise of the new medical-industrial complex. Perhaps the most basic element that all the changes share is simply that health care has become oriented more toward economic performance. Yet, not all parties—particularly the uninsured, the vulnerable ill, and payers—are well served by such an orientation.

A curious and important aspect of the change is that, notwithstanding the fact that health care is now a major public policy concern, much of the shift has been the incidental by-product of federal policy initiatives rather than an intended result. Although there are exceptions—such as the federal government's HMO program in the 1970s—most of the governmental policies and programs that stimulated these changes did so inadvertently. The payment methods used in the first twenty years of the Medicare program were a major factor behind the creation and growth of investor-owned hospital companies. The Comprehensive Health Planning Program created opportunities for nonhospital providers (for example, of diagnostic imaging services) by restricting hospitals' growth plans, and the education-financing programs that increased the supply of physicians also helped create the pressure underlying the growing commercial activities of physicians. The phasing out of the federal Hill-Burton program for hospital construction funds forced hospitals to turn to private capital markets, thereby making them accountable for economic performance to an unprecedented extent.

Because many changes were accidental, debates about advantages and disadvantages of most elements that have transformed health care were largely external to the policy process and occurred while the changes were taking place, not before they began. Thus, there was no standard of positive and negative effects against which developments could be measured. Nor could they be studied on a pilot basis before being adopted. They simply happened, with researchers and policy makers playing a constant game of catch-up in trying to understand the nature, cause, and significance of one development before the next one occurred.

Even so, the successes of researchers in building a body of

theory and empirical findings about the behavior of health care professions and institutions contributed in several ways to the transformation of the health care system. Research findings have had much influence on policy and have contributed to shifting perceptions about the fit (or lack of fit) between the needs of patients, individually and in the aggregate, and the performance of many elements of the health care system. Among other things, our understanding of the behavior of professionals and institutions has contributed to dissatisfaction with the idea of trust as a substitute for more rigorous mechanisms of accountability.

## Controversial Issues

This book is an attempt not only to document important changes that have occurred and are continuing to occur in the health care system but also to bring empirical information to bear on the many controversies that have been spawned by the transformation of that system. Indeed, many aspects of the change in health care from a community service to a major economic sector have been controversial.

Much of the controversy has been attached to the development that for many observers best symbolizes the transformation: the rise and proliferation of *for-profit* health care organizations. Investor-owned and proprietary organizations that provide health care have been criticized for the values connoted by their for-profit orientation and for the behavior that is thought to result from it. Health care, it is said, should be guided by a higher principle (even though obvious discrepancies have long existed between reality and the highest ideals of nonprofit organizations and of medical professionalism).

For-profit health care, of course, has its defenders. Some of their arguments are based on the mixture of ideology and economic theory that holds that for-profit firms will accomplish more, pay more attention to the patient as customer, and provide services more efficiently than will organizations operated by individuals who have no vested interest in the profitability of the organization.[8] Other arguments rest on the practical point that the government's unwillingness to use tax money to provide capital for health care facilities makes the use of private financial markets necessary. Furthermore, it is argued that the availability and use of investor capital provides alternatives for communities and institutions that are experiencing difficulty in raising capital or in operating their facilities in an economically sound fashion. Some advocates of more profit-oriented health care also rest their case on values of freedom and pluralism. They contend that the burden of argument should be on those who object to change, not on those who advance it.

Much of the worry about the sweeping changes in health care comes from the fear that the concept of health care will be changed from that of a community service to that of a marketplace commodity.[9] There is fear that, as a consequence, economic goals will be pursued at the expense of more humanitarian goals and values. The assumption that the for-profit provider's economic interest and the patient's interest are in conflict is sometimes stated explicitly, as when it is asked whether the purpose of health care is "profit for investors or better health for the public."[10] Arguing that health care is different from other goods and services, critics contend that providers who are more interested in profit than in ideals of services will be more likely to ignore needs that cannot be met profitably, to cut quality if this would be difficult to detect, and to exploit the vulnerabilities of payment systems. These arguments are generally rejected by for-profit advocates, who argue that traditional ideals are largely mythical, that for-profits do not behave much differently from nonprofits (or, alternatively, that they behave better), and that existing problems lie in incentives that fail to reward (or that actually punish) institutions that follow the highest standards of social responsibility.

Nonprofit hospitals, too, have been criticized—for seeming to ape the behavior of the for-profits, for failing to live up to their charitable mission, and, more mundanely, for not justifying their tax exemptions. But more than simple imitation may contribute to the similarity of for-profit and nonprofit facilities. Both regulatory constraints and economic pressures reduce degrees of freedom, and declining surpluses brought about by competitive pressures may reduce the ability of nonprofit hospitals to engage in such forms of discretionary behavior as providing care to patients who lack the means to pay.[11]

Other concerns stem from the increase in centrally managed, multi-institutional arrangements—particularly the growth of the large investor-owned health care companies—which, it is feared, will attenuate the linkage between health care institutions and the community and reduce the responsiveness of the institution to the needs of both the community and the medical staff. In addition, there is concern that the rise of multi-institutional arrangements complicates the task of monitoring the behavior—particularly regarding costs—of individual institutions. There are also worries about the economic and political power that accompany the growth of the multi-institutional systems that provide health care, the declining relative power of the physician, and the impact that billion-dollar organizations may have on public policy.[12]

Opponents of profit-oriented health care also wonder how all of these developments may affect the moral or ethical position of the medical profession itself. Do certain types of investments by physicians or arrangements with institutions create new conflicts of interest, perhaps reducing the likelihood that the physician will adhere to the fiduciary ethic under which the patient's interest is always supposed to come first? Many critics inside and outside the profession believe so.

Finally, the new forms of financial accountability to third-party purchasers have also been controversial, with advocates asserting that these methods are a sound way to try to eliminate unnecessary, costly services and critics expressing concern about interference in the doctor-patient relationship, bureaucratic costs, and quality of care.

## The Problem of Accountability

Perhaps the broadest common denominator shared by the seemingly diverse elements in the transformation of the American health care system is that they all affect the basic structure of accountability of health care—either by introducing new elements, changing old elements, or rendering less plausible the informal alternatives to formal accountability. These developments have potential implications for all important aspects of our health care system: the extent to which it meets the needs of individual patients and of communities, its cost, and the quality of care.

Accountability is, to coin an oxymoron, a dull buzzword—something that everyone believes in but that few can get excited about. This is, in part, because the term is often used rather unspecifically in critiques about the failure of health care institutions to fulfill their social responsibilities.[13] Thus, calls for increased responsiveness to the needs of patients, the community, or traditional values are often couched in calls for more accountability. Such critiques tell us something about the social expectations attached to health care, but it is not the sense of the term *accountability* that I wish to use.

Nor is my use of the term limited to the complex set of regulatory mechanisms with which individual and institutional providers of health care cope daily—the 174 regulatory bodies with which New York hospitals reportedly dealt in the 1970s,[14] the 64 inspections undergone and the 85 reports made by single hospitals studied by the U.S. General Accounting Office in 1980.[15] This web of externally imposed requirements is an important part of the overall structure of accountability that applies to providers of medical services, but it is not the whole set.

Accountability, as I use the term, refers to the mechanisms by which individuals and organizations are held responsible for their behavior. Used thus, the term refers to a relationship of power and authority and can be defined empirically: organizations or individuals are accountable to the parties that control access to the resources they seek.[16] Some such mechanisms are internal to organizations; others can be found in the linkage between an organization and its environment. In a hospital, for example, access to needed resources (capital, revenues, charitable contributions) may be controlled by the trustees, the physicians who admit paying patients, purchasers of care (patients and third-party payers), and the licensure and credentialing bodies that control eligibility to offer (and charge for) services.[17] Accountability, therefore, is concerned with questions of for what and to whom a party is responsible and with the ways in which that responsibility is brought to bear.

For several basic reasons accountability is a particularly difficult and absorbing problem in health care. The use of private-sector organizations to provide publicly financed services presents one set of issues. The fact that services are commonly paid for by parties who are not physically present to oversee what is being purchased presents a second. A third set of problems stems from the fact that patients are vulnerable emotionally, and typically have much less knowledge than the party (the physician) who defines their problem and provides advice.

The complex regulatory structure that has developed in health care is a response to these problems. Economists have long understood that in health care, market forces will work particularly imperfectly.[18] Something is needed to supplement the forces of the marketplace.

In the context of the changes with which this book is concerned, two aspects of the overall structure of accountability in health care are particularly significant. First, providers of health care are subject to multiple mechanisms of accountability, on several dimensions, and to a diverse set of parties. Broadly speaking, the mechanisms pertain variously to financial matters, quality of care, and provision of needed services.

The financial matters for which an organization is (or could be) held accountable include the price of services, the efficiency with which they are provided, assurance that services billed for were delivered, and the overall financial performance and economic health of the organization. Issues of quality range from the treatment of particular patients (here the mechanism of accountability when things go awry is the lawsuit)[19] to the more than 2,400 structural and procedural items on which accreditation by the Joint Commission for the Accreditation of Healthcare Organizations (JCAHO) is based, and from the requirements of state Life Safety Codes to such statistical indicators as mortality rates.[20] Issues of access include the availability of particular services (such as offering a twenty-four-hour emergency room) to convenience of hours and location and willingness to serve patients who lack the means to pay.

In addition to being held accountable on different dimensions, health care institutions are accountable to multiple parties— patients, payers, physicians, their own boards, communities, the providers of capital, and the various public and private monitoring organizations that accredit, certify for eligibility, or otherwise ensure that services are being provided properly. Significantly, the matters for which an institution is accountable to patients differ from those for which it is accountable to payers, or physicians, or providers of capital, or regulatory agencies. Moreover, the mechanisms of accountability vary substantially in their formality, ranging from the detailed contractual arrangements that are part of the capital acquisition process (for example, the issuance of bonds) or the minutiae of the accreditation process to the informal influence on hospitals of physicians and patients via the accountability of the marketplace. (By this I refer to the basic reality that an institution's access to a continued flow of funds depends on continued usage by physicians and their patients. This means that in a very real sense hospitals are informally accountable to the physicians and other parties who decide where patients will be admitted.) Part of the complexity of the accountability structure of health care thus comes from the fact that the institutions (and physicians) are accountable to several parties, through various structures and mechanisms, on different matters.

Moreover, because issues of finance, quality, and access are intertwined, trade-offs inevitably arise. Efforts to satisfy one party may detract from the ability to meet the requirements of another party. For example, a hospital's acquisition of an expensive new technology that pleases its medical staff may increase the financial burden on payers. Or a hospital's willingness to provide care to patients who lack the means to pay may be detrimental to the economic interests of the investors who provide the institution with capital.

An organization's performance can thus be seen as a series of compromises among the interests of the various parties to which the organization is accountable.[21] This is of key importance in grasping the significance of major changes in matters of to whom, for what, and with what degree of formality the individuals and organizations that provide health care are held accountable.

In addition to the matter of diversity and trade-offs, a second aspect of accountability in health care is of central importance to my analysis. There is an unusual juxtaposition that begs for explanation. Institutional providers of care have traditionally been expected to behave in ways that do not serve their short-term economic interests, but autonomy and self-regulatory mechanisms have been prominent. The reason for this, I believe, lies in three basic elements that were *not* formal mechanisms of accountability.

These elements, which, in effect, substituted for formal mechanisms of accountability, were (1) the nonprofit status of health care institutions, particularly the "voluntary" hospital; (2) local control of such institutions by volunteer trustees who, though not publicly accountable, played an important oversight role while also helping to raise capital; and (3) medical professionalism. Notwithstanding the social importance of medical care and the presence of such formal mechanisms as licensure and certification requirements, there has been heavy societal reliance in health care on assumptions about and trust in these elements. Trust has in many ways substituted for more formal mechanisms of accountability.

These elements—and the ideals they represent—fit the widely held values and expectations about the way health care should be provided. As an alternative to more elaborate and formal modes of public accountability, it was left to nonprofit institutions and their volunteer trustees, and to the professionalism of physicians, to ensure that community needs would be met, that the organizations that provide medical care would operate differently from businesses (for example, that they would try to meet patients' needs even in circumstances in which no economic gain would be possible), and that the vulnerabilities of patients and of payment systems would not be exploited.

## Basic Themes

This book will examine the nature and consequences of a series of basic changes in health care: the growing prominence of for-profit organizations in the provision of services; parallel changes occurring among nonprofit organizations; alterations in the conditions of medical professionalism; and the rise of utilization management by third parties. In examining these diverse developments, I will apply two strategies.

First, the significance of these changes will be sought in an account of how the structures or mechanisms of accountability have been affected. The concern will not only be with formal internal lines of authority, although shifts in the formal control of health care organizations are among the most important aspects of the transformation of health care. Mechanisms of accountability also exist outside formal organizational charts, as with the need for hospital administrators to satisfy influential physicians, even though physicians have not traditionally served on hospital boards and have no official authority over the administrators. Also outside of formal lines of authority is the fact that providers of medical services are increasingly subject to the accountability of the marketplace, with the flow of dollars on which organizational survival depends coming more and more from the organization's success in selling services and less from its ability to attract charitable contributions.

Second, the changes will be considered in terms of their implications for the previously described elements of trust, which have long substituted for formal paths of accountability. My analysis suggests that as the system becomes more heavily oriented toward economic incentives, the plausibility of reliance on trust comes into increased doubt.

In addition to describing changes that pertain to accountability, I will bring available empirical data to bear so that we can narrow the range of speculation about the significance of changes in the structure of accountability. While empirical research can shed much light on the controversies that were mentioned earlier in this chapter, some issues can never be fully resolved in empirical terms because they stem from value positions. Because health care involves important issues of public policy, the behavior of health care providers, individually and in the aggregate, must be viewed from several standpoints. These include not only questions of how the interests of patients and payers, both of whom have their own particular vulnerabilities, are served. They also include the evaluation of performance in terms of the broader standpoint of public interest, and particularly contributions to the overall equity of the health care system.[22]

Neither the creation of for-profit health care organizations nor the need for health care organizations to attend to the economic bottom line is a wholly new development. Nonetheless, there has been a change in the explicitness and pervasiveness of profit-seeking behavior. It has become the focus of the very structures of accountability that are built into health care organizations.

The problem of accountability has never been adequately resolved. The system in which these economic transformations have occurred was not one in which cost-effective, high-quality care was being provided to everyone who needed it. The question is not whether a satisfactory system is threatened but whether persistent shortcomings of the system are being mitigated or exacerbated by the economic and organizational changes that are sweeping over health care and replacing traditional forms of responsibility with new structures of accountability.

This question can be answered only if we examine these structures of accountability in American health care and understand what it means if for-profit organizations replace nonprofits, if conditions of medical professionalism are changed, and if third-party purchasers of care assume a dominant role in determining which services patients should receive. What is the nature and effect of the changes that are transforming health care? Is it true that there is little today that distinguishes nonprofit health care organizations from their profit-oriented competitors? Do reasons still exist for public policies that are supportive of a strong nonprofit presence in health care? And is the fiduciary ethic of the medical profession a thing of the past, or does it still have a leading role to play? These are the matters to which this book is devoted.

Chapters 2 and 3 describe the growth of the for-profit sector among providers of health services and the distinctiveness of their internal structures of accountability. Chapter 4 documents a series of parallel developments that have occurred among nonprofit hospitals. Chapters 5, 6, and 7 show that, some similarities notwithstanding, significant differences remain in the behavior of for-profit and nonprofit health care organizations. Chapters 8 and 9 examine important changes in the conditions of medical professionalism, and Chapters 10 and 11 document the effort by third-party payers to impose new forms of accountability on providers of medical services. Chapter 12 offers an assessment of these various changes in the accountability structure of health care and argues that nonprofit organizations and medical professionalism should continue as key elements in the structure of accountability of American health care.

# Accountability for Profitability: Proprietary and Investor-Owned Health Care Organizations

The growing prominence of for-profit health care providers is the most visible and symbolically powerful of the changes that have swept American health care in the past twenty years. This is not only because the label *for-profit* suggests a purpose quite distinct from traditional ideals, but also because these organizations' internal accountability structures differ from those of nonprofit organizations. Their accountability for profit has important implications for the behavior of the organizations and the stability of the health care system of which they are a part.

## The Extent of For-Profit Health Care

For-profit ownership has become prominent among all types of health care facilities, including:

- 14 percent of community hospitals, including 10 percent of the beds and a daily average of 8 percent of the patients (If the nonprofit and public hospitals that are *managed* by for-profit organizations are added in, the percentage of hospitals under the control of for-profit firms approaches 20 percent. These hospitals are concentrated in relatively few states, mainly in the South and West.)[1]
- 34 percent of all psychiatric hospitals (but only 10 percent of psychiatric hospital beds), including 66 percent of *private* psychiatric hospitals (1984)[2]
- 81 percent of nursing homes (1980)[3]

- 66 percent of HMO plans and 45 percent of HMO members (1987)[4]
- 57 percent of the preferred provider organizations (1985)[5]
- 32 percent of Medicare-certified home health agencies (1985)[6]
- 90 percent of freestanding surgery centers[7]
- 93 percent of primary care centers[8]
- 42 percent of dialysis facilities, including 79 percent of *freestanding* dialysis centers (1984)[9]
- 63 percent of blood banks[10]

In addition, an undocumented but presumably large percentage of cardiac rehabilitation, physical rehabilitation, and diagnostic imaging centers are for-profit. For-profit ownership is even reported among hospices and birthing centers.

In light of the growth in recent years of home health agencies, ambulatory care centers, preferred provider organizations (PPOs), and HMOs, Arnold Relman's 1980 estimate that for-profits account for 20 to 25 percent of health care dollars is probably an understatement today.[11] Moreover, the emergence of publicly traded, investor-owned health care companies has increased the size and power of for-profit organizations, as has the growth in vertical integration, by which the same organization controls suppliers and customers.

## Proprietary and Investor-Owned Organizations

To understand the internal accountability structures of for-profit health care organizations, it is useful to distinguish between proprietary and investor-owned organizations. As the name suggests, *proprietary* institutions are characterized by direct involvement of the owners in the management and operation of the facility. Proprietary organizations thus tend to be small and locally controlled. Through much of this century there has been a substantial proprietary sector among hospitals and nursing homes. In recent years new proprietary organizations have developed on a very broad front—particularly among numerous kinds of ambulatory care and diagnostic facilities and home health agencies. With hospitals and, to a lesser extent, nursing homes, however, proprietary ownership has come to be substantially replaced by investor ownership.

*Investor-owned* health care companies are managerially operated organizations that own multiple facilities and whose owners are connected with these facilities only by virtue of holding shares in the parent company. The shift from proprietary to investor-owned institutions is part of a broader change in the internal accountability structure of health care organizations: the rise of multi-institutional systems and the associated decline in local control.

Multi-institutional systems have been defined as "organizations in which a number of separate institutions are under a single corporate management that has overall authority for operating decisions and for policy formulation."[12] As we shall see in Chapter 4, however, the extent of centralized control is more properly understood as something that varies from organization to organization than as a matter of definition. Multi-institutional systems, which can be of for-profit, nonprofit, or public ownership, now exist among virtually all types of facilities.[13] For example, a 1985 survey by a trade publication identified 175 hospital chains (including 1,976 hospitals—almost one-third of all hospitals in the United States), 28 psychiatric hospital chains (166 hospitals), 54 nursing home chains (2,596 homes), 20 HMO organizations owning 213 multiple plans, 10 surgery-center chains (150 facilities), 9 renal dialysis chains (302 facilities), and so forth.[14] There were also numerous examples of facilities run by another type of chain—for example, 281 nursing homes and 44 HMOs were being run by multihospital systems.

Multihospital systems under religious and government ownership have existed for decades, although their numbers were always small.[15] It was the dramatic rise of the investor-owned hospital chains, however, that called attention to the fact that the accountability structure of health care was being changed.

In view of the concern that accompanied this change, it is worth noting that multi-institutional arrangements have long been favored by reformers ("corporate rationalizers," in Robert Alford's term),[16] who sought a better and more efficient health care system through regionalization, interinstitutional cooperation and coordination, and greater integration of facilities and resources. Over the past half-century, multi-institutional arrangements have been an ideal advanced by such distinguished bodies as the Committee on the Costs of Medical Care in the early 1930s and by government programs such as the Regional Medical Programs of the 1960s, the Comprehensive Health Planning Act, and the Health Resources Planning and Development Act of 1974. Multi-institutional arrangements were seen as a solution to such problems as duplication of services, discrepancies between the need for and availability of services in some areas, and lack of coordination between different levels of service (primary, secondary, tertiary, and long-term care).

The rise of multi-institutional systems over the past twenty years has little to do with centralized planning or government programs to reduce duplication and improve coordination of services; it stemmed instead from decisions made in the private sector by individual institutions and entrepreneurs. The government played an indirect role, however, since one underlying force was the institutions' difficulty in coping with the growing complexities of regulatory requirements and reimbursement rules and with the essential task of raising capital after the phase-out of federal support for hospital construction. Moreover, as I shall discuss, the growth of systems through the purchase of existing facilities or the construction of new ones was encouraged by Medicare's payment policies.

*Accountability and Proprietary Organizations*

Small size, management by owners, and the direct and immediate impact of the organization's economic performance on the owner make the internal accountability structure of proprietary organizations simple and straightforward. Plainly stated, the day-to-day operation of the organization is controlled directly by the person or persons who own the organization and its profits. Relatively little is known, however, about the operation and performance of proprietary health care organizations, which are in general reluctant to respond to surveys and are not subject to the reporting requirements that apply to publicly traded companies.

The pace of change and the development of new types of organizations have been so rapid that it is difficult for regulatory and licensure processes to keep abreast in developing standards and reviewing compliance with those standards. Moreover, there are disputes about whether new mechanisms of external accountability—such as licensure and certification—are needed for some types of proprietary organizations. Some centers are subsidiaries of other organizations, such as hospitals, and operate under those organizations' licenses. The National Association for Ambulatory Care has argued vigorously that primary care facilities and urgent care centers should not be licensed as such but should be seen as augmented physicians' offices and thus as covered under existing licensure requirements for physicians. Few states have licensing requirements for such centers, particularly if the word *emergency* is not used in their names. The development of separate regulatory mechanisms may also have been retarded by the suspicion that some calls for licensure, accreditation, or certification-of-need requirements were little more than attempts to protect existing institutions from competition.

Notwithstanding these problems, the key regulatory mechanisms of accountability for various types of ambulatory and home care organizations are state licensure, which applies only to some types of organizations and whose requirements vary greatly from state to state, and certification by Medicare or other third-party payers. There is much room for doubt about the adequacy of these mechanisms in the absence of more elaborate and effective monitoring procedures than now exist.[17] Voluntary accreditation procedures are being developed by the Joint Commission on Accreditation of Health Care Organizations and the Accreditation Association of Ambulatory Health Care. These efforts have progressed slowly because the process of developing standards and processes for accreditation is complicated and the reimbursement system has generally not provided enough incentive for ambulatory care facilities to undergo a voluntary accreditation process that they must finance themselves.[18]

### Accountability and Investor Ownership

The change in accountability that has resulted in the shift from a proprietary to an investor-owned for-profit sector has had several results in addition to the reduction in local control. The size—and therefore the potential power and influence—of the investor-owned corporations completely changes the scale of the for-profit sector. At its zenith the Hospital Corporation of America owned or managed more than 450 hospitals, and a number of other companies have had annual revenues in excess of $1 billion. In contrast to proprietary organizations, companies whose stock is publicly traded must adhere to disclosure and reporting requirements established by federal laws governing the sale of securities. Yet, although compliance with those reporting requirements provides investors with important information about a company's performance, it offers little insight into such matters as the cost or quality of services in company-owned facilities or service to patients who lack the means to pay. Information about these matters sometimes comes to light through the work of investment analysts, who often learn much that is otherwise not made public by companies.[19] (Privately held companies are not subject to reporting requirements that apply to publicly traded firms; indeed, it can be difficult to obtain any information about these companies, even about their numbers. It is thus significant that several hospital companies went private in the late 1980s.)

Accountability for making a profit is deeply embedded in the ways in which these organizations are controlled and in how they maintain access to capital. Publicly traded corporations have many more shares and shareholders than do other for-profit organizations, and their internal structure of accountability is much more complicated and indirect than in smaller, proprietary organizations. Although these organizations come increasingly under the control of professional managers, who have their own interests,[20] the underlying organizational goal or purpose is nevertheless to generate a return on the owner's investment. This is emphasized in several aspects of the organizations' functioning.

Because ownership of company stock by employees is often encouraged by companies and is facilitated through stock options and incentive plans, management often has a direct stake in the organization's profitability. Although the interests of management and stockholders may diverge under certain circumstances (for example, in a hostile takeover attempt), stock ownership gives employees an interest in the economic performance of the organization. Despite the fact that even the largest such employee-stockholders usually own only a small percentage of a publicly traded company's stock, the value of their stock is affected by their own decisions and actions, which affect the company's profitability. Some investors consider this factor so crucial to economic performance that they base decisions to buy or sell the stock of a particular company in part on the extent of stock ownership (or, conversely, large sales of stock) by top company management.

Profitability is, of course, the key indicator by which these companies are evaluated by investors and for which management is held accountable. The penalties that managers pay for disappointing earnings range from a decline in the value of their own stock, to the loss of their jobs, to the possibility that the company itself will cease to exist as an independent entity (and, again, the likely loss of their jobs).

Although corporate management is hired and fired by a board of directors whose members are elected by stockholders, the accountability of top corporate officials to stockholders is generally more indirect than this suggests. The number of stockholders militates against the organization of effective opposition to management. The simplest and most ordinary expression of stockholder dissatisfaction is the decision to sell stock. Stockholder dissatisfaction translates into decreases in the price of stock on the market, presumably to a level that is justified by prospects for future earnings. Also, if the stock price per share becomes too low in relation to the company's assets, the danger of a corporate takeover attempt increases. In recent years there have been several takeover rumors and attempts involving health care companies.[21]

The general corporate takeover phenomenon that has grown in the wake of declines in earnings and associated reductions in stock prices has increased the amount of attention managers give to financial goals. As the sociologist Paul Hirsch wrote in 1986:

> During the past decade, professional managers have been sharply reminded that they are hired agents for the owners of the corporation. Top management and boards of directors of large business firms have experienced a loss of power and autonomy to set the firm's future course. As the corporation itself is increasingly defined as a salable bundle of liquid assets, rather than as a producer of goods and services, top executives' incentives and orienta-

tion are channeled to accord priority to . . . financial and share price goals, over and above a commitment to the firm's product or products.[22]

When the product is health care, this dynamic raises some special concerns.

Although various elements influence investors' decisions to buy or sell stock (or investment analysts' recommendations to buy or sell),[23] past earnings, trends in earnings growth, and expectations regarding future earnings are clearly major factors. The most important investment decisions are made by institutional investors (for example, mutual fund and pension fund managers) who are themselves held accountable for their financial performance. The volatility of the relationship between expected earnings and stock prices is dramatically illustrated by events in the history of the Hospital Corporation of America (HCA), the largest and, thus, presumably the most stable of the investor-owned health care companies.

In the fall of 1983 HCA was generally held in high regard by the investment analysts who followed the health care companies.[24] HCA's earnings per share had increased at an average compound annual rate of 25.6 percent over the previous ten consecutive years; its stock sold at a premium, trading in late August of that year at about nineteen times the previous year's earnings. This was approximately one and a half times the average price-to-earnings ratio of the Standard and Poor's 500 stocks, an indication that the market believed that the company's future earnings would be above average.[25] When this confidence was shaken, however, the translation into declining value of ownership shares was immediate.

On November 1, 1983, a rumor circulated about a forthcoming report by the General Accounting Office that was said to be critical of the accounting procedures used in HCA's 1981 acquisition of Hospital Affiliates International.[26] Panic selling of the company's stock was triggered by speculation about the possible negative effect of this report on comparing profits. The price per share had plummeted that day $5 per share on a volume of 369,100 shares before HCA requested that the New York Stock Exchange temporarily suspend trading of its stock.[27] The value was later recovered, but the incident demonstrated how brutally the market could treat a company whose earnings were threatened.

This point was illustrated again two years later when HCA announced at a meeting of industry analysts that its longtime pattern of uninterrupted earnings growth was ending—that earnings would flatten. As the *New York Times* described it, "panic selling began, pushing down the price of the company's shares and those of the rest of the industry as well. It is estimated that the industry group lost more than $1.5 billion in market value in one day."[28]

Because of the link between profitability and the financial rewards to executives, and because investors who purchase equity in a company are seeking returns substantially above what they can receive from secured debt, strong pressures exist for consistent growth in earnings and for short-term economic performance. Obviously, such pressures are no guarantee that a company will be able to perform as well as managers and stockholders might desire, but they inescapably influence managerial decisions. It is clear that the primary responsibility of management is to enhance the value of investors' equity, and this depends on profitability more than any other factor. Management will ultimately be held accountable by the board of directors and by the stock market for its ability to generate satisfactory returns on investment.

## Accountability within Companies

The investor-owned hospital companies are hierarchical organizations in which lines of authority descend from the chief executive officer (CEO) of the company to the hospital level—specifically to the CEO of the hospital. The degree of centralized control differs markedly among the major investor-owned chains. At Humana, Inc., described in a Harvard Business School case study as "a highly centralized company, characterized by centralized decision-making and stringent financial and operating controls,"[29] many key functions are carried out at the corporate level, not at individual hospitals. These functions include financing, personnel recruitment and development, accounting, data processing, consulting, purchasing, pricing of services, and patient billing. Policies and procedures in many areas, such as staffing-level guidelines, are developed in the corporate offices. Other companies allow their hospitals more autonomy, but all retain the authority to develop specific goals for the financial performance of individual hospitals.

Those goals are generally spelled out in budgetary documents that are developed among administrators of hospitals, the next management level, and ultimately the corporate level of the company. The process varies to some extent from company to company. At Humana the company's operating budgets are formulated in the corporate office on the basis of corporate goals and past performance and then transmitted to regional offices, which prorate and transmit financial goals to individual hospital CEOs, who in turn must develop their hospitals' budgets accordingly. (Capital budgets, by contrast, start with proposals from the hospital level that are then reviewed and adjusted at higher levels.) Among other, more decentralized companies the operating budget process is initiated at the local level and is channeled upward. Within HCA targets that reflect corporate goals are not dictated to the hospitals. Instead, budgets are negotiated in a consultative process that begins with the hospital and moves up the corporate ladder. As described in 1984, the process begins with the development by the hospital administrator of a service demand budget for the next year and projections for the following three years.[30] After the budget is approved by the regional division, it serves as the framework for the development of the operating budget. (Capital budgets are also developed from the bottom up at HCA.)

Although details vary, the companies' budgetary processes effectively provide individual hospitals with goals and targets on various matters: number of admissions, amount of revenues, level of bad debt and average age of receivables, staffing ratios, capital expenditures, and expense levels for purposes such as marketing.

Data systems are in place to enable higher executives to monitor the performance of each institution and to receive regular reports regarding the relationship between performance and goals. In National Medical Enterprises, regional managers have monthly meetings with each hospital's CEO to review operations, and they are accountable to the corporate office for expense control, profitability, Medicare and Medicaid utilization rates, age of accounts receivable, and program development. Monthly budget and performance review meetings are conducted in regional and corporate offices. Humana's data systems allow continuous monitoring of the performance of its hospitals on many financial (and patient satisfaction) dimensions, and hospitals report monthly on various matters, including reimbursement, bad debt, balance sheet reconciliation, income statement reviews, and explanations of budget variances. Humana's monitoring focuses on five basic areas: patient census, accounts receivable, profit margins, full-time equivalents (FTEs) of employees per occupied bed, and pretax profit. For example, through the patient billing system, patient census can be monitored and compared to that of previous years and previous weeks so that emerging trends can be seen.

Monitoring by divisional and corporate officials is not confined to matters that pertain to expenses, revenues, and profits, however. Humana uses a system of checks and balances that is meant to ensure that key functions are not neglected in the interests of short-term institutional profits. For example, since a hospital CEO could increase the short-term profitability of a hospital by deferring maintenance or letting equipment age, Humana conducts engineering quality assessments periodically in every facility. If equipment is needed, action can be taken. Humana's administrators are responsible for ensuring that the hospital maintains accreditation, and the company also reviews patient questionnaires (mailed out by and returned to the *corporate* office after the patient is discharged) and provides periodic summaries to hospital administrators. Procedures also exist for physician evaluations of facilities and for the usual quality assurance and utilization review functions within the hospitals.

At HCA an important part of the internal accountability structure is the voluminous management plan submitted annually by hospital administrators to divisional offices. The plan, which includes goals and objectives, detailed budgets, and demographic and competitive analyses, provides a baseline against which the hospital and the corporate offices can evaluate a hospital's progress during the year. The plan also includes comparisons of the previous year's performance against goals and objectives. The plan includes detailed financial objectives measured by earnings, margins, cash flow, pretax return on assets, hospital utilization, manpower development, and identification of new projects. The plan also states quality assurance objectives such as accreditation, positive patient evaluations, and monitoring of medication and patient incidents. Also included are projections of service demand for the upcoming year, based on trends in the socioeconomic, political, and competitive environment of the hospital, as well as strategies for meeting the demand. Data analyses are included on service areas, hospital utilization (inpatient, outpatient, emergency department), patient mix, and other aspects of operations. The ability of the hospital's physicians to meet the service needs of the hospital is evaluated on the basis of data on physicians' ages, admissions, and specialization. This information may prompt physician recruitment efforts. HCA's centralized computer system enables the hospital and corporate offices to monitor many factors at any time—trial balances, department revenues, and other performance indicators.

The accountability structures within the investor-owned companies go beyond detailed goals and systems for monitoring performance in relation to those goals. They also include the reward system within the organization. The investor-owned companies make much more extensive use of incentive compensation than do nonprofit hospitals.[31] Humana, for example, ties a significant portion (as much as 50 percent of the base salary) of a hospital administrator's compensation to the hospital's performance on goals regarding census, accounts receivable, profit margins, employees (full-time equivalents) per occupied bed, and pretax profit. The reward structure also includes advancement in the career path provided by the structure of large-scale multihospital systems. It is common for managers of hospitals to reach that position after having gained experience in lower-level positions in different hospitals within the organization, for successful managers of small hospitals to be promoted to larger ones, and for managers at regional or corporate levels to be drawn from those who have performed well at the hospital level.

The combination of explicit performance goals and criteria,

monitoring systems, economic incentives, and career paths provides a structure that powerfully translates the companies' economic goals and imperatives to the individual institutions.

## Profitability and Other Aspects of Performance

Although most of the goals and projections that are built into the budget documents of these organizations either are financial or have direct financial implications (for example, number of admissions), it would be erroneous to conclude that the managers of investor-owned hospitals ignore other matters. I have already mentioned that in companies such as Humana and HCA, hospital CEOs are expected to maintain the hospital's accreditation. But more generally, hospitals operate in a complex field of forces which may affect economic performance—sometimes in unexpected ways.

For example, an investor-owned hospital that I visited in 1984 as part of a case study for the Institute of Medicine had recently opened an emergency room, even though it was understood that this would increase the number of nonpaying patients who would have to be treated.[32] This step was taken not because the CEO wanted his hospital to do its part in caring for the city's uninsured population but because he believed that the paying admissions that would be generated by the emergency room (he expected 25 percent of emergency room visits to turn into admissions) would outweigh the additional bad debts.

Many steps that a hospital CEO might take to increase the hospital's profitability could instead have a negative effect. Reducing expenses by making cuts that affect quality could increase the risk of lawsuits, jeopardize accreditation, and alienate physicians who admit patients. Turning away patients who lack the ability to pay is the profit-oriented practice that has probably generated the most concern, and even this strategy must be used carefully because it could bring the hospital afoul of the law, create negative publicity, or, if the patient happens to have a physician, jeopardize relations with the medical staff. Thus, the administrator of one of the investor-owned hospitals that I visited during the Institute of Medicine study of for-profit health care stated (and staff physicians confirmed) that in the interest of both good public relations and good staff relations, patients of a staff physician would never be refused admission on grounds of inability to pay.[33] (The costs of this policy were undoubtedly made more acceptable by the fact that people who lack the means to pay often do not have a private physician and thus have no one to support their admission to the hospital.)

It is clear, however, that the budgetary process and accountability structure of these organizations provide mechanisms that can be used to implement such steps as cutting staff, deferring maintenance or capital expenditures, and eliminating unprofitable services should these steps be deemed economically beneficial. Nevertheless, hospital CEOs are held indirectly accountable for maintaining good relationships with the medical staff and a good image in the community, since such factors can affect the hospital's ability to attract patients. Indeed, because of very poor relationships between the hospital CEO and the staff physicians in one of the investor-owned hospitals visited in the Institute of Medicine study, the hospital was virtually empty. Doctors were admitting their patients to other hospitals. The CEO was subsequently fired.

My point is not that a hospital accountability structure that leans strongly toward profitability will never have negative implications for such aspects of a hospital's performance as quality of care or service to patients who lack the means to pay. Yet, many elements can influence overall economic performance and organizational behavior, and all hospitals face economic constraints. Does the accountability structure of investor-owned hospitals lead to organizational behavior that systematically differs from that of nonprofit institutions? Do they cut corners on some matters for which health care institutions are—or could be—responsible, such as maintaining quality of care, responding to the needs of the community or of individual patients even in the absence of an economic return, or maintaining integrity in providing and billing for services? Or does the orientation toward profitability create pressures for better service and more efficiency?

Whether there are systematic differences in the behavior of investor-owned and nonprofit hospitals is properly regarded as an empirical question, not as a matter to be answered with definitions and logic. The empirical relationship between ownership and the behavior of health care organizations will be a recurrent theme over the next several chapters.

# · 3 ·

# The Evolution of Investor-Owned Hospital Companies

The history of investor ownership of hospitals over the past two and a half decades or so illustrates many of the dynamics that result from accountability structures oriented toward profitability. Both the companies' responsiveness to economic incentives and a lack of stability in the ownership of particular institutions are important parts of the story.

Although the investor-owned hospital companies emerged in the mid-to-late 1960s, for-profit health care organizations were by no means new. In fact, early in the twentieth century half of U.S. hospitals were small proprietary institutions,[1] mostly established by doctors to provide facilities for themselves and for the community. The number of these proprietary hospitals declined throughout the century. Many closed, while others became non-profits.[2] This decline has continued in recent years even as for-profit ownership has become more common elsewhere in health care. By 1989 only 258 independent proprietary hospitals remained in the United States, an enormous decrease from the estimated 2,400 proprietary institutions in 1910.[3]

Although the difficulty of generating profits in health care before the advent of Medicare and Medicaid undoubtedly contributed to the decline of the proprietary hospitals, other factors were also involved. Many, perhaps most, proprietary hospitals were established before technological change and improving standards (reflected, for example, in more stringent Life Safety Codes for buildings) dramatically increased the amount of capital required to establish hospitals and keep them up to date. In addition, the life span of some proprietary hospitals was linked to the professional careers of their physician-founders. In explaining the decline of proprietary hospitals in the 1940s, the American Hospital Association's director of research noted that their small size (an average of thirty-seven beds at that time) limited their ability to offer the services and facilities that modern practice demanded. He also mentioned two other explanatory factors that resonate in today's marketing-oriented, cost-competitive health care system: "the patients' appreciation of the advantages of a large, well-equipped, specialist-staffed hospital, [and] tax freedom and other immunities that give the voluntary hospital a competitive cost advantage."[4]

It is not clear, however, just how important the tax advantages of the nonprofits were in explaining trends among for-profit hospitals. Much of the decline of proprietary hospitals took place at a time when corporate taxes (and, therefore, the nonprofits' advantages) were comparatively low, and much of the growth of the investor-owned hospital companies occurred during a period of relatively high corporate taxes.

## The Rise of Investor-Owned Hospital Companies

In the late 1960s and 1970s the continuing decrease in the number of independent proprietary hospitals came to be mirrored by the rise of hospitals owned by investor-owned companies. The companies that came to assume dominance—American Medical International (AMI), Hospital Corporation of America (HCA), Humana, Inc., and National Medical Enterprises (NME)—either had their origins in the late 1960s or began their period of rapid growth at that time. The willingness of investors to put equity capital into health care companies was one of many consequences of the enormous infusion of federal dollars into the health care system by way of the Medicare and Medicaid programs. When added to the existing employment-related health insurance coverage, Medicare and Medicaid meant that 80 to 90 percent of the population had hospitalization insurance that either paid on the basis of hospitals' charges for services provided or reimbursed hospitals for allowable costs of services to beneficiaries.[5] It became possible for hospitals to make a great deal of money.

The growth of the hospital companies was facilitated by key details in the ways that Medicare and other "cost-paying" purchasers of care (primarily Blue Cross plans) determined allowable costs, most notably capital costs. Medicare's payments to hospitals included reimbursement for the cost of interest on borrowed funds, depreciation expenses, and, for for-profit institutions, return on equity.[6] Cost payers covered their share of institutions' capital costs; the remainder was included in the charges for which other payers reimbursed hospitals.

One consequence of Medicare's payment rules was that the flow of dollars to an institution generally increased when it was acquired by a new owner.[7] Some of this cash flow was just reimbursement for out-of-pocket expenses (interest), but much of it was for a noncash expense—depreciation—which was calculated on the basis of the purchase price. Return-on-equity payments also created additional cash flow. All of this meant that hospitals became more valuable to new owners than to sellers and stimulated acquisition activity.

The reimbursement environment from the late 1960s until the early 1980s made it difficult *not* to make money operating hospitals, so long as they were located away from concentrations of low-income populations and in states that did not regulate hospital income. As the companies prospered in this environment, their ability to grow was limited primarily by their ability to find suitable hospitals that could be acquired or locales where necessary governmental approval could be obtained for construction of new hospitals. The companies' attraction to areas with relatively high rates of population growth and low levels of regulation[8] resulted in a concentration in particular states, mainly in the South and the West. The willingness of the investor-owned hospital companies to acquire struggling hospitals and to build new hospitals even when the need for beds was marginal helps to explain why their occupancy rates have persistently been 10 to 15 percent lower than those in nonprofit hospitals.

The acquisition patterns of the hospital companies changed over time as the targets of opportunity for growth shifted. The purchase of proprietary hospitals was the primary source of the early growth of investor-owned companies.[9] Such hospitals had long been the least stable type, opening and closing with particular frequency.[10] They had been established by physician-owners

for a variety of reasons—sometimes as a business venture, sometimes as a response to disputes with other hospitals, sometimes
because needed facilities were not conveniently available. Given
an opportunity to obtain a good price for their investment, many
owners of proprietary hospitals were willing to sell.

By the early 1970s the construction of new facilities emerged
as a second source of growth. Overall, 20 percent of the growth of
the six largest hospital companies was eventually due to construction.[11] In some instances the opportunity for entry into a
new market was a result of physician dissatisfaction with existing hospitals.[12] Construction as a source of growth peaked in the
period 1970–1974.[13] The decline thereafter was probably a result
of both new regulatory restrictions on entry, such as certificate-
of-need requirements, and competing demands on capital which
resulted from the next growth strategy—acquisition of entire
companies rather than individual institutions.

The acquisition of other companies was the largest single
source of growth of the surviving investor-owned firms after the
mid-1970s. Some of the largest companies were acquired by
others—most notably when Humana acquired American Medicorp in 1978 and when the Hospital Corporation of America
(HCA) acquired Hospital Affiliates International (HAI) in 1981.
Making wholesale acquisitions of operating hospitals was
inadvertently encouraged and facilitated by the Medicare capital-
payment methods described earlier. The HCA-HAI transaction
brought governmental attention to those policies and, as later
discussion will show, led to their change in the 1980s.

The final source of hospitals for the investor-owned companies
was nonprofit and public hospitals. The six major companies,
which had acquired only thirty-one such institutions between
1965 and 1980, bought sixty-five between 1980 and 1984.[14] The
fact that there were relatively few such acquisitions during the
early growth years of the investor-owned companies was probably due less to the fact that the companies had little interest in
such institutions than in the fact that such institutions were not
available for sale. There was much suspicion of for-profit ownership among trustees of nonprofit hospitals and local government
officials. Also, the reimbursement environment meant that the
institutions that were financially strained tended to be small
rural hospitals or hospitals that, because of mission or location,

treated large numbers of uninsured patients. Even in a generous reimbursement environment, such hospitals were not attractive to acquisition-oriented hospital companies. Legal complications presented by the sale of nonprofit organizations' assets to for-profit organizations were also a barrier. In some cases, however, paths were found around this problem, for example, through the creation of a new nonprofit organization with the proceeds of the sale. (For example, the Wesley Foundation in Wichita, Kansas, was created with $200 million of the proceeds of the sale of Wesley Hospital to HCA in 1985.)

By the 1980s mergers and acquisitions had resulted in consolidation of many of the investor-owned companies, and few independent proprietary hospitals remained. If the growth of such companies was to continue, nonprofit or public hospitals would have to be acquired. Some such institutions were finding the regulatory and reimbursement environments to be increasingly complex and difficult, and some had capital needs that could not readily be met. The same forces led certain institutions into management contracts or multi-institutional arrangements and caused others to consider closure or sale of the facility. The investor-owned companies were still interested in growth, had capital, and had become less of an unknown factor. For the first time the companies were able to acquire institutions of real prominence in their communities.[15]

By 1983 the investor-owned hospital companies owned more than 13 percent of the general hospitals in the United States and managed another 6 percent.[16] The Hospital Corporation of America alone owned or managed 7 percent of the hospitals in the United States at one point. The merger and acquisition activity of the late 1970s and early 1980s had concentrated ownership in a handful of companies. As of September 30, 1984, 59 percent of the investor-owned hospitals were owned by six chains—Hospital Corporation of America (200 hospitals), American Medical International (115 hospitals), Humana (87 hospitals), National Medical Enterprises (47 hospitals), Charter Medical Corporation (41 hospitals), and Republic Health Corporation (24 hospitals). Many of those companies had extensive other holdings as well, such as hospital management subsidiaries, nursing homes, and ambulatory care centers.

The major companies had experienced consistent earnings

increases of 20 percent or more per year, attracting large amounts of relatively inexpensive equity capital as a result. Medicare's reimbursement rules for interest expenses and depreciation effectively made debt capital cost-free. Various companies successfully sought and obtained capital through means that had never been seen before in health care—sale of stock, convertible debentures, the Eurodollar market.

The merger and acquisition activity fueled by the availability of capital created the impression that those few chains might take over the entire health care system, a prospect that many found alarming.

Executives from the investor-owned companies spoke with considerable certainty about two matters. One was that their steady increases in earnings and corporate growth were due to the managerial ability and incentives that came from their organizational form. The other was that the bulk of their business came from sources of payment that were solid and predictable. The federal government, it was said, would never be able to walk away from the Medicare program, and labor unions would never relinquish the health benefits that they had won. This meant, investors were told, that the for-profit hospital business was about as solid as anything could be.

Moreover, it was suggested that for-profit hospitals gained economic protection from the fact that most hospitals were nonprofit. This was so, the argument went, because nonprofit hospitals were less "efficient" than for-profits, and the payment environment would always have to be generous enough to accommodate them. Congress could never withstand the political heat that would come from taking actions that would harm large numbers of these important if inefficient entities. The investor-owned hospitals were swimming in the same protected waters, so investment in them could hardly be safer.

Forgotten by the early 1980s was the fact that hospitals had historically been unprofitable institutions. When the American Hospital Association (AHA) began its National Hospital Panel Survey in 1963, the average community hospital was losing $6 for every $100 of patient care revenue that it took in.[17] Even though implementation of Medicare and Medicaid reduced the loss, the average community hospital continued to report that patient care expenses exceeded patient care revenues throughout the 1960s and 1970s.[18] During that period the average hospital was able to report a positive *total* margin only because it had nonpatient revenues with which to offset the losses on patient care. The financial picture for hospitals improved steadily, if slowly, after the passage of Medicare and Medicaid, but it was not until the 1980s that the AHA reported that the average hospital generated more revenues than expenses from patient care. By 1984, when the average net patient margin reached the unprecedented level of 2 percent, the total net margin had increased to 6.2 percent of revenues.

Thus, the growth period for the investor-owned hospital sector was one of unprecedented prosperity for hospitals. As might have been expected, however, annual double-digit increases in health care costs finally produced multiple reactions by public and private third-party purchasers of care. What had not been understood before then became apparent: these companies had grown not because of managerial magic but as a result of the skilled use of the incentives that had been built into payment systems for hospitals. As those incentives were changed in the early 1980s, it became clear that the companies' growth strategies were now obsolete.

## The End of the Golden Era

By the early 1980s the federal government's interest in controlling health care expenditures had led to significant changes in the flow of money to health care providers. Medicaid programs in various states also adopted methods to reduce the amounts paid for care of their beneficiaries. And, as the decade moved forward, employers began to take a wide variety of steps to control their health care costs (see Chapters 10 and 11). Attention focused particularly on hospitals as the major source of expenditures. As the payers' reforms started to hit, the largest investor-owned companies began to diversify into new lines of business and to sell more hospitals than they acquired.

Three changes in reimbursement rules and methods in the federal Medicare program contributed most heavily to these changes in strategy. The first pertained to depreciation expenses, a significant source of cash flow under Medicare's payment rules.

The immediate stimulus for the change was HCA's 1981 acquisition of the third-largest hospital chain, Hospital Affiliates International, in a complex merger transaction. HAI's fifty-four hospitals, eighteen nursing homes, and ten office buildings, a subsidiary that managed almost one hundred hospitals, and some forty other corporate entities were purchased by HCA from HAI's parent company, the Insurance Company of North America, for $425 million in borrowed cash, 5.39 million shares of stock valued at $190 million by HCA, and $270 million of HAI debt assumed by HCA. Although other large-scale acquisitions had previously taken place among the hospital companies, the HCA-HAI deal generated serious questions. After learning that Medicare costs had risen by $50 a bed per day at an HAI hospital in Richmond, Virginia, after its acquisition by HCA, Congressman Willis Gradison asked the General Accounting Office (GAO) to study the impact of HCA's acquisition of HAI on health care costs.[19] The resulting study revealed much about how Medicare capital-reimbursement policies had been fueling the growth and consolidation of the investor-owned hospital companies.

The GAO found that the interest and depreciation expenses associated with the HCA-HAI transaction had raised costs in the acquired hospitals by $55 million for the first year alone, over and above any costs that might have been associated with improvements or changes in hospitals' services or facilities.[20] HCA disputed several aspects of the GAO's analysis and conclusions[21] and argued that Medicare was paying too little for depreciation, not too much. Nevertheless, legislation was quickly passed to change the rules that had based Medicare's payment of depreciation expenses on the cost of the asset to the organization that acquired it rather than on the original cost of the asset.[22] Henceforth, Congress decided, Medicare would pay only once for the depreciation of an asset no matter how many times it changed hands.[23] This reduction in payments for depreciation expenses diminished the attractiveness of making acquisitions.

The second change, which also reduced the flow of dollars to for-profit hospitals, was in Medicare's return-on-equity (ROE) payments. The ROE formula paid hospitals a percentage of their equity each year. The percentage was originally set at 1.5 times the rate of return earned by Medicare's Hospital Insurance Trust Fund on its investments. Though long a bone of contention for nonprofit hospitals, which did not receive such payments, return on equity became a political issue when the annual percentage rate for ROE payments exceeded 20 percent owing to the high interest rates in the early 1980s. Legislation ensued that reduced the formula by one-third—to the equivalent of the rate of return on the Trust Fund.

The third change was the passage in 1983 of Medicare's so-called prospective payment system (PPS), which replaced the cost reimbursement system that was widely seen as the primary culprit in the persistent inflation of hospital costs. Under PPS, the most significant change in the health system since the passage of Medicare, hospitals are paid on the basis of prospectively set per-case rates. Cases are defined in terms of the patient's diagnosis and other patient-related factors that affect cost (such as the patient's age or presence of complications). When paid a set amount based on which diagnosis-related group (DRG) a patient fits into, hospitals have an economic incentive to reduce their expenses, since they can keep the difference between their costs on a case and the DRG payment for that case.

The level at which the rates were first set, and the hospitals' initial success in reducing their expenses, largely by shortening hospital stays, produced an increase in the margin of profits for the average hospital.[24] With experience and mounting budgetary pressure, however, it became apparent that the PPS system not only had reversed the inflationary incentives of cost-based reimbursement but also was a vehicle of unprecedented effectiveness for Congress and the Health Care Financing Administration (HCFA) to limit Medicare's expenditures by squeezing hospitals economically.

Once PPS was implemented, the profitability of hospitals quickly became a policy concern in a way that it had never been as long as Medicare was reimbursing for allowable costs. By early 1987 several congressional hearings had been held on hospital profitability, and analyses had been carried out by the Office of the Inspector General, the Prospective Payment Assessment Commission, the American Hospital Association, and the Congressional Budget Office, among others.[25] Hospital margins on Medicare patients in the initial year under prospective payment were reported in different analyses and for different subgroups of hospitals to have ranged from 12 to 18 percent. The direct relationship between one year's decision on adjustments of Medicare payments and the next year's hospital profitability figures was there for the Health Care Financing Administration, the Office of Management and Budget, and Congress to see.

Hospital associations argued that the profitability picture had already changed in the two to three years that it had taken to compile the data. They also argued that to base yearly rate adjustments on past profitability figures would violate the spirit of the prospective payment system under which hospitals were supposed to be allowed to benefit from the profits that they could generate when paid a fixed price. Nevertheless, Congress inevitably found things on which it would rather spend tax revenues than on paying hospitals amounts that exceeded their costs by 15 or 20 percent. To justify this decision, it was argued that the high profits were never intended, that they resulted from flaws in the ways that the rates were originally set, and that they were partly a result of past inefficiencies that hospitals were only now correcting.

In any event, the reports of initially high profit margins among hospitals were an invitation for the federal government to adjust payment levels accordingly, and annual payment rate increases thereafter trailed inflation. Thus, the 30 to 40 percent of revenues from Medicare that were once seen as providing a highly secure source of income for the hospital industry became a problem with which hospitals had to cope. Rate adjustments began to constrict the profit that could be made in serving Medicare patients in acute care hospitals. The American Hospital Association reported that profit margins in the hospitals studied in its National Hospital Panel Survey had begun to "dip sharply" by 1986.[26] A study released by the Healthcare Financial Management Association in early 1987 said that patient care margins for services to all patients had dropped by 75 percent in the four years since the onset of Medicare's PPS system. The study also projected that the average hospital would lose money (down 1.1 percent) on Medicare patients in 1988.[27] (The political uses of the data on hospital profits may explain why the AHA had difficulty in collecting such data from hospitals and why it finally stopped trying to do so in its annual survey of hospitals.)

At the same time that hospital profits began to attract the attention of federal budget cutters, many other payers were developing and implementing new approaches to limiting their own expenditures for hospital care, either by reducing the use of hospitals or by cutting the amount they paid to hospitals, for example, by negotiating discounts. (Some of the most significant of these changes—embodied in the rise of managed care—are the subject of Chapters 9, 10, and 11.)

The results of those actions by payers in both the public and private sectors, as well as of technological changes and changes in physicians' practice patterns, quickly became apparent in reduced hospital admissions, shorter lengths of stay, and, as a consequence, sharply lower hospital occupancy rates. Within a very few years a hospital-controlled economic environment was becoming an environment characterized by administered Medicare prices and price competition for the business of other payers.

## Responses of the Investor-Owned Hospital Companies

As early as the fall of 1985 announcements began to emerge from one investor-owned hospital company after another that previously declared profit expectations were being revised downward. Since most of these companies had never reported anything but increases in earnings, this was shocking news indeed. Furthermore, as quarterly report followed quarterly report, companies announced declines from the previous year's earnings, and in some cases even showed losses. By mid-1986 the clear consensus among observers was that the era of high profitability in the business of running general hospitals had passed.

In anticipation of, or in response to, the changes in the hospital market, the major investor-owned companies all developed new strategies. Although these strategies varied from company to company, they all shared one purpose: to lessen company reliance on hospital ownership for income. Broadly speaking, two approaches have been used—the sale of hospitals and entry into new lines of business.

### Sale of Hospitals

By 1987 the four major companies (HCA, AMI, Humana, and NME) had all become net sellers of hospitals, owning fewer hospitals in the United States than in earlier years. Humana's net sales of hospitals began in the early 1980s. The other three companies became net sellers in 1985.[28]

Some hospitals were sold outright, usually to smaller and newer investor-owned companies. (Several of these companies subsequently experienced severe financial problems; a few have gone bankrupt.) Such sales were usually explained as reflecting a decision that a particular hospital did not fit into the company's overall plans, although it is likely that few were profitable. In some cases the hospitals that were sold had been acquired as part of the purchase of another company, but because of local competitive factors they seemed to hold little promise of profitable operation. In other cases (particularly with Humana), the hospitals that were sold were not of the suburban hospital type on which the company had decided to concentrate.

Another method of selling hospitals (adopted by NME and AMI) involved the creation of separate organizational entities, called real estate investment trusts (REITs), to which hospitals were sold and then leased back by the company. This approach allowed the company to pull its capital out of hospitals while continuing to operate them.

A third method, announced by HCA in 1987, involved the "transfer" of 104 hospitals to a new company owned by employees (through an employee stock ownership plan) and by certain members of HCA's top management. This transaction left HCA with 80 acute care and 50 psychiatric hospitals, plus its management contracts in 215 hospitals.

The results of the efforts of the hospital companies to extract themselves from hospital ownership can be seen in Table 3.1. Companies that had owned a total of 519 hospitals in the early 1980s owned only 320 by late 1987. With one exception (Charter Medical), the companies were smaller still by 1989.

### Shift to Psychiatric and Substance Abuse Treatment

The growth of Charter Medical Corporation in the late 1980s was part of another general trend in the investor-owned hospital sector—its growing concentration in specialty hospitals, particularly psychiatric and substance abuse facilities. In the late 1980s

*Table 3.1.* The declining size of the major investor-owned hospital companies

|  | Maximum number of hospitals owned | Number owned late 1987 | Number owned late 1989 |
| --- | --- | --- | --- |
| Hospital Corporation of America | 202 (1982) | 82 | 78 |
| American Medical International | 115 (1984) | 86 | 54 |
| Humana, Inc. | 90 (1981) | 81 | 81 |
| National Medical Enterprises | 47 (1982) | 38 | 36 |
| Charter Medical Corp. | 41 (1984) | 14 | 90 |
| Republic Health Corp. | 24 (1984) | 19 | 18 |

Sources: Directories of the Federation of American Hospitals (now Federation of American Health Systems); corporate annual reports.

the number of for-profit hospitals grew very slowly (for example, from 1,114 in 1987 to 1,134 in 1989, according to figures published by the major trade association FAHS, the Federation of American Health Systems). Concealed in the stable figures, however, was a marked decline in the number of general acute care hospitals owned by the companies.

According to the FAHS, the number of specialty hospitals—mostly psychiatric and substance abuse facilities—increased from 469 in 1986 to 618 in 1989. The percentage of for-profit hospitals that were specialty facilities doubled—from 27 percent to 54.5 percent—between 1984 and 1989.[29] Since the total number of for-profit hospitals remained about constant, the change had to come from the conversion of existing facilities and/or through the construction of new facilities and the disposal of others. It is clear that some of the growth came from new institutions (the 1990 FAHS directory mentions that fifty new investor-owned psychiatric hospitals were built in 1989). It is also clear that a substantial number of the investor-owned general acute care hospitals that existed in 1986 were no longer functioning as such by 1989, although it is not clear how many simply closed, how many were sold to new owners that were not investor-owned companies (there have been sales to both nonprofit groups and individual proprietors), and how many were converted to psychiatric or other specialty facilities. Whatever the composition of the change, it involved roughly 20 to 25 percent of all investor-owned hospitals in just five years, a shift whose magnitude far exceeds the amount of change that was occurring among nonprofit institutions.

An increase in the incidence of the problems treated by psychiatric and substance abuse facilities does not appear to be the major reason for the shift of investor capital in that direction. Three other factors are involved. First, since many states have mandated that employers' health benefits must provide coverage, third-party payment based on facilities' billed charges has become more widely available. Second, psychiatric services and facilities are explicitly exempted from the prospective payment system, so these facilities are not subject to the economic squeeze from Medicare. Third, because there is a comparatively low level of professional agreement on indications for treatment and on the efficacy of different treatment modalities, it is hard for payers and reviewers to assess the necessity and appropriateness of treatments provided. The money-making opportunities are obvious when third parties are mandated to provide benefits for services that are difficult to monitor.

Meanwhile, the explosive growth in the cost of psychiatric benefits—as well as suspicions that some providers were exploiting third-party payment systems by providing services that were not really needed or were not efficacious—led many employers to take steps to stem the flow. Their responses have included both reduction in coverage of psychiatric services under their benefit plans and the implementation of utilization management programs (see Chapters 10 and 11) aimed at reducing costs. By early 1990 there were suggestions that the golden era for private psychiatric care might prove to be brief, with Wall Street analysts predicting a "shakeout" among the for-profit psychiatric chains because of a slowdown in the growth of admissions.[30]

## New Lines of Business

Another strategy adopted by the major hospital companies was to enter new lines of business. To date, the major initiatives have been in the health care field—in insurance, medical equipment, or provision of services—although, unlike nonprofit hospitals, the hospital companies are under no obligation to keep their capital in health care. Some of the new ventures have been largely independent of the company's hospital operations; others have involved lines of business that had some potential for coordination with hospital operations. For example, NME, long the most diverse of the companies, was heavily involved in both nursing homes and home care. Although in theory the operation of hospitals, nursing homes, and home care could be part of an organized system of care, in NME's case most such facilities were acquired separately and operated through separate administrative structures. Nevertheless, vertical integration is a strategy that all of the companies have pursued in one way or another.

*Vertical integration* refers to the "linking of enterprises at immediately related stages of production," as when a merger takes place between a company and a supplier or customer.[31] It can result from mergers and acquisitions, from creation of new facilities or organizational entities, or from creation of new capacities within an organization.

Vertical integration in health care has historically been a vision of reformers. Early examples, such as prepaid health care plans, rested heavily on ideals about continuity of care and rational organization of different levels of care.[32] The 1932 plan by the Committee on the Costs of Medical Care called for organized groups of physicians, dentists, nurses, pharmacists, and other health care personnel to be organized around a hospital so as to be able to provide home, office, and hospital care.[33] In the 1970s the idealistic conception of vertical integration turned up in such places as the Robert Wood Johnson Foundation's demonstration program on hospital-based primary care.[34]

In the 1980s vertical integration acquired a different flavor as the major hospital companies entered new lines of business intended not only to make money in themselves but also to funnel patients into the company's hospitals. One approach involved the creation of primary care or urgent care centers, either from scratch or by purchasing physicians' practices. Although the use of such centers as a feeder system for hospitals was in no way confined to the investor-owned companies, the most notable example of urgent care centers as an important line of business was Humana's MedFirst clinics. Humana's experience was notable in three regards.

The first was its magnitude: at one time Humana owned more than 150 centers. The second was its exploratory nature. The question was whether such clinics should be operated as independent entities, with no relationship to a Humana hospital, or whether they should be located in the service areas of Humana hospitals and generate business for the hospitals. Both of these uses of MedFirst clinics involved difficulties. For independent centers, the question was whether they could generate sufficient return on investment on their own without the function of supplying patients to a company-owned hospital. But establishing primary care centers as feeders for hospitals put the company into competition with the physicians on whom its hospitals already depended for referrals. Those physicians sometimes responded by reducing their use of the company's hospitals in favor of other hospitals. In some instances physician retaliation became a serious problem for Humana hospitals, for example, in San Antonio, Texas.[35]

The third notable aspect of Humana's MedFirst experience was the speed with which the company entered the market and, when economic losses began to mount, left it by selling the lot in two or three large transactions.[36] This is but one of many examples that illustrate how quickly investor-owned organizations can undertake a new line of business or enter a new marketplace, and how quickly they can exit.

Another major approach to vertical integration among the hospital companies was the development of financing capability to go along with provision of services. Again, although this approach was not confined to the investor-owned companies,[37] all of the major investor-owned hospital companies moved in this direction in the early and mid-1980s. Humana, which was the first to enter the insurance business, was unique in developing its own insurance program. A second approach was to purchase or make a joint venture with an existing insurance company. In

1985 HCA purchased the New Century Life Insurance Company and later established Equicor in a joint venture with the Equitable Life Assurance Society. The third approach, the acquisition or establishment of HMOs and PPOs, was tried by Humana, HCA, AMI, and NME, as well as numerous nonprofit organizations.

The hospital companies' efforts to combine insurance and hospital services were slow to pay off, and most companies largely abandoned the strategy, with Humana being the notable exception.[38] (The joint financing ventures of nonprofit hospitals have also struggled.)[39] Disadvantages of these arrangements include pricing problems, difficulty in achieving the desired degree of utilization control, and conflicts in goals between the insurer and provider sides of the organization. The success of one side comes at the expense of the other.

It should not be surprising that a hospital company's ability to prosper and grow during the lush reimbursement period of the 1970s and early 1980s provided no assurance that the company could succeed in a different economic environment or a different business. Under difficult economic conditions the pursuit of high returns on investment can lead to rapid entry into and exit from new ventures.

### Changing Ownership of Investor-Owned Hospital Companies

A final trend that grew out of the financial turmoil through which the investor-owned hospital companies passed in the late 1980s was a reflection of larger trends in the American corporate sector: the threat of corporate takeovers and leveraged buyouts by management groups. Three of the major companies—American Medical International, National Medical Enterprises, and the Hospital Corporation of America—were the subjects of takeover attempts by outside investors. AMI, although not succumbing to the first such attempt, was eventually purchased by an investor group and taken private. HCA was eventually purchased by a management-led investor group and taken private. (Two other major hospital companies, Charter Medical and Republic Health Corporation, were also taken private by management-led groups in the late 1980s.)

What the effects of these actions will be is difficult to foresee. Ownership by a relatively small group will strengthen the link-

age between the organization's economic performance and the
financial status of management. Accountability moves in a
much narrower circle. On the one hand, opportunities for mischief may develop (as is implied in the analysis presented in
Chapter 6). On the other hand, the organization is freed to some
extent from the pressure to keep quarterly returns high and, thus,
can perhaps take a longer-term view. That perspective may lead
to more responsible behavior. The implications of taking the
health care companies private are complex and poorly understood.

### Implications of the Hospital Companies' Experience

The major lessons from the past twenty years' experience with the
hospital companies concern responsiveness to incentives. The
capital payment methods of Medicare were a congressional
response to the lobbying of both the largely nonprofit American
Hospital Association, which sought inclusion of interest and
depreciation as reimbursable costs, and the largely for-profit nursing home industry, which successfully pressed for inclusion of
return-on-equity payments to for-profit providers. Medicare and
Medicaid also contributed to additional demand for hospital
sources because of the large increase in numbers of people with
third-party coverage. The development of the hospital companies
into an important force was a consequence.

This responsiveness to the availability of funding has been
seen among other types of for-profit health care as well. Table 3.2
shows the market shares of different types of for-profit firms
before and after funding became available through public programs. The increase of the for-profit sector among hospitals was
less dramatic than among other types of providers, perhaps
because such an extensive number of providers (mostly nonprofit
hospitals) already existed, as a result of almost twenty years of
federal subsidies for hospital construction under the Hill-Burton
program.

The willingness of entrepreneurs to invest capital when they
perceive opportunities in the market is, of course, one of the
advantages of the free enterprise system. The fact that Medicare's
payment methods not only increased demand but also limited

*Table 3.2.* Public programs and the growth of for-profit health care

| Type of facility | Change in coverage | Market share of for-profit ownership (%) | |
|---|---|---|---|
| | | 3–5 years before | 3–5 years after |
| Acute hospitals | Medicare enacted, 1965 | 5 | 7 |
| Nursing homes | Medicaid enacted, 1965 | 60 | 70 |
| Dialysis centers | Medicare covered, 1972 | 4 | 21 |
| Home health agencies | Medicare coverage provisions changed, 1981 | 7 | 25 |
| Psychiatric hospitals | States mandate private insurance coverage, 1975–1980 | 1 | 6 |
| Residences for mentally impaired | Title XX enacted, 1974 | 10 | 38 |

Source: Data in Theodore R. Marmor, Mark Schlesinger, and Richard W. Smithey, "Nonprofit Organizations and Health Care," in Walter W. Powell, ed., *The Nonprofit Sector: A Research Handbook* (New Haven: Yale University Press, 1987), p. 227.

most of the risk helps explain how HCA, a company that was founded in 1968, could own or manage one out of every fourteen U.S. hospitals fifteen years later. Although HCA and, to a greater extent, Humana received recognition as well-managed companies, without question the payment environment was friendly to growth. But of all the companies, only Humana has shown the ability to carry out a coherent strategy even as the payment environment has changed. Although its MedFirst clinics did not succeed, Humana has not experienced the other companies' large reduction in numbers of hospitals owned or rapid entry into and exit from the HMO or managed care field.

The ability of for-profit organizations to move rapidly to meet demand can be a significant advantage, particularly when the nonprofit or public sectors are slow to react. Yet, although the hospitals owned by the investor-owned companies are located predominantly in regions in which population growth occurred, responsiveness to unmet demand was not, by and large, the dynamic that accounted for the rise of investor-owned hospital companies. They grew primarily by purchasing existing facilities. Nevertheless, there are parts of the health care system in which the responsiveness of for-profit organizations to unmet demand has been a key factor. Stated differently, a health care system made up exclusively of nonprofit and public facilities might be less responsive to the changing demands of payers, patients, and physicians.

At the same time, the past twenty years have revealed two important drawbacks of investor ownership. First, for-profit organizations are free to sell assets and to move their capital into other lines of business. Consequently, some for-profit hospitals have experienced multiple changes of ownership. Two California hospitals—Community Hospital of Sacramento and Laurel Grove Hospital—went through the following sequence. They were physician-owned proprietary hospitals until being purchased by Beverly Enterprises in the early 1970s. In the mid-1970s Beverly sold them to AID, Inc., a subsidiary of the Insurance Company of North America (INA). INA subsequently acquired Hospital Affiliates International (HAI), and moved the AID hospitals into HAI. HAI was bought by HCA in 1981. The two hospitals were among eight hospitals that HCA sold in 1983 to Republic, a company that had been started by four former HAI executives. One can only speculate on the consequences of a hospital's being under six different owners in twelve years. While this example is no doubt extreme, large numbers of hospitals have undergone several changes in ownership as a result of acquisitions, divestitures, mergers, and reorganizations among the investor-owned hospital companies.

The propensity for change in the investor-owned sector can be seen in Table 3.3, which shows one year's listings of transactions involving medical and health services companies. The data are derived from the 1987 edition of *Predicasts F&S Index of Corporate Change*, a reference publication that compiles headlines from news, financial, and trade publications. More than 150 different events—ranging from startups to takeovers to bankruptcies—were reported among the "medical and health services" companies.

The events themselves are listed in the appendix to this chapter. They included the formation of 8 HMO or preferred provider firms; takeover attempts of HCA, AMI, and Beverly Enterprises

*Table 3.3.* Predicasts *F&S Index* summary of a year's activity in the for-profit medical and health services sector, 1987

| | |
|---|---|
| Companies created and joint ventures started | 16 |
| Takeovers/sales of companies, divisions, units | 114 |
| Partial acquisitions of company stock | 19 |
| Company acquisitions described as to happen[a] | 20 |
| Company sales/acquisitions | 26 |
| Acquisitions/sales of divisions | 14 |
| Acquisitions/sales of multiple units | 20 |
| Acquisitions/sales of individual units or HMOs | 15 |
| Failed attempts to acquire companies | 6 |
| Bankruptcies/Chapter 11 filings/ending business | 5 |
| Restructuring/reorganizations/spinoffs | 6 |
| Name changes | 5 |

Source: Predicasts *F&S Index of Corporate Change, 1987 Annual Edition*
(Cleveland: Predicasts, 1988), pp. 512–516.

Note: A few listed transactions with no apparent relationship to health services delivery have been excluded.

a. Often the only entries about transactions were in advance of the transaction. In cases in which subsequent entries showed the transaction did not occur, the entry is included in the "failed attempts" category. The transactions listed in this section appear to have actually taken place.

(the largest nursing home firm); the sale of home care and medical management divisions by National Medical Enterprises; the sale of two subsidiaries by AMI; the creation of a real estate investment trust by AMI to which 7 hospitals were sold and leased back; the purchase of 69 nursing homes in one transaction by Beverly Enterprises; HCA's sale of 104 hospitals to Health-Trust, a new company created by means of the tax advantages of employee stock-ownership plans; the purchase by Humana of International Medical Centers, the nation's largest Medicare HMO, which was virtually bankrupt when sold; and the bankruptcies of American Healthcare Management and Westworld Community Healthcare, Inc. (which owned, respectively, 33 and 36 small hospitals, according to the 1987 directory of the Federation of American Health Systems).

This one-year listing conveys a sense of the volatility in ownership and control that is part of the movement of capital among
investor-owned firms. What can only be imagined is how these
changes are reflected at the level of the individual organizations
where patient care services are provided. Effects range from
rumor and speculation to actual changes in management, data
systems, budget procedures, and policies.

The other drawback of for-profit ownership of hospitals is the
propensity to go out of business. All studies of hospital closures
have found a disproportionate representation of for-profit hospitals. This was once a matter affecting only individual hospitals,
but the replacement of proprietary ownership by investor ownership created the possibility of numerous hospitals' being affected
simultaneously by firms' financial woes. Indeed, bankruptcies
occurred among several small investor-owned hospital companies in the late 1980s.[40]

This brief review of the evolution of the investor-owned hospital
companies shows that in the for-profit world, capital can move
quickly from areas of low return to areas where higher returns are
expected (or hoped for). This goes far beyond the examples that
can be cited on the nonprofit side and appears to result from the
accountability structure of for-profit organizations. This characteristic may be an advantage in some circumstances, but it can be
a disadvantage in situations in which patient populations or
groups of physicians have become dependent on the organization.

Because government will continue to be a vital source of
income for providers of health services, the government's policies as payer (and also as regulator) deeply affect the return on
capital invested in health care. Just as policies in public programs
inadvertently created the circumstances that led to the formation of investor-owned hospital companies with billions of dollars in revenues, public policy has more recently stimulated
moves in other directions. In neither case was an impact on
investor ownership the goal of the policy.

The growth of investor-owned hospital companies stimulated
much of the concern in the early 1980s that for-profit organizations might take over the health care system. By the middle of
the decade they had halted their aggressive pattern of acquisi-

tions, and by the end of the decade they were no longer the object of much discussion in health policy circles.

Understanding their behavior nevertheless remains vital. For-profit enterprise plays a large role in health care, with for-profit ownership either predominant or growing among many types of health care organizations. The mid-1980s found all of the major investor-owned health care companies making major strategic changes in a search for new sources of revenues. Companies continue to emerge and to seek their own niches.

Despite the difficulties encountered by the hospital and HMO companies, it is far too early to write off the investor-owned companies on the grounds that their rapid growth has ended. Humana, Inc., returned to investor analysts' lists of good investment opportunities in 1989, with Seth Shaw and Mark Banta of Prudential-Bache waxing enthusiastic: "Even after a 55% spurt in its stock price this year, Humana still represents one of the most attractive values in our universe. We feel that higher ground lies ahead. We see plenty of momentum in earnings growth this year and next. We believe Humana is the right investment in today's stock market."[41] Other companies, particularly in the home health care business, continue to be admired by analysts.

Most of the major companies have survived and continue to operate, along with a significant number of smaller companies. Moreover, the need for health services will not disappear, and some financial analysts see serious problems of long-term viability in the nonprofit sector:

> The passage of Medicare and Medicaid both forced and facilitated the adoption by nonprofit hospitals in the short run of patterns of financing asset growth which probably cannot be sustained in the long run. The persistence of the nonprofit form over the past twenty years is therefore not convincing evidence of its long run viability. This will depend, in part, on the magnitude of future investment opportunities. While this is difficult to predict, the best available estimates suggest that the problem will grow more serious in the future rather than less.[42]

Finally, the experience with for-profit hospitals has had a number of spillover effects—most obviously on the behavior of nonprofit hospitals and, arguably, on the assumptions of payers and regulators about the extent to which providers can be trusted.

The economic pressures on hospitals have led to a widespread search for new revenues. Will the pressures of a more difficult economic environment stimulate for-profit institutions to become the most cost-effective providers of care, as their proponents have long predicted, or to become less socially responsible, as their critics have long feared? Clues can be found not only by examining accountability structures and understanding the economic incentives that are at work but also by comparing the past behavior of for-profit and nonprofit institutions. That is a topic to which we will turn in subsequent chapters.

## Appendix: Activity in the For-Profit Medical and Health Services Sector in 1987

The following transactions were listed in *Predicasts F&S Index of Corporate Change, 1987 Annual Edition* (Cleveland: Predicasts, 1988), pp. 512–516.

*Companies Created and Joint Ventures Started    16*

Aetna joint-venture HMOs with Voluntary Hospitals of America off to slow start

Biodecision Labs forms to support clinical research

Biotherapeutics jointly establishes cancer research lab with Scripps Clinic

Blue Care Network established to combine 6 HMOs

Blue Cross (Missouri) forms HMO in joint venture with U.S. Healthcare

California Biotechnology to form jointly Karo Bio, medical research and development (R&D)

CAPP CARE PPO founded as joint venture among 5 insurers

Chase Medical Group sells initial public offering of 1.2 million shares

Genetics Health Ventures forms joint venture to develop treatment for cancer-based immune system products

Group Health Corporation to launch jointly long-term health-care HMO for elderly with Metropolitan

HLS Holding, medical management services company, formed by merger of Health Learning Systems

J&J Health Management subsidiary created by J&J to market
health promotion programs
MD Health Plan to be formed by Connecticut State Medical
Society
NeoRx forms joint venture to develop immune system–based
cancer treatment products
Pacific Mutual forms HMO Alliance Health Plan
Superior Dental Care—first for-profit dentist-owned HMO plan


*Takeovers/Sales of Companies, Divisions, Units*  114

PARTIAL ACQUISITIONS OF COMPANY STOCK  19

Alternacare: 6.43% purchased
American Health Services: 6% purchased by Glen International
American Medical Buildings may be partially bought by Unicorp
American
Canning executives buy 60% of MedServe
Century Healthcare sells 4% to Healthcare International
Continental Medical: 21% bought by W. C. Anderson
First American Health sells 5.2% to Massey Group
Health Care Services—40% bought by Mediq
Healthcare International buys 4% of Century HealthCare for $1
million
Home Intensive Care: 8% bought by investment firm
Lifetime Corporation to buy 16.5% of Nippon Lace
Lifetime Healthcare: 27% sold by Glen International to 2 execu-
tives
Lincoln National buys share of HealthWin Insurance from U.S.
Healthcare Systems
Medical Sterilization partly acquired by Sumimoto Heavy Indus-
tries
National Medical Enterprises sells 17% share in National Health
for $20.6 million
National Heritage Parent Southmark sold 18% at public offering
National Medical Care: W. R. Grace increases holdings from
49.9% to 80%
Southmark sells 18% stake of National Heritage at initial public
offering
United HealthCare: 39.5% bought by Warburg Pincus

Often the only entries about transactions were in advance of the transaction. In cases in which subsequent entries showed the transaction did not occur, the entry is included in the "failed attempts" category. The transactions listed in this section appear to have actually taken place.

AMI rumored to consider spinoff of some hospitals to employees
Beverly Enterprises to be acquired by MedServe Health Company
Care Enterprises may be acquired by Southmark
Care Plus to buy Professional Care for $19 million
Central Texas Health to be bought by Physician Corporation of America
CoMed to be acquired by Total Health Systems for $19 million
Digital Diagnostic Systems to be bought by LINC Financial Services
Edgerton Trust (nursing homes) to buy Emeral Concrete Company
Healthcare Services America to sell to Paul Ramsey Group for $27 million
Heritage Health Systems to buy Omnicare (HMO)
HMO/Alliance to sell to Keystone Health Plan West
HMO America to be acquired by union of Chicago M.D.s
Maxicare Health Plans may buy Complete Health (HMO)
Medical Imaging Center to acquire MIL/IML Imaging care company
Mediq may acquire 40% of Health Care Services
Medlab to be sold to Nichols Institute for $5.3 million
MIL Imaging to be bought by Medical Imaging Centers
PrimeCare Health to buy TotalCare (HMO)
Professional Care may be bought by investor group
Westworld to be sold to Gateway

COMPANY SALES/ACQUISITIONS DESCRIBED
AS HAVING TAKEN PLACE   26

AlternaCare bought by Medical Care International
American Care (HMO) bought by Ramsey Health Care
American Medical Centers bought by Partners for $41 million
American Medical Services acquired by Trans World for $93 million

Belmar bought by National Medical Enterprises

Care IV (home care) acquired by Medical Personnel Pool

Care Mark (home care) bought by Baxter

Charter Medical: leveraged buyout by management

CliniShare bought by Health West Foundation

Florida Life Care (healthcare facilities) bought by Trizec

Healthcare Services America to be sold to Paul Ramsey Group

Healthsouth Rehabilitation buys Neurorehabilitation Rehabilitation

Humana buys International Medical Centers (HMO company) for $40 million

Hunt Research buys Quest Blood Substitute

Inhalation Therapy Services acquired by Medserv

Inland Health Care bought by Partners National Health Plans

Lifetime Corporation buys Quality Care hospital firm from GrandMet

Medical Research Assoc (R&D) sold to Concept

Mediplex Hospital Company sold to Meditrust for $30 million

Mediq Mobile Services acquires Syncor International mobile medical scan business

Mental Health Management (psychiatric service company) sold to Mediq

New England Critical buys NPO therapies (home care)

Partners Health Plans buys American MedCenters for $41 million

Senior Health Plan bought by Northwestern National Life for $1.1 million

TakeCare (HMO) bought by investor group

Tender Loving Care bought by Staff Builders from Norrell

ACQUISITIONS/SALES OF DIVISIONS    14

AMI to sell Inhalation Therapy Services to MedServ

AMI Diagnostic Services being sold to Mediq

Basic American Medical sells Data Scan Service to MMI Medical

Baxter Healthcare to sell home respiratory business to Glasrock Home Health Care for $60 million

Corning Glass Works sells Metpath to JS Pathology

Eckerd Drugs sells Eckerd Med-Cure to Markka Healthcare Centers

HMO America to sell North Florida operations to Metlife

Intracorp's ACORN Division sells to MS Goldsmith to form
ACORN PsycMgmt.

Jung sells home health business to Kendall Health Care

Medserv to buy durable medical equip. unit from Beverly Enterprises

NME sells home health services division to Kimberly Services

NME sells Curacare, medical management services division, to
American Shared Hospital Services

NME sells National Medical Homecare in leveraged buyout

Pearle Health Services sells Primacare ambulatory care chain to
Presbyterian Healthcare

ACQUISITIONS/SALES OF MULTIPLE UNITS    20

AMI forms American Health Properties to buy and lease back 7
AMI hospitals

American Health Care sells 2 of their 7 hospitals

Beverly buys 69 nursing homes from Stevens for $100 million

Crown buys 4 nursing centers, 3 retirement communities

Genesis Health Ventures sells 4 long-term-care facilities to
Health Care Property Investors

Greenery Rehabilitation selling and leasing back 3 nursing
homes to Health and Rehabilitation Properties

Health Care REIT sold 6 nursing homes for $13.9 million to limited partnership

HCA to sell 2 hospitals pursuant to Federal Trade Commission
order

HCA sells 104 hospitals to HealthTrust, an ESOP

HEI sells 2 hospitals to Missouri Baptist Hospital for $26 million

Humana selling 35 MedFirst centers to Health Stop

Humana sells 102 MedFirst centers to Health Stop

Humana to sell 68 MedFirst units to Primedical

John Hancock to sell 5 HMOs

National Health to sell 8 healthcare centers to ESOP for $40 million

NuMed sells 2 acute care hospitals

Republic sells 2 hospitals to Health Management for $21 million

Rite-Aid sells 6 freestanding home care units to D. Seeley

Southmark to buy 28 nursing homes from Bybee Associates for
$70 million

Whittaker sells 4 HMO operations to Travelers for $48 million

ACQUISITIONS/SALES OF INDIVIDUAL UNITS
OR HMOS    15

NME sells hospital to Affiliated Medical Enterprises

Beverly sells Durham Care to Greenery Rehabilitation for $3.3 million

Blue Cross California selling TakeCare HMO to investor group

Delaware Valley HMO acquired by QCC

GH selling Miami General Hospital to C&S Health for $18 million

Group Health Plan sells HMO to Principal Health Care

Healthcare International sells Eastwood Hospital to HealthVest

Heritage Health Systems acquires Omnicare

Humana buys Sunshine Health Plan

Maxicare sells Alabama HMO to Complete Health

Mediplex Group sells 172-bed facility to Meditrust

MetLife HealthCare buys HealthCare Network HMO

National Hospital Health sells Network Health Plan to Partners National Health Plans

Partners buys 50% of Health Master HMO

PruCare selling NorthCare Med Group to Michael Reese Health Plan


*Failed Attempts to Acquire Companies*    6

AlternaCare: Medical Care International (outpatient surgical centers) fails to buy

American Medical International: Dr. Pesch and Alpha Health Systems try to buy AMI

Hospital Corporation of America: 2 former executives and lawyer attempt takeover

Inhalation Therapy Services to be bought by W. Canning

National HMO cancels merger with Prime Medical Services

Prime Medical: potential buyout of medical facilities management firm hits snag


*Bankruptcies/Chapter 11 Filings/Ending Business*    5

American Healthcare Management files for protection from creditors under Chapter 11 of Bankruptcy Code

American Medical Services to be sold by Trans World in liquidation move

HMO America shutting down unprofitable HMOs in Detroit and Miami

WellCare Healthplan (HMO) to be liquidated

Westworld Community Health files for protection under Chapter 11

*Restructuring/Reorganizations/Spinoffs*   6

American Medical Services to be spun off by Transworld to jointly form TW Services

Beverly Enterprises to restructure operations and sell some assets

CareUnit created by spinoff of Comprehensive Care specialty care operations

Community Psychiatric modifies proposal to reorganize into a master limited partnership

HealthCall to franchise home health services

McKesson combines 3 home health businesses into 1 division

*Name Changes*   5

American Health Services is new name of NMR Centers

HealthCall is new name of Sickroom Service

Meridia Health System is new name of Strategic Health Systems

Primedica is new name of Inhalation Therapy Services

Staff Builders is new name of Tender Loving Health Care Services

# Accountability in Nonprofit Hospitals: How Distinctive from Investor-Owned?

In Chapter 2 the examination of the accountability structure of for-profit health care organizations implied a distinction with their nonprofit counterparts. Yet a now commonplace criticism of nonprofit hospitals is that their behavior is indistinguishable from that of for-profits. These criticisms are not wholly unfounded, as this chapter and Chapter 5 will show. Yet, differences of public policy importance remain.

Historically, many nonprofit hospitals have roots as charitable institutions,[1] and the funds with which they were originally established and constructed typically came from governments and philanthropy. Although existing in the private sector, and not always as responsive to public needs as critics would have them be, these organizations have historically had an aura of community service rather than profit seeking and have, accordingly, benefited from fund-raising drives and service by volunteers. Doctors have also contributed their services, and a willingness to provide care for charity patients was once a condition of hospital privileges in many institutions. The continuing strength of these charitable roots varies today from hospital to hospital.

## Legal and Economic Distinctions

The difference between for-profit and nonprofit hospitals is not only historical. Significant legal and economic distinctions are summarized in Table 4.1. For-profit corporations may be chartered for any legal purpose; nonprofit organizations are chartered

*Table 4.1.* Basic legal and economic differences between for-profit and nonprofit hospitals

| For-profit | Nonprofit |
| --- | --- |
| Corporations owned by investors | Corporations without owners or owned by "members" |
| *Purpose:* Management has legal obligation to promote wealth of shareholders within the boundaries of law; does so by providing services | *Purpose:* Has legal obligation to fulfill a stated mission (provide services, education, research, etc.); must maintain economic viability to do so |
| Can distribute some proportion of profits (net revenues less expenses) to owners | Cannot distribute surplus (net revenues less expenses) to those who control the organization |
| Management ultimately accountable to owners (stockholders) | Management accountable to voluntary, often self-perpetuating boards |
| Sources of capital include: Equity capital from investors Debt Retained earnings (plus depreciation and deferred taxes) Return-on-equity payments from third-party payers (e.g., Medicare) | Sources of capital include: Charitable contributions Debt (generally tax-exempt) Retained earnings (plus depreciation) Government grants |
| Revenues derived from sale of services | Revenues derived from sale of services and from charitable contributions |
| Pay property, sales, and income taxes | Generally eligible for exemptions from most taxes |

Source: Bradford H. Gray, ed., *For-Profit Enterprise in Health Care* (Washington, D.C.: National Academy Press, 1986, p. 6.

only for charitable, religious, educational, or scientific purposes that are deemed to be in the public interest.

For-profit organizations are accountable to owners who want to see returns on their investment and who are entitled to their proportional share of the organization's profits, whether those profits are paid out as dividends or reinvested as additional equity in the company. A nonprofit has no owners as such and is legally forbidden to distribute surplus revenues to its board of directors, administrators, doctors, or anyone else. Although salary increases and other prerequisites may have a similar effect, Internal Revenue Service regulations for tax-exemption purposes have put nonprofits on notice that incentive compensation must be "reasonable," "not dependent principally upon incoming revenue," and must not produce "abuse or unwarranted benefits."[2] The nonprofit's surpluses must be used for the purpose for which the organization was legally chartered.[3]

Nonprofit health care organizations generally enjoy exemptions from several types of taxes paid by for-profit organizations—notably, corporate income taxes and local property taxes. Furthermore, they benefit from federal laws that permit the issuance for capital financing of bonds that are tax exempt to the holder and therefore entail payment of lower interest rates than would otherwise be the case.[4]

A legal distinction that has now largely disappeared concerns *tort liability*, from which nonprofit hospitals enjoyed immunity as charitable institutions in many states. The immunity was created by the courts, and its decline was brought about by an accretion of court decisions rather than any single policy decision by a legislative body. The change is a reflection of how the courts have viewed the charitable aspects of the activities of nonprofit hospitals. Charitable immunity from tort liability is a doctrine that today holds in only a very few states.[5]

The doctrine originated in a Massachusetts court in 1876,[6] but "in the past few decades, impelled by the availability of insurance at reasonable cost and the greatly improved financial condition of many charitable institutions, the trend has been sharply toward elimination of immunity."[7] The decline in charitable immunity for nonprofit hospitals thus reflects changes in the financing of hospitals.

Several legal theories and policy arguments have provided support for charitable immunity. The oldest held that payment of tort damages from a trust fund would be a breach of the trust. Another held that a charity was not responsible for the negligent acts of an employee (the doctrine of *respondeat superior*) because the organization derives no "profits" from the actions of the employee. A third maintained that one who accepts charitable services implicitly promises not to hold the charity liable for its negligence. Still another found the basis for tort immunity in the restrictions on the use of the charity's assets for purposes other than those for which the charity was organized. One final argument is that exemption from liability acts as a stimulus to socially desirable charitable activity.

These arguments have slowly been swept aside in court decisions over many years. Edith Fisch, Doris Freed, and Esther Schacter, in *Charities and Charitable Foundations,* find the best (and certainly most colorful) statement of the reasoning in a 1961 dissenting opinion by a Pennsylvania judge, Michael A. Musmanno, in a case involving a Philadelphia hospital. He wrote:

> It is historically true, and it is a tribute to the soundness of the human heart that it is true, that there was a time when good men and women, liberal in purse and generous in soul, set up houses to heal the poor and homeless victims of disease and injury. They made no charge for this care. They felt themselves richly rewarded in the knowledge that they were befriending humanity.
>
> Hospitals then were little better than hovels in which the indigent were gathered for the primitive cures available. The wealthy and the well-to-do were cared for in their homes. The hospital or infirmary was more often than not part of the village parish. Charity in the biblical sense prevailed. And if it happened that some poor mortal was scalded by a sister of mercy, who exhausted from long hours of vigil and toil, accidentally spilled a ladle of hot soup on a hand extended for nourishment, there was no thought of lawsuits against the philanthropists who made the meager refuge possible. But if, following such a mishap, litigation should have been initiated in the courts, it is not difficult to understand why judges would be reluctant to honor such a complaint, convinced on the basis of humanity, that an enterprise utterly devoid of worldly gain should be exempt from liability. A successful lawsuit against such a feeble structure might well have demolished it and have thus paralyzed the only helping hand in the world of unconcern for the rag-clothed sick and the crutchless disabled.
>
> The situation today is quite different. Charitable enterprises are not housed in ramshackly wooden structures. They are not mere storm shelters to succor the traveler and temporarily refuge those stricken in a common disaster. Hospitals today, to a large extent, are mighty edifices, in stone, glass and marble. They maintain large staffs, they use the best equipment that science can devise, they utilize the most modern methods of helping themselves to the noblest purpose of man, that of helping one's stricken brother. But

they do all this on a business basis, and properly so . . . And if the hospital is a business for the purpose of collecting money, it must be a business for the purpose of meeting its obligations.[8]

Moreover, the availability of insurance changed the issue from the potential awarding of a charity's assets to, less threateningly, the "cost of reasonable protection against liability." By 1974 Fisch, Freed, and Schacter were labeling the doctrine of charitable immunity a "crumbling anachronism."[9]

## Growing Similarity of Nonprofit and For-Profit Hospitals

Notwithstanding the basic legal distinctions, nonprofit hospitals have undergone several changes that increase their similarity to investor-owned hospitals. In this chapter I will discuss four major aspects of this growing similarity: (1) the heavy reliance on revenues from the sale of services, (2) hospitals' dependence on economic performance for gaining access to capital, (3) the decline of local control resulting from the rise of multi-institutional systems, and (4) the proliferation of hybrid for-profit–nonprofit organizations. These changes have implications for the premise on which accountability in health care has traditionally rested: that health care institutions as nonprofit organizations have been animated primarily by goals of community service, not by economic aims, and that local control provided needed accountability.

### Sources of Revenue

The words *for-profit* and *nonprofit* call up sharply contrasting images having to do, respectively, with business and charity. Indeed, nonprofit hospitals once depended on charitable contributions for much of their funding. But from the early twentieth century, hospitals have found it necessary to generate revenues by charging patients who had the ability to pay for the services that they received. In fact, Rosemary Stevens traces the practice of accepting paying patients back to the founding of Pennsylvania Hospital in 1751.[10] By 1904 paying patients were providing almost three-fourths of the revenues of religious-based hospitals and about half of the revenues of other nonprofits, and payment was the "true scientific plan" for hospital charity.[11]

As the growth of third-party payment systems reduced the numbers of people who lacked the means to pay, the share of hospitals' revenues that came from charges for services increased. By the 1980s, 95 percent of the revenues of nonprofit hospitals was coming from the sale of services to patients, and, as Table 4.2 shows, the sources of revenues for nonprofit and for-profit hospitals looked very similar.

Even so, nonprofit hospitals (and government hospitals) have greater access to other sources of revenue than do for-profits, which obtain more than 98 percent of their revenues from the sale of services to patients. Though small, this difference between sectors may become more significant as price competition increases in the health care industry.

The growing reliance of nonprofit hospitals on the sale of services to patients as a source of revenue makes them subject to what can be called the accountability of the marketplace. It has become necessary for nonprofit hospitals to seek to attract patients and to provide services that will encourage patients and physicians to use their hospital instead of another. Failure to

*Table 4.2.* Sources of revenue for community hospitals, by ownership, 1983 (millions of dollars)

| | Nonprofit | | For-profit | | State/local government | |
|---|---|---|---|---|---|---|
| | $ | % | $ | % | $ | % |
| Total net revenue | 89,632.6 | 100.0 | 10,231.1 | 100.0 | 22,050.4 | 100.0 |
| Net patient revenue | 84,955.3 | 94.8 | 10,070.5 | 98.4 | 18,813.8 | 85.3 |
| Other operating revenue | 2,623.5 | 2.9 | 124.8 | 1.2 | 2,402.5 | 10.9 |
| Tax appropriations | 53.1 | a | — | 0.0 | 1,931.9 | 8.8 |
| Other | 2,570.4 | 2.9 | 124.8 | 1.2 | 470.6 | 2.1 |
| Nonoperating revenue | 2,053.8 | 2.3 | 35.9 | 0.4 | 834.1 | 3.8 |
| Contributions | 370.9 | 0.4 | 1.1 | a | 220.5 | 1.0 |
| Grants | 160.8 | 0.2 | — | 0.0 | 92.2 | 0.4 |
| Interest | 1,155.4 | 1.3 | 12.6 | 0.1 | 212.0 | 1.0 |
| Other | 366.7 | 0.4 | 22.2 | 0.2 | 309.5 | 1.4 |

Source: American Hospital Association data in Bradford H. Gray, ed., *For-Profit Enterprise in Health Care* (Washington, D.C.: National Academy Press, 1986), p. 100.
a. Less than 0.1 percent.

attract and maintain an adequate patient population results in poor economic performance and, thus, lack of access to sources of capital (see the discussion in the next section of this chapter).

Economic dependence on the sale of services is part of the incursion of the money economy into health care—a process Eli Ginzberg calls *monetarization*.[12] Because of the rising availability of reliable sources of third-party payment and the failure of philanthropic contributions to match the growth in the cost of providing care, all parts of the health care system have for many years been increasingly dependent on payments received for services provided. Although some institutions still obtain substantial philanthropic support, charitable grants and contributions now make up less than half of 1 percent of the revenues of the average hospital.

Reliance on the sale of services for economic survival has important consequences. Not the least of these is the possibility that nonprofit status can become more of a convenience than a necessity (as it was before third-party payment became prevalent) or an expression of philosophy. Business terminology and business thinking have pervaded the nonprofit hospital world. Eyebrows are no longer raised when the president of a nonprofit hospital chain proclaims, "We need a new breed of management trained in the entrepreneurial spirit of things."[13]

Marketing and the use of advertising are now commonplace in the nonprofit as well as the for-profit hospital sector. Trade sources report that hospitals spent $1.1 billion on marketing in 1986, of which $500 million was for advertising (up from $313 million in 1985 and $101 million in 1984).[14] The same sources reported that 91 percent of hospitals advertised in 1986, up from 64 percent in 1985. Nevertheless, advertising appears to be more prevalent among the for-profits (where it apparently began) than among the nonprofits. For example, the two biggest spenders on television advertising in 1985 were Humana ($5 million) and Comprehensive Care Corporation ($4.2 million), the investor-owned hospital and alcohol treatment companies.[15] In response to a researcher's query about eight for-profit and eight nonprofit multihospital systems in 1980, the trade publication *Modern Healthcare* reported that the former had taken out sixty-four ads and the latter only one.[16] That for-profit health care organizations advertise more than nonprofits is not surprising since so many of the for-profits are new organizations that are seeking to break into established markets. Also, advertising is much more often compatible with the ethos of a for-profit than a nonprofit organization. Yet one need only look at television or open a newspaper in many—perhaps most—cities in the United States to observe that nonprofit hospitals do advertise.

Although advertising by hospitals was still uncommon enough in the mid-1980s to have some news value,[17] major trade publications developed regular sections on marketing. The American Hospital Association, which first published guidelines on hospital advertising in 1977, now offers various types of assistance to hospitals, including a publication entitled "Fifty Effective Print Ads for Hospitals."

Success in the competitive marketplace is a major determinant of the survival of institutions. It underlies hospitals' varied efforts to maintain or increase their market share, to think in competitive terms (for example, by opening primary care centers near other hospitals), to spend money on the latest technologies so as to attract the physicians who admit patients, to develop new sources of revenue to make up for declines in the use of inpatient services, and to enter into joint ventures, alliances, and preferred-provider arrangements.

*Sources of Capital*

Access to capital is the lifeblood of any medical institution that aspires to keep its facilities modern and its technological capacities current, or that seeks to expand its range of services. Capital costs account for between 5 and 10 percent of the expenses of the average hospital. Chapter 2 traced the demanding accountability structure that stems from for-profit organizations' unique source of capital: owners' equity. The for-profit organization's drive for economic performance, which stems from owners' property rights in a firm's profits and growth, is the factor commonly assumed to differentiate for-profit from nonprofit organizations.

Such an assumption could not have been challenged in earlier eras in which nonprofit hospitals relied heavily on charitable contributions and government funds (initially local, but later federal) to meet their capital needs. But nonprofit hospitals' sources of capital today sharply depart from that historical pattern.

In the late 1960s, the same period in which the investor-owned hospital companies began to emerge and grow rapidly (and for the same causes), a market developed in hospital debt. A convenient milestone for marking the beginning of the trend is 1968, when Standard & Poor's rated its first health care bond. Standard & Poor's later explained its decision: "The Medicare system, then in its infancy, assured the solvency of most facilities by providing a steady stream of revenues. In addition, CON [certificate of need] legislation limited competition and provided hospitals with relatively stable markets. The benefits of cost-based reimbursement and restraints on competition, combined with those of a growth industry, assured success and were instrumental in S&P's decision to rate health care financing."[18]

Medicare provided more than a stream of revenues: as a result of heavy lobbying efforts by the industry, it treated hospitals' capital costs (the interest and depreciation expenses of nonprofit hospitals) as reimbursable expenses. Accordingly, hospitals have come to rely overwhelmingly on debt to meet their capital needs. By the early 1980s nearly 80 percent of construction funds for nonprofit hospitals came from borrowing, up from about 40 percent in the late 1960s, when government grants, primarily from the now extinct Hill-Burton program, provided more than half of their capital.[19] The federal government's contribution to the capital needs of hospitals now takes the form of reimbursement for expenses associated with past capital outlays (primarily interest and depreciation) and of tax revenues forgone because of the use of tax-exempt bond funding, which increased from 16 percent to 56 percent of nonprofit hospitals' construction funds between 1973 and 1981.[20] By 1981 philanthropy and government grants combined had declined to less than 8 percent of the capital funding of hospital construction projects.[21]

Thus, the sources of capital of for-profit and nonprofit organizations are much more similar than they were in the days when the nonprofits depended primarily on charity and government. In fact, although Chapter 2 emphasized equity contributions as a source of capital in for-profit firms, several surveys between 1969 and 1981 showed that from 40 to 80 percent of the capital for construction among investor-owned hospitals came from debt.

The expectations and demands of investors who lend capital are quite different from those of nonprofit hospitals' traditional sources of capital, which had at least some concern for the institutions' charitable activities and community services. Indeed, Hill-Burton grants specifically entailed legal obligations regarding community service and free care.[22] By contrast, lenders' primary concerns are risk and expected return. As was the case with ownership of companies' stock, much of the investment in the debt of nonprofit hospitals comes from institutional investors who are themselves accountable for their performance in investing the funds that are entrusted to them.

For-profits and nonprofit do differ in their access to tax-exempt borrowing.[23] This creates an interesting paradox in the provision of capital. Because the nonprofits' tax-exempt bonds pay lower rates of interest, they are attractive investments primarily to tax-paying organizations and individuals. The opposite is also true: for tax-exempt nonprofit investors (such as pension funds and endowments), the higher-interest bonds of investor-owned organizations are a much more attractive buy than are tax-exempt bonds. As a result, those who invest in the debt of for-profit health care companies are disproportionately, perhaps predominantly, nonprofit organizations, while those who buy the tax-exempt bonds of nonprofit hospitals are taxpaying, for-profit organizations.

The cost of funds for borrowing institutions is a function of the lenders' evaluation of the risk of the loan. Lenders generally rely on the assessments by national rating agencies, such as Moody's and Standard & Poor's, which rate borrowers' economic soundness and creditworthiness. The higher an institution's rating, the lower its cost of borrowing.[24] It is said that a substantial proportion of U.S. hospitals could probably not obtain an investment-grade rating.[25] A hospital that needs capital in such circumstances may have to pay very high interest rates for debt financing, seek bond insurance, find another source of financing such as a local bank, join an alliance or a multihospital system, find a purchaser, or close its doors. The basic point is that the creditworthiness of a hospital influences its access to, and the cost of, capital.

The factors that rating agencies consider in evaluating the creditworthiness of hospitals are thus a significant part of the accountability structure of nonprofit hospitals. The better the hospital's economic situation, the more creditworthy it is, as is shown in Table 4.3. Ratings of creditworthiness are based on site visits to the hospital by the rating agencies, meetings with key parties (representing the hospital's management, board, medical staff, and financial advisers), and review of extensive documentation, including a feasibility study by a nationally recognized firm. Such a study, which considers past performance and future projections, usually involves an examination of the hospital's market situation—demographic and utilization trends and competing institutions—and a financial analysis.[26]

The evaluation of creditworthiness penalizes the provision of unprofitable services and care for uninsured patients, creating a double bind for institutions that try to adhere to the charitable

*Table 4.3.* Key operating characteristics of hospitals with various Standard & Poor's bond ratings, 1982

| | Average values for hospitals with bond ratings of: | | | | | |
|---|---|---|---|---|---|---|
| | BBB | BBB+ | A− | A | A+ | AA+ |
| *Service variables* | | | | | | |
| Number of occupied beds | 88.90 | 139.99 | 157.50 | 235.87 | 414.48 | 803.47 |
| Percentage of Medicare and Medicaid patients | 49.47 | 48.11 | 44.96 | 43.21 | 39.56 | 38.13 |
| *Financial variables* | | | | | | |
| Net income ($000) | 199.47 | 400.11 | 514.62 | 849.99 | 1,791.54 | 3,766.0 |
| Cash flow ($000) | 431.53 | 768.42 | 1,000.05 | 1,674.91 | 3,257.52 | 6,621.1 |
| Current ratio[a] | 2.19 | 2.43 | 2.74 | 2.72 | 2.20 | 2.75 |
| Long-term debt/equity (%) | 88.88 | 70.62 | 69.53 | 64.06 | 59.64 | 50.13 |
| *Coverage variables* | | | | | | |
| Available for debt service ($000) | 672.13 | 936.42 | 1,260.57 | 2,110.21 | 3,839.12 | 7,526.6 |
| Debt service/gross patient revenue (%) | 8.76 | 7.13 | 7.58 | 5.28 | 4.53 | 3.28 |
| Maximum debt service coverage | 1.60 | 1.95 | 2.23 | 2.30 | 2.64 | 3.46 |

Source: Blyth Eastman Paine Webber Health Care Funding, "Health Care Policy: The Crisis in Capital Formation" (1982), p. 5.

a. Ratio of current assets to current liabilities.

aspects of the traditional mission of hospitals. Furthermore, the creditworthiness of rated organizations is regularly monitored. Hospitals rated by Standard & Poor's must submit an annual financial audit and provide data about the past year's performance: number of admissions, occupancy rates, outpatient services, payer mix, bad-debt level, and so forth. Such data can affect the ratings and the market value of the hospital's bonds.

Even so, the relationship between the bond price and anticipated earnings is not nearly so close as the relationship between stock price and earnings. In this sense debt financing does not create as much pressure for earnings growth as the pressure that stems from equity financing in investor-owned organizations. In some ways, however, bondholders have stronger leverage over institutional decision making than do stockholders, who ordinarily exercise their influence primarily through decisions to buy and sell stock (see Chapter 2). The rights of bondholders and obligations of the borrowing authority or institution are detailed in a bond indenture, which not only specifies the interest rate and date of maturity of the bonds but also sets forth information such as past financial data and projections and conditions designed to protect the lender.[27] Because debt service on revenue bonds is paid from the hospital's earnings, the hospital's ability to generate those earnings is monitored by a trustee, frequently a bank, which is appointed to act on behalf of the bondholders. If the hospital's ability to generate sufficient income for debt service comes into question, the trustee has the power to intervene directly to protect the bondholders' interests. Under some circumstances the hospital could be compelled to make changes in policies and methods of operation. If the hospital actually defaults on its debt, the trustee can take possession of the hospital and institute whatever measures are to the best advantage of the bondholders, although such actions have been rare.

Even if some observers see these circumstances as making nonprofit hospitals very similar to for-profit hospitals,[28] such a view probably makes too little of the investor-owned organization's drive toward earnings growth. Nevertheless, nonprofit hospitals' dependence on and accountability to private providers of capital undoubtedly explains, at least in part, why the average margins (revenues minus expenses as a percentage of revenues) of nonprofit institutions and the after-tax profit margins of investor-owned hospitals have been similar (around 5 or 6 percent of revenues in the early 1980s).

### Growth of Nonprofit Multi-Institutional Systems

Another parallel development in both the for-profit and nonprofit hospital sectors is the growth of multi-institutional systems. The number of nonprofit hospitals that are part of multihospital systems grew from 331 in 1960, to 472 in 1970, to 981 in 1983.[29] Multi-institutional arrangements allowed nonprofit institutions to gain needed help in coping with increasingly complex reimbursement systems and regulatory requirements and in obtaining access to funds from private capital markets.[30] In the late 1970s and early 1980s, the number of multi-institutional systems and of hospitals that were members of such systems grew more rapidly in the nonprofit than the for-profit sector,[31] a trend that has continued.[32] (By the late 1970s, it should be noted, most for-profit institutions were already part of a system.)

There are several important points of comparison in the growth of multihospital systems in the for-profit and nonprofit sectors. In contrast to the growth of investor-owned systems, which resulted largely from acquisitions and new construction, the nonprofit systems grew primarily through mergers and voluntary agreements among institutions. The latter path to the creation and growth of multihospital systems required much less capital and did not generate the same increased flow of dollars between cost-based payers and hospitals because interest and depreciation expenses were not created.

Even with the growth of nonprofit multihospital systems, membership in such systems did not come to typify the nonprofit sector as much as it did the for-profit sector. Unlike the for-profits, a substantial majority of nonprofit hospitals remain independent. Furthermore, although nonprofit systems are more numerous, they are also much smaller, averaging fewer than five hospitals per system (compared with the for-profits' nineteen hospitals per system) in 1983.[33] Larger size may enable organizations to achieve economies of scale, to undertake projects that would be beyond the capacity of smaller organizations, and to bring more resources to bear to meet the needs of patients, physicians, and communities. But it may also create a kind of indifference to local needs, particularly if size is accompanied by centralization of decision making and by distance and the existence of multiple organizational levels between institutions and corporate offices. In that sense, size itself could create some problems of accountability for meeting individual and community needs.

By some measures investor-owned hospital companies do not appear to be the most highly centralized of the multihospital systems. The only available study found them to be in an intermediate position between the more centralized public and secular nonprofit systems and the less centralized religious nonprofit systems.[34] This finding may be misleading, however, because the study measured centralization in terms of the presence of a local board, not the amount of authority vested in it. Of the investor-owned systems that had local hospital boards, half reported that those boards were only advisory.

The two sectors differ substantially in the accountability of hospital administrators (or chief executive officers, as they are increasingly called), whose role affects many key aspects of the institutions' operations.[35] Hospital administrators have traditionally been formally accountable to a local board.[36] The formal accountability of the hospital administrator in multihospital systems clearly differs from that of independent institutions, as can be seen in Table 4.4, in the responses of hospital administrators to questions about who employs them and who evaluates their performance. Hospital administrators in nonprofit systems appear to be more locally oriented than administrators in investor-owned hospitals. Only a small number (16 percent) of administrators of investor-owned hospitals report that the hospital is their employer, and most (86 percent) indicate that a corporate officer is their immediate supervisor. By contrast, at nonprofit hospitals most of the administrators who do not describe themselves as employees of the hospital are employees of religious orders (probably most are nuns).

It is clear that the growth of multi-institutional systems—particularly investor-owned ones—can have profound implications for the accountability of hospital administrators. In many instances the system, and not the institution, controls the hospital administrator's paycheck, performance evaluation, salary increases, and promotions. Indeed, the fact that career ladders

*Table 4.4.* Relationship of hospital administrators to employer and to immediate supervisor, by type of hospital

| | % of administrators responding | | | | | | |
| | Investor-owned | | Nonprofit | | State and local | Federal | All |
| | System | Freestanding | System | Freestanding | | | |
|---|---|---|---|---|---|---|---|
| **"Who is your employer?"** | | | | | | | |
| Hospital | 16 | 57 | 49 | 89 | 68 | 49 | 72 |
| Management firm | 63 | 33 | 11 | 5 | 24 | 0 | 14 |
| Religious order | 0 | 0 | 28 | 4 | 0 | 0 | 7 |
| Other | 21 | 10 | 12 | 1 | 8 | 51 | 7 |
| (Est. number) | (257) | (83) | (569) | (2013) | (737) | (121) | (3870) |
| Chi square = 306.8 df[a] 15; p < .0001 | | | | | | | |
| **"Who is your immediate supervisor?"** | | | | | | | |
| Board of directors | 9 | 71 | 69 | 90 | 76 | 4 | 75 |
| Executive committee | 2 | 5 | 1 | 7 | 1 | 2 | 4 |
| Corporate officer | 86 | 19 | 26 | 2 | 11 | 15 | 14 |
| University officer | 0 | 0 | 1 | 2 | 7 | 0 | 2 |
| Public official | 0 | 0 | 0 | 0 | 4 | 76 | 3 |
| Other | 3 | 5 | 3 | 0 | 0 | 3 | 1 |
| (Est. number) | (266) | (83) | (569) | (2001) | (746) | (125) | (3790) |
| Chi square = 585.8 df[a] 25; p < .0001 | | | | | | | |

Source: Foundation of the American College of Hospital Administrators, *The Evolving Role of the Hospital Chief Executive Officer* (Chicago, 1984), pp. 50–51.
a. df = degree of freedom.

exist *within* systems is often cited as a competitive advantage in recruiting managerial talent.

The broad move toward multihospital systems appears to have had much less impact on the tradition of local accountability in the nonprofit sector than in the for-profit sector. This, in turn, may affect an institution's responsiveness to local needs. Because hospitals serve local rather than national populations, local accountability may also influence how successfully institutions can operate in an increasingly competitive environment.

### Hybridization and the Blurring of Distinctions

Notwithstanding the legal distinctions between for-profit and nonprofit hospitals that were shown earlier in this chapter (see Table 4.1), the line between sectors has been blurred somewhat by hybridization. Several of the investor-owned companies have started nonprofit foundations with the donation of stock, but these foundations, though important, are clearly peripheral to the company's operation. The hybrid arrangements that have developed in the nonprofit sector are much more significant in that they are more commonplace and typical and in many cases have an observable relationship to the operation of the institution. Nonprofit hospitals are now involved in at least five different types of hybrid arrangements, affecting hospital management contracts, departmental leases and management contracts, corporate restructuring, joint ventures, and hospital alliances.

*Management contracts.* One of the oldest types of for-profit–nonprofit hybrids, going back at least to the early 1970s, is the nonprofit hospital that is managed under contract by an outside firm, a pattern that also occurs among public hospitals. By the early 1980s more than six hundred hospitals (almost 11 percent of the community hospitals in the United States) were contract managed,[37] although not all of the managing organizations were for profit.[38]

Among the reasons why hospitals enter into management contracts is the complexity of the reimbursement and regulatory mechanisms that they face.[39] A management contract provides such hospitals with access to expertise in establishing modern accounts and records systems, billing procedures, inventory controls, and so forth.[40] Large multihospital systems can often send much better trained managers to a small-town hospital than the hospital could attract on its own. For the young manager who works for a multihospital system, the management of such a hospital may be an initial step on a career path leading to more responsibilities in larger hospitals. Such a manager may also have access to many more backup resources than does the administrator of an independent small-town hospital.

Studies of contract-managed hospitals have shown that management firms (both for-profit and nonprofit) seek to improve hospitals' financial control systems, reduce staffing and other costs, recruit new medical staff, and improve community relations.[41] Yet, most studies have found the impact of contract management to be modest,[42] although there is some evidence of improved financial performance.[43] Not surprisingly, the best-documented step that can be taken to improve fiscal performance is also the simplest: raising charges for the hospital's services. Nevertheless, contract managers seem to satisfy the boards of the hospitals that hire them.[44]

The for-profit management of nonprofit hospitals raises some problems of accountability. For example, the separation of ownership and management introduced several complications into the auditing of costs under cost-based reimbursement systems. Among those were determining the reasonableness of management fees, figuring the cost base of services and supplies obtained through the management firm rather than through arm's-length transactions, and facing fairness problems that arose when payers found it necessary to sanction a hospital for actions taken by a management firm. (In extreme situations, as we shall see in Chapter 6, the nonprofit organization can become little more than a fig leaf for a for-profit entrepreneur who has found some advantage in managing an organization that has been incorporated as a nonprofit rather than incorporating the organization as a for-profit. This advantage may lie in the property-tax exemption or in evading restrictions built into a government program. Fraud, however, does not appear to be the underlying motivation behind most management contracts.)

Diffusion and confusion of responsibility can result from the use of contract management. The separation of ownership from control by means of a management contract can create uncertainty about whose will is being worked and who should be held accountable for actions taken by the hospital. Indeed, this is sometimes part of the appeal of management contracts for hospital boards that are considering taking steps that could prove unpopular in their communities. For example, in "Coast Town," a community studied by the Institute of Medicine's Committee on For-Profit Enterprise in Health Care, a contract management firm closed the emergency room in the public hospital and absorbed much of the criticism that would otherwise have gone to the county council, which hired the contract management company and tacitly approved the closure as part of the effort to reduce the hospital's drain on the county treasury.

More generally, however, the relationship between existing governance structures and contract managers appears to be quite varied, as is suggested by William Shonick and Ruth Roemer's study of contract management in seven public hospitals: "In some cases the introduction of the management firm enabled the Board of Supervisors to remove itself from the hospital's problems and pay little attention to how it was fulfilling its mission. In others, the advent of the management firm increased the involvement of the Board in the hospital's affairs. Because they were paying a far from negligible fee for service, some supervisors listened to the firm's administrator with greater care than they had to their own."[45]

The for-profit firms that manage nonprofit hospitals undoubtedly use many of the same techniques and procedures that are applied in their own hospitals, so that managed hospitals would seem to be more like for-profit than nonprofit hospitals. Yet, the contract manager is accountable to the hospital's governing authority, which has power over renewal of the contract. In this respect these hospitals would seem to be closer to nonprofit hospitals than for-profit institutions. Such are the paradoxes and ambiguities introduced by a hybrid.

*Departmental contracts.* Another type of hybrid arrangement is the contract management of particular departments within hospitals. Such contracting has increased rapidly in recent years, in part because of changes in reimbursement systems.[46] The largest areas of contract management—food service and housekeeping, which are contracted out in 20 to 25 percent of U.S. hospitals—do not involve patient care and thus are not hybrids as far as medical care is concerned. Nonetheless, many clinical departments in hospitals are managed by for-profit firms. Data from a trade survey of seventy-eight firms that manage clinical departments in hospitals are presented in Table 4.5. Although the data were not broken down by type of hospital ownership, these numbers provide an indication of how common this particular type of hybrid has become.

Hospitals may sign departmental management contracts for several reasons: to gain access to an efficiency that theoretically results from the management of similar departments in multiple institutions; to offer a new service (for example, treatment for alcohol abuse or chemical dependency) quickly and with minimal complications, and often with sophisticated marketing and advertising as part of the package; to generate new revenues; and to deal with chronic personnel problems, such as the staffing of emergency departments. Like management contracts, departmental contracts blur responsibility and accountability. The size, visibility, and influence of managed departments (particularly if

*Table 4.5.* Hospital departments managed under contract, 1985

| Department managed | Number of hospitals | % increase from 1984 | Number of contractors |
|---|---|---|---|
| Chemical dependency | 160 | 21 | 7 |
| Eating disorder clinics | 14 | 40 | 3 |
| EEG diagnostics | 375 | 0 | 1 |
| Emergency | 577 | 19 | 6 |
| Freestanding urgent/primary | 53 | 104 | 5 |
| Home health care | 45 | 36 | 9 |
| Occupational therapy | 29 | 61 | 7 |
| Physical therapy | 286 | 7 | 13 |
| Psychiatric | 117 | 67 | 4 |
| CT scanner | 67 | 72 | 2 |
| Rehabilitation | 34 | 240 | 4 |
| Respiratory therapy | 155 | 87 | 7 |

Source: *Modern Healthcare,* August 29, 1986, p. 49.

there are several within a single hospital) can affect the character of an institution. Patients may not understand that a program in which they have sought care is not run by the hospital (with which they may have had experience and which may have strong charitable or religious traditions) but by a strongly profit-oriented company. Programs that market directly to the public frequently advertise both the registered trade name of the program (for example, CareUnit) and the name of the hospital. Thus, in a variety of ways for-profit departmental management contracts in nonprofit hospitals blur the distinction between for-profits and nonprofits and diminish the reasons to expect behavioral differences between the two.

*Restructuring.* A third type of hybrid was created by the process known as corporate restructuring, which came into vogue in the late 1970s and early 1980s and resulted in the transformation of many nonprofit hospitals into much more complex organizations that included both for-profit and nonprofit entities. Although arrangements varied, the restructuring process usually created a holding company (or perhaps two) that had both nonprofit subsidiaries, such as the hospital itself or a charitable foundation, and for-profit subsidiaries engaged in a wide variety of businesses. Those businesses were often—but not always—health related. In many instances, they were joint ventures with medical staff members, other hospitals, or other organizations.

The main goals of hospitals in restructuring were to increase the organization's flexibility in responding to changing conditions and new opportunities, to escape regulatory constraints, and to increase income. For example, the pursuit of certain money-making opportunities could jeopardize a nonprofit hospital's tax-exempt status unless conducted through a for-profit entity. In some instances, reimbursement rules might result in reduced payments to a hospital to offset income earned from activities unrelated to patient care, including fund-raising. Such considerations led hospital consultants to suggest creating more complex organizations that made separate organizational entities out of the hospital, the fund-raising unit, and the various for-profit businesses and joint ventures. Efforts were sometimes made to pair for-profit activities that made money with activities that lost money to reduce or eliminate tax liability.

The process of corporate restructuring does not necessarily

change the accountability structure of the hospital because the same board could be put in charge of the overall holding company. As a practical matter, however, it seems likely that the corporate restructuring process could sometimes alter institutional governance and increase the profit orientation of the nonprofit hospitals that were restructured. The creation of a new corporation involves the creation of a new board, which may have different members than the board of the hospital. The hospital becomes one of several subsidiaries of the new corporation. The whole restructuring process is aimed at maximizing the organization's income within the limits set by tax law, reimbursement rules, and various legal constraints such as restrictions in debt covenants. It seems unlikely that a hospital's ethos and mission would be unaffected by such organizational changes. At the very minimum, the subsidiaries create new demands on the time and attention of the board.

*Joint ventures.* Many hospital restructurings involve more than moving existing functions into new organizational forms. New entities have often been created through joint ventures between the hospital and other corporate entities. "The joint venture is a protean concept encompassing almost any collaborative enterprise deemed to be of mutual benefit by two parties whose interests otherwise would be either divergent or overtly competitive."[47] Unlike earlier shared-service arrangements among hospitals for such activities as laundries, data processing, and purchasing, joint ventures are typically involved in services offered to the public.

Although it is difficult to estimate the number of joint ventures involving hospitals, trade publications in recent years have been full of examples, and the level of professional activity (such as conferences and consultant-sponsored seminars) has been high. Many hospitals enter into joint ventures with other hospitals for the purchase of expensive technologies, such as radiological diagnostic equipment.[48] Joint ventures have been reported between for-profit and nonprofit multihospital systems, as with a hospital jointly owned by National Medical Enterprises and Methodist Health Systems, Inc., of Memphis, or the joint venture between Intermountain Health Care and Hospital Corporation of America. These arrangements are for the ownership and operation of particular institutions. More complex are joint ventures between major commercial insurance companies and large alliances of nonprofit hospitals, such as Voluntary Hospitals of America, Inc., and American Healthcare Systems, discussed in the next section of this chapter.

Finally, many joint ventures between hospitals and organizations include some, although not necessarily all, medical staff members. An American Hospital Association survey in 1984 showed only 12 percent of hospitals to be involved in such joint ventures, but they appear to have become more common.[49] Joint ventures of this kind have several attractions for the parties concerned. They can be used to capitalize an activity and ensure a flow of patients, to minimize the competition between hospital and staff members, or to help the hospital gain access to capital by giving it some indirect benefit from the tax advantages that accrue to physicians as investors. Typically, physicians contribute patient referrals and capital to the venture; the hospital makes administrative, managerial, and marketing contributions.

Such joint ventures are of several types. One type, constituting a large subset, is designed to generate new revenues by offering laboratory or ambulatory care services: home care, primary care, diagnostic testing, ambulatory surgery. The idea is to increase referrals, to provide more services to the institution's patients, and to capture a larger share of the revenues generated by the physician-patient or hospital-patient relationship.[50] A joint venture frequently has the advantage of starting with an existing business rather than having to begin from scratch.

Another subset of joint ventures between hospitals and medical staff members involves creation of alternative delivery systems, such as an HMO or preferred-provider organization (PPO). The joint venture becomes the vehicle for essential administrative functions, utilization controls, and marketing. Some joint ventures have the more limited purpose of creating an organizational entity that will align the hospital's and physician's economic incentives, which come into conflict when the hospital, but not the physician, is being paid on a price-per-case basis, as under Medicare diagnosis-related groups (DRGs).[51]

Joint ventures raise several issues of accountability. First is the creation for physicians of incentives that could affect their fiduciary obligation to patients. Even in such an unlikely place as a book of "winning strategies" for hospitals, the discussion of joint ventures is accompanied by this concern: "Can organizations designed to capture increasing percentages of any patient's health care expenditures, and do so to a large extent by internalizing referral patterns, accomplish their goals without compromising the physicians' (and the hospital's) primary allegiance to the patient?"[52] (This issue is part of a larger topic that is examined in Chapters 8 and 9.)

Second are matters having to do with control. The hospital is but one party—sometimes a minority partner—in the control of the joint venture. Highly entrepreneurial individuals are probably an essential ingredient in any successful joint venture. Tension between such individuals and others who adhere to traditional ideas of the role or mission of the nonprofit hospital seems inevitable: "It is noncontroversial to observe that successful operation of a for-profit endeavor mandates a managerial style substantially different from that animating the typical nonprofit hospital."[53] Thus, the joint venture is another example of the hybridization process that is altering the traditional nonprofit orientation of health care institutions.

*Alliances.* "We structured an organization that blends the basic strengths of voluntary health care with entrepreneurial innovation."[54] So stated Voluntary Hospitals of America (VHA) chairman Don L. Arnwine in describing the hybrid nature of his organization in 1986. In contrast to multihospital systems, which are defined by an organization's ownership of more than one hospital, alliances are entities that are owned *by* the hospitals that have formed the alliance. Alliances are for-profit organizations that operate and are taxed as cooperatives. The profits from the alliance's various ventures can either be reinvested or be paid out to the stockholding organizations.

Although some alliances include only a few hospitals, there are two giants. In 1986 VHA comprised more than six hundred hospitals, including many of the nation's largest, reporting more than $24 billion in annual revenues and accounting for 13 percent of U.S. hospital beds, treatment of one in six patients, and affiliations of one in four practicing physicians.[55] The thirty-three nonprofit multihospital systems that made up American Healthcare Systems in 1985 had $14 billion in revenues.[56] (For comparison, the Hospital Corporation of America, the largest investor-owned health care company, had 1985 revenues in excess of $4 billion and owned or managed about four hundred hospitals.)

In a typical alliance each member (which can be either a hospital or a multihospital system) purchases an ownership share in the organization and is represented on the board. Thus, hospitals in an alliance retain more autonomy than do hospitals in multihospital systems. In addition, the hospital has the power to sever the relationship if it becomes dissatisfied. Nevertheless, tensions regarding centralization of control have arisen in some alliances.

Alliances were originally conceived to give affiliated hospitals the advantages of membership in a multihospital system—with regard to group purchasing, shared services, and access to capital—without yielding institutional autonomy. Nothing was to be done to alter member hospitals' essential nature as locally controlled, nonprofit organizations. In the increasingly competitive environment of the mid-1980s, however, alliances developed new strategies. Although the various alliances are at different stages and are pursuing different strategies, certain activities and approaches are making alliances much more like true multihospital systems. Moreover, certain similarities to *investor-owned* systems have become unmistakable.

The first was the move toward increasingly hierarchical structures. For example, the six hundred hospitals that made up VHA were organized into twenty-eight regional systems, which were in turn organized into six divisions.

The second was the practice of raising capital for hospitals at the system level, which made it necessary for the system to develop methods for holding individual hospitals financially accountable. At least four alliances issued pooled tax-exempt bonds in 1985, and several became involved in borrowing in taxable markets.[57] Most radical was VHA's stock offering of $40 million to finance a joint venture with Aetna Life and Casualty Company. Other capital-raising vehicles explored by alliances include real estate investment trusts. The question is how hospitals' own goals fare when their alliance is raising capital from equity investors, real estate investors, and venture capitalists.

A third similarity was the trend toward combining hospitals and insurers to sell broad health care plans to employers and other large purchasers of care. Just as various investor-owned hospital companies sought to enter the insurance *and* health care markets, several alliances developed insurance/health care plans to be marketed to large purchasers.

These changes in the organization and functions of alliances signify an important shift in the relationship between hospitals and alliances. Member hospitals were pressured to give up much more autonomy than was originally contemplated. Tensions can result between the requirements of the alliance and the autonomy of institutions. The activities of the two largest alliances illustrate the changing role of such groupings and the resulting conflicts.

Voluntary Hospitals of America was founded in 1977 as "a company cooperatively owned by 30 of the nation's most successful and highly respected nonprofit health care organizations." By 1986 the number of shareholder hospitals was approaching ninety, including many of the nation's most eminent hospitals: Abbott Northwestern Hospital in Minneapolis, Barnes Hospital in St. Louis, Baylor Health Care System in Dallas, Cedars-Sinai Medical Center in Los Angeles, Henry Ford Hospital in Detroit, Mary Hitchcock Memorial Hospital in Hanover, New Hampshire, The Johns Hopkins Hospital in Baltimore, Pennsylvania Hospital in Philadelphia, Massachusetts General Hospital in Boston, and Yale-New Haven Hospital. The VHA system (which also included hundreds of affiliate hospitals) had grown to "more than 600 hospitals and 135,000 physicians in 48 states."[58]

The goal of the organization had undergone a major shift along the way. Its 1983 annual report, "The Future of America's Health Care," had only the following words on the first page: "The goal of Voluntary Hospitals of America is to strengthen the voluntary hospital sector and improve their competitive position by providing systems' advantages while maintaining local autonomy and control." In short, the organization was to assist the autonomous hospitals that were its shareholders and their affiliates. To this end, VHA had created a group of organizations—some in joint ventures with other corporations such as the Mellon Bank and ServiceMaster Industries—that provided services to VHA hospitals, including management assistance, a vehicle for raising capital, assistance with marketing, group purchasing, and so forth. Most of the organizations in the "VHA Circle of Com-

panies," like the VHA itself, were for-profit, clearly making the
VHA a hybrid organization. But the hospitals themselves remained autonomous.

By 1986 a shift had taken place in the organization's orientation.
Both the title of its 1986 report, "Building America's Preeminent
Health Care System," and the statement of goals contained
therein signaled that the creature established to help its shareholders was now determined to act as a system: "Our goal as a
national system—our Common Vision—is to achieve national
preeminence as a fully integrated health care system through
uniting the technological, economic and human resources of VHA
hospitals and their medical staffs to meet the health needs of
people across the nation." The vision of the future that had led to
this change of orientation was stated on the first page (where the
statement about local autonomy had appeared three years previously):

> As consolidation in the nation's health care industry progresses,
> the majority of services will be provided by a handful of large
> systems. The most successful of these will unite leading health
> care organizations, physicians, advanced technologies, and innova-
> tive insurance programs into a single marketing force with finan-
> cial resources and service depth to meet total health care needs
> locally, regionally, and nationally . . . Voluntary Hospitals of Amer-
> ica has led the industry in redefining the possibilities for such a
> fully integrated health care system.

To this end, VHA joined with Aetna to form Partners National
Health Plan, which is described as follows: "Partners links the
skills, services, and delivery capabilities of VHA hospitals and
their physicians with Aetna's insurance marketing, administration, and customer-service strengths. The company develops,
finances, manages, markets, and owns innovative health care
plans utilizing VHA hospitals and their related providers. The
plans include both HMOs and PPOs for group and individual buyers
in local, regional, and national markets."[59]

The success of this approach was limited, at best. Initial losses
were substantial, even if expected, and some key top executives
were replaced. It became clear that if Partners were to market
such plans, significant pressure for more centralized control of
the hospitals would result. VHA's public position in mid-1986

was that the issue of hospital autonomy was "not a problem."[60] Partners was eventually sold in 1989.

The experience of another alliance—American Healthcare Systems—demonstrates the difficulties that arise in the transformation of an affiliation organization from servant to master of its member hospitals.

American Healthcare Systems (AHS) was formed in August 1984 through the merger of two other large alliances, Associated Health Systems of Phoenix and United Healthcare Systems of Kansas City. Shareholders were nonprofit multihospital systems with at least $100 million in annual revenues. AHS touted itself as the "nation's largest nonprofit network," and its president proclaimed that "this merger will make our shareholders even more competitive with large, for-profit chains without losing their identity as community hospitals."[61] In the view of its chairman, AHS was setting out to become one of the "15 to 20 vast health care companies" of which most American hospitals would be a part in the future.[62] Among AHS's operating subsidiaries were a shared-service organization (which had affiliations with 933 hospitals in 1984), American Healthcare Ventures, which was to develop new businesses, and American Healthcare Capital, which, like a comparable VHA firm, was "charged with seeking fresh capital using multihospital bond issues and stock offerings as vehicles."[63] AHS also announced its intent "to take part in or create large hospital [sic] maintenance organizations (HMOs) and preferred provider organizations (PPOs)."[64] This last strategy, which was consistent with a broad trend among large multihospital systems, created strong pressure for changing an alliance's role from serving its members while preserving their autonomy to serving the organization's collective interest through activities that require shareholders to yield a significant degree of their autonomy.

By early 1986 the move into the world of managed care was under way. Joint ventures with two insurance companies had been signed, and a subsidiary called American Healthcare Plans, Inc., had been formed. In March, however, the president, the chief operating officer, and the vice president of finance all resigned. The most visible issue was the tension between the corporate officers' vision of how to get from here to there and the reluctance of many shareholder systems to make the requisite sacrifice of autonomy. A trade source described the situation within AHS: "The leaders of American Healthcare Systems and other alliances of nonprofit hospitals and chains say they want to stop acting like, and being thought of as, old boys' clubs. They seek the credibility of *Fortune 500* corporations, but they aren't ready to give up all of the characteristics of voluntary boards of nonprofit hospitals or trade associations. Their need to manage by consensus is generally considered a weakness by investor-owned competitors, but some observers think it may prove to be a major strength."[65]

Thus, strategies that led to the creation of hybrid organizations into which huge sums of private capital were poured clearly intensified pressures for centralized (or perhaps regionalized) control. It seems inevitable that the character of the institutions that are caught up in these trends will change.

The activities and strategies of alliances have had striking similarities to those of the for-profit sector. There is more than a little irony in a trade publication advertisement by an investor-owned hospital firm which touts its services as offering nonprofit hospitals "an alternative to participation in alliances."

The nonprofit sector has long been predominant among American health care organizations. It is often glibly asserted that for-profit and nonprofit organizations have different goals: one seeks to make money while the other seeks to provide service. As we have seen in this chapter, the lines distinguishing the for-profit from the nonprofit sectors of today's health care industry have become blurred. The developments that have been examined in this chapter are making the accountability structures of the nonprofit hospital world more similar to those of the investor-owned world. The heavy reliance on the sale of services for revenues, the dependence on private capital markets, the rise of multi-institutional systems, and the hybridization phenomenon are significant developments for the traditional, locally controlled nonprofit hospital.

It is probably not surprising that spokespersons from the for-profit sector have commonly responded to hostile criticism with arguments about similarities across sectors. Every organization, whether for-profit or not, must make a profit if it is to survive, they say, suggesting that those who believe otherwise are naive or hopelessly idealistic. And, indeed, some of the idealists have expressed deep disquiet about the changes they see happening in nonprofit hospitals: "Voluntary hospitals, unable to cross-subsidize expensive but essential clinical services because of cost competition, are becoming ever less distinguishable from the proprietary hospitals as they 'market' and 'demarket' (rid themselves of money-losing clinical services), diversify, 'unbundle,' 'spin-off' for-profit subsidiaries, develop 'convenience-oriented feeder systems,' attempt to adjust case mix, and triage admissions by their ability to pay."[66]

Yet some basic legal and economic differences remain between for-profit and nonprofit organizations—even those that operate in the same competitive field. Nonprofits continue to be "organizations without owners," and most are still governed by local volunteer boards. Moreover, in recent years there has been a rise in self-conscious attention to the question of institutional "mission" on the part of nonprofit hospitals.[67]

Modern nonprofit hospitals obviously must be concerned with financial performance and cost control, and many have adopted marketing and other accoutrements of the health care "business." Hybridization is commonplace. Does all this mean that their behavior as organizations will be indistinguishable from the behavior of profit-maximizing business corporations? Researchers have developed a considerable body of empirical evidence that bears on this question, and it is to this evidence that we turn in the chapters that follow.

## · 5 ·

# The Performance of For-Profit and Nonprofit Health Care Organizations

In the previous two chapters I described the growing general prominence of for-profit health care organizations and some parallel developments within the for-profit and nonprofit sectors of the hospital industry. I have emphasized the hospital sector because of its centrality and economic significance in our health care system, because of the size and importance of the investor-owned hospital companies, and because the hospital field embodies most of the issues involved in the increasing profit orientation of the health care system. Also worth noting is the fact that developments in the hospital field have produced criticism not only of for-profit ownership (criticisms, incidentally, that are very similar to those made of other types of for-profit health care organizations) but also of the *nonprofits*—pertaining both to social responsibility and to justifications for tax exemptions. More so among hospitals than other types of health care organizations, the comparative behavior of for-profit and nonprofit organizations has public policy implications for *both* sectors.

This chapter focuses on comparative evidence about the performance of for-profit and nonprofit hospitals and the implications of changing economic conditions in the industry. Yet, the empirical literature on the effects of form of ownership is not limited to hospitals. This chapter will also consider the implications of evidence about the comparative performance of other types of for-profit and nonprofit health care organizations.

## Differences Associated with Property Rights

The material contained in earlier chapters could be used to support three different arguments about the comparative behavior of for-profit and nonprofit health care organizations: that for-profit ownership is worse in some respects, that it is better, or that type of ownership makes little real difference. The first two arguments rest on a key distinction between the two types: the presence in for-profit organizations, as opposed to nonprofit organizations, of owners who have a property right to their share of the organization's profits.

To critics this means that for-profit providers of health care will tend to respond poorly in some crucial situations, such as when a patient who lacks the means to pay requires care, when there is a need in the community for a service that cannot be provided profitably, or when decisions must be made whether to invest in activities such as clinical research and education that are substantially public goods.[1] The advocates of for-profit health care argue that socially responsible behavior is not limited to any one type of institution,[2] and that the owners' interest in the profits of for-profit organizations provides incentives that make these organizations more efficient than nonprofits.[3]

The question of who is entitled to any income generated by the organization may not, however, be as crucial in shaping organizational behavior as is the environment in which the organization operates. As Paul DiMaggio and Walter W. Powell have observed, organizations in the same field tend to take on a degree of similarity (isomorphism).[4] This occurs because organizations in the same field may face similar competitive conditions, because they may have to meet common requirements (for example, accreditation or certification), and because of imitation.

There are reasons, therefore, to predict either differences or similarities in the behavior of for-profit and nonprofit organizations, differences that could affect patients, physicians, payers, and public policy. In the remainder of this chapter, I will examine evidence about hospital ownership and questions of cost, quality, and access; consider the meaning of the growth of multi-institutional systems and of the growing economic squeeze on hospitals; and, finally, discuss the implications of ownership-related differences in other types of health care institutions.

## Hospitals and the Cost Question

The comparative economic behavior of for-profit and nonprofit hospitals has been more extensively studied than any other aspect of their activity. Research on the theoretically interesting question of whether for-profits are indeed more efficient than nonprofits has produced answers that range from equivocal to negative. Research making the more practical comparison of the direct cost to purchasers of care shows clearly that it has cost more to buy hospital services from for-profit hospitals than from nonprofit hospitals.

### Studies of Expenses

The Institute of Medicine's (IOM) 1986 report, *For-Profit Enterprise in Health Care*, reviewed eight studies of hospital expenses in the production of services. These studies used various methods and sources of data and controlled for many potentially confounding factors (including distinguishing investor-owned from independent proprietary hospitals). The results of all but one of the studies contradicted the hypothesis of the efficiency of for-profit organizations, finding that expenses incurred per day in investor-owned hospitals were from 3 to 10 percent higher than in nonprofit hospitals.[5] Studies that examined expenses per *stay* found smaller or negligible differences between investor-owned and nonprofit hospitals because average lengths of stay were shorter in investor-owned hospitals.[6] None of the studies provided support for the efficiency hypothesis.

Some studies identified reasons for higher per-day expenses in investor-owned hospitals. One was the higher capital expenses (interest and depreciation), a result of the companies' growth strategies under cost-based reimbursement. Investor-owned organizations grew primarily by means that required substantial outlays of capital (either the purchase of existing organizations or new construction).[7] By contrast, much of the growth of nonprofit multihospital systems came through mergers that did not require cash outlays. Other factors resulting in higher expenses in investor-owned hospitals were central office costs, greater use of ancillary services, lower occupancy rates, and taxes.[8]

The initial studies that documented investor-owned hospitals' higher expenses were criticized for failing to make all of the adjustments that would be needed for a truly fair test of the efficiency hypothesis.[9] Although no studies have been able to make all the suggested adjustments, several have gone beyond the simple comparisons of the early studies.

One adjustment that the critics called for pertains to the treatment of taxes paid by the for-profits. In a well-designed study that made adjustments for taxes, however, higher expenses in for-profit hospitals were again found.[10] In another study that was done by the Vanderbilt University economist Frank Sloan, one of the chief critics of the cost studies, and the Hospital Corporation of America's Robert Vraciu, adjustments were made not only for taxes but also for the public subsidies and charitable contributions received by nonprofit hospitals; no difference was found in expenses per stay between for-profit and nonprofit hospitals in Florida, but per diem expenses averaged 2 percent higher in for-profits.[11] (Serious questions have been raised about the validity and generalizability of these findings.)[12]

In a study by Regina Herzlinger and William Krasker, a third type of adjustment was made—for the way capital expenditures were accounted for—as well as adjustments for taxes.[13] They argue that the expenses reported by an institution that has an old physical plant and old equipment appear artificially low because those assets are being depreciated in terms of their cost at the time of purchase without any adjustment for what it would cost to replace those assets; interest expenses may be affected similarly. The usefulness and validity of the empirical analysis that applied this argument were obscured by a number of methodical problems with the study, as well as its polemical tone.[14]

In sum, comparative studies of expenses incurred by hospitals in the care of patients have either provided no support for the efficiency hypothesis or produced results that are tainted by methodological flaws.

### Cost to the Payer

In constructing their measures of hospitals' "costs to the community," neither Sloan and Vraciu nor Herzlinger and Krasker addressed the matter of cost to the payer, which is different from an institution's expenses in providing services. Even if there are good methodological reasons for researchers who are interested in the efficiency hypothesis to "adjust" the nonprofits' expenses upward to compensate for the effects of taxes not paid and charitable contributions received, and to adjust the for-profits' expenses downward to correct for the distorting effects of their high capital expenses, those adjustments are irrelevant to the payer. Payers' expenditures until recent years were based either on their reimbursing hospitals on the basis of conventionally accounted-for costs, as with Medicare's cost-based reimbursement, or on their paying the hospital's charges for services it provided.

The six studies of hospital prices (that is, of the cost to the payer) that were reviewed in the IOM report found that the cost to payers that reimbursed hospitals for allowable costs was from 8 to 15 percent higher in investor-owned chain hospitals than in nonprofit hospitals. These higher costs stemmed not only from the previously mentioned factors (for example, the for-profits' acquisition patterns), but also from the Medicare reimbursement formula that included a return-on-equity payment only for for-profit institutions. As a result of this formula, for example, the Congressional Budget Office projected Medicare capital reimbursement *per bed* in fiscal 1984 at $7,170 in for-profit hospitals (of which $3,410 was the return-on-equity payment), compared to $3,360 in nonprofit hospitals and $2,230 in public hospitals.[15]

It might be assumed that Medicare's move from a cost-based system to a system based on price (per case) would have hurt the for-profits, with their higher accounting costs, or that in any case the question of comparative cost to that particular payer would no longer be an issue. Available evidence suggests, however, that the earlier picture regarding comparative costs to Medicare may not have changed. Despite their higher historical costs, for-profit hospitals initially had higher profits under the prospective payment system than did nonprofits.[16] The reasons for this probably include the following: (1) artifacts of the period of transition from cost-based to prospective payment and the fact that investor-owned hospitals were concentrated in parts of the country where average lengths of hospital stay were comparatively short even prior to the new system; and (2) the fact that capital costs—a major source of revenues for for-profit hospitals in Medicare's ostensibly cost-based system—continued to be paid under the old cost-based system. Thus, it seems likely that Medicare's cost of purchasing care continues to be higher in for-profit hospitals than in comparable nonprofit hospitals, although no new studies have as yet been done.

For purchasers who pay billed charges, their cost disadvantage in buying services from an investor-owned hospital has been even more pronounced because investor-owned hospitals have higher markups than nonprofit hospitals.[17] Studies found the price per admission for charge-paying patients to be from 17 to 24 percent higher in investor-owned hospitals than in nonprofit hospitals.[18] On a per-day basis the difference was even more dramatic, with charges 23 to 29 percent higher in investor-owned hospitals than in nonprofits.[19] It is not known how growing competitive pressures in the 1980s affected these price differences.

Thus, available evidence does not support the notion that for-profit hospitals are more efficient than nonprofits, and there is strong evidence that from the purchaser's standpoint, for-profit hospitals have been substantially more expensive. It is worth noting here, however, that data about comparative costs in hospitals cannot be generalized to other types of health care organizations. Important variations in the regulatory and payment environments, as well as historical factors, undoubtedly affect the comparative costliness of for-profit and nonprofit organizations in different fields. Among HMOs, for example, the only available study shows for-profits to have higher expenses than nonprofits.[20] The nursing home field presents a different, more complicated story.

Studies have shown that expenses are lower in for-profit nursing homes than in nonprofit homes.[21] Nonetheless, this is not necessarily evidence of efficiency. There appears to be a wider range in the quality of care among nursing homes than among hospitals, and it is not clear that nursing homes of comparable quality are being compared in the cost studies. Furthermore, on average, nonprofit nursing homes have higher revenues, in part because many receive support from sponsoring organizations, such as religious groups. This is one reason why nonprofit nursing homes are generally better able to attract private-pay residents and, therefore, to serve fewer patients covered by the relatively low-paying Medicaid program. These factors explain why nonprofit homes tend to have higher per-patient revenues per day and why it is difficult to interpret the differences in expenses in terms of efficiency.

## The Quality-of-Care Question

Is the quality of care better or worse in for-profit than in non-profit institutions? Although clear theoretical reasons can be offered to support the expectation that for-profits would be more efficient or would provide less charity care, it is less clear why people expect a difference between for-profits and nonprofits in quality of care.

One answer to why profit status might affect quality has been offered by Burton A. Weisbrod and Mark Schlesinger, who observe that there are aspects of quality that the market can detect and aspects that it cannot.[22] For-profit organizations, they hypothesize, may perform better than the nonprofits with regard to the tangible aspects of quality care but worse on those aspects of care in which quality is more subtle and, thus, difficult for the recipient to evaluate. This intriguing hypothesis faces two difficulties, however. First, testing it would require that researchers find measures of quality that the market cannot detect; if such measures were readily available, presumably the market would be making use of them. Second, in hospitals the most direct customers are physicians, and they *do* have the ability to assess the quality of hospital services. If physicians act in the best interests of their patients, there would seem to be little competitive advantage accruing to hospitals that reduce quality in ways that are unacceptable to physicians.

This may explain why studies have generally found no substantial differences in quality of care between investor-owned and nonprofit hospitals. Two early studies of malpractice cases in the 1970s found no evidence of any overrepresentation of for-profit hospitals.[23] The Institute of Medicine examined a much larger body of evidence on such indicators of quality as hospital accreditation, board certification of staff physicians, numbers of nursing personnel, and mortality from several elective surgical procedures. Differences were small and did not consistently favor either ownership form; the IOM committee concluded that there is "no overall pattern of either inferior or superior quality in investor-owned chain hospitals as compared to not-for-profit hospitals."[24]

The rise of the investor-owned hospital companies may actually have improved quality in the hospitals they acquired. Some hospitals were available for acquisition because of their unsound financial situation, a factor that could detract from quality.[25] Many hospitals purchased by investor-owned companies were subsequently renovated or replaced. Also, most hospitals that were bought by these companies had previously been independent proprietaries, which were often undercapitalized and did not have to compete for the patients of their physician-owners.[26] Accreditation rates are much lower among proprietary hospitals than hospitals owned by investor-owned chains.[27]

The incentives in the era of cost-based and charge-based payment systems gave hospitals no reason to compromise on quality, particularly since they were competing for the allegiance of admitting physicians. But with Medicare shifting to a per-case payment system, and with competition growing among hospitals for the business of charge-paying purchasers of care, hospitals have been given powerful incentives to cut costs. Might the new incentives be so powerful—particularly at for-profit hospitals— as to overwhelm the factors that encourage high quality (scruples, fear of liability, the continuing need to satisfy physicians)? One study suggests not—at least in three of the largest investor-owned chains. Using a variety of quality indicators, such as accreditation data and mortality from elective surgery, Stephen Shortell and his colleagues found no quality differences between investor-owned and not-for-profit multihospital systems in the early post–prospective-payment era.[28]

Another study, however, which examined hospital characteristics associated with high death rates among Medicare patients in 1986, found that for-profit hospitals had significantly elevated mortality.[29] (Public hospitals also had higher mortality rates than private nonprofit hospitals.) The reasons for the increased rates in for-profit hospitals were not clear. The researchers, however, made many adjustments to ensure that the hospitals studied were comparable in terms of the severity of illness of patients. Other findings from the study support an interpretation of the mortality rates as indicators of quality, not just statistical artifacts of some sort. For example, mortality rates were found to be inversely related to the percentage of physicians who were board certified, the percentage of nurses who were certified, occupancy rates, and payroll expenses per bed.[30]

Two earlier studies had failed to find a relationship between type of hospital ownership and patient mortality.[31] The reasons for the differences in results is not clear. They could be due to methodological variations among the studies—particularly the fact that the researchers in the most recent study were able to make more adjustments to control for the effects of cross-hospital differences in the severity of patients' illnesses. It could also be possible that the association between mortality and ownership developed only after the Medicare prospective-payment system changed the incentives faced by hospitals. If so, this could be a hint of a possibly troublesome aspect of for-profit ownership as the health care system becomes more cost driven and competitive.

The earlier studies suggest that investor ownership is not incompatible with quality of care. Were those results due to a particular economic environment and a particular kind of relationship between hospitals and physicians? The factors that lead to high quality at a medical institution are not well understood. In nursing homes, where quality standards vary widely, the most serious problems tend to appear in for-profit facilities.[32] Is this because of the chronic underfunding of nursing homes? If so, as economic pressures on hospitals mount, might problems of quality appear first among for-profits? Or are the problems due to the comparative absence of physician-advocates in nursing homes? If so, quality problems might be associated with hospitals' finding ways to divide the physician's loyalty when it serves the hospital's economic interests to do so. The methods by which hospitals have been able to bring about changes in physician-controlled patterns of care (for example, shortened lengths of stay) in the wake of prospective payment thus assume importance.

It is clear that continued improvement is needed in the measurement of quality of care, and additional analyses of ownership-related differences in quality are called for. Past absence of differences cannot be projected into the future with confidence, particularly since the circumstances that caused them are so poorly understood.

### Provision of Uncompensated or Unprofitable Services

As recipients and dispensers of charitable contributions and government support, hospitals have long helped fill gaps in the financing of medical services. Various estimates over the last decade have shown that 31 million to 37 million Americans lack health insurance, and hospitals that serve them often lose money in the process. Furthermore, some services offered by hospitals generate costs that exceed revenues.

The most common objection to for-profit health care is the presumed unwillingness of for-profit organizations to serve patients who cannot pay for care or to provide necessary but unprofitable services. Some critics have been content to assume that a striking contrast with nonprofit organizations exists. As Chapter 4 showed, however, nonprofit hospitals, like investor-owned hospitals, are under strong pressure to perform well economically.

The presumption that for-profit hospitals do not provide uncompensated care or unprofitable services is clearly not correct. American Hospital Association data show that the uncompensated care (bad debt plus charity) in for-profit hospitals amounts to approximately 3 or 4 percent of revenues,[33] and a national survey in the early 1980s showed that 6 percent of the patients admitted at the average for-profit hospital were uninsured.[34] In a few for-profit hospitals (3.1 percent) more than one-fifth of the patients were uninsured.[35] Documented cases of refusal to provide services to patients who need care but who lack the means to pay have not been peculiar to investor-owned hospitals and have involved only a very small proportion of them.[36]

Regarding presumed unprofitable services, there are numerous examples of for-profit hospitals' providing virtually any service that can be cited.[37] Many investor-owned hospitals have neonatal intensive care centers, and more than 90 percent of investor-owned hospitals with more than fifty beds have emergency departments. In the early 1980s even the investor-owned hospitals' lack of involvement in teaching and research activities underwent a change.[38]

Yet, a listing of the unprofitable activities of for-profit organizations should not obscure their basic for-profit purpose: to generate a return on investment. The pursuit of profit does not require—and may not be facilitated by—an attempt to make a profit on each and every service or patient. Other factors also play a role. Under some circumstances a hospital may risk civil liability or expulsion from the Medicare program if it refuses to provide urgently needed care. Moreover, hospitals' concern for their reputation and image in the community sometimes encourages behavior that cannot be justified solely on short-term economic grounds. The need to maintain good relations with the physicians who admit paying patients may sometimes make it expedient for a hospital to offer certain services that are not themselves profitable, or may make it prudent to allow a staff physician to admit a patient who lacks the means to pay. Also, a certain level of bad debt is inevitable in a business in which services often must be provided in advance of payment. Some services that a hospital offers may generate both bad debt and revenue. For example, an emergency room will inevitably bring in some bad debt, but a hospital may nevertheless find it profitable to have an emergency department because one-half of hospital admissions commonly come by that route.

For such reasons it makes little sense to analyze the behavior of for-profit hospitals by comparing them with hypothetical models of expected behavior. Comparisons with nonprofit hospitals are much more useful because the nonprofits predominate and are expected to behave in some measure as charitable institutions.[39] When comparisons are made, however, they raise as many questions about the nonprofit sector as about for-profits. This occurs, in part, because the consequences of using *national* data for such comparisons are not always recognized.

Analyses of two sources of national data on hospitals' service to patients who lack the means to pay have found differences that are surprisingly small in light of common perceptions about for-profit and nonprofit organizations. In 1982 the Office for Civil Rights in the Department of Health and Human Services (DHHS) conducted a national census of hospitals, which were asked to report admissions by payment source for a two-week period. As Table 5.1 shows, although nonprofit hospitals had a larger percentage of uninsured and Medicaid patients than did for-profit hospitals, the differences were small. The contrast with public hospitals makes the similarity between the for-profits and the nonprofits more striking. The other source of national data—surveys by the American Hospital Association—have shown similarly minor differences.[40] For example, in 1983 uncompensated care (bad debt and charity) in nonprofit hospitals amounted to 4.2 percent of gross patient revenues, compared to 3.1 percent in for-profit hospitals. In 1982 the difference was even smaller, and in nonmetropolitan areas for-profit hospitals reported slightly *higher* levels of uncompensated care than did nonprofits.

Figures such as these have contributed to the widespread perception in health policy circles that there is little or no difference between for-profit and nonprofit hospitals beyond their tax status. These data, however, do not actually measure the extent to which hospitals serve patients who lack the means to pay,[41] and the AHA data—voluntary and self-reported as they are—are subject to many sorts of bias. Investor-owned hospitals tended not to respond to the financial portions of the AHA survey on which uncompensated care percentages were based.

Another national study, published in 1990, showed more substantial national differences between nonprofits and for-profits. Richard Frank, David Salkever, and Fitzhugh Mullan analyzed the data on the approximately 200,000 patients who were discharged annually from the hospitals participating in the National Hospital Discharge Survey between 1979 and 1984.[42] The numbers pertain to *patients* discharged from these hospitals, rather than *dollars* from different sources of payment. In the six years covered by the study, nonprofit hospitals (reported separately for church affiliated and nonchurch affiliated) served from 3 to 4 percent more uncompensated and Medicaid patients than did the for-profits (see Table 5.2). A contrast with public hospitals is also apparent.

Because investor-owned hospitals are heavily concentrated in certain states, national comparisons of for-profit and nonprofit hospitals inevitably mean that hospitals operating under different circumstances are being compared. This is an important point, because on at least two highly relevant matters—the pres-

Table 5.1. U.S. inpatient admissions, by source of payment and type of hospital ownership, 1981 (millions of admissions)[a]

| Type of hospital | Uninsured | | Medicaid | | Medicare | | Private and other | | Total | |
|---|---|---|---|---|---|---|---|---|---|---|
| | Number | % | Number | % | Number | % | Number | % | Number | % |
| For-profit | 0.2 | 6.0 | 0.3 | 8.7 | 1.0 | 30.7 | 1.9 | 54.6 | 3.4 | 100.0 |
| Nonprofit | 2.1 | 7.9 | 2.5 | 9.4 | 7.8 | 28.5 | 14.7 | 54.2 | 27.2 | 100.0 |
| Public | 1.3 | 16.8 | 0.9 | 11.9 | 2.0 | 27.0 | 3.4 | 44.3 | 7.6 | 100.0 |
| Total | 3.6 | 9.5 | 3.7 | 9.8 | 10.9 | 28.5 | 20.0 | 52.2 | 38.2 | 100.0 |

Source: Bradford H. Gray, ed., *For-Profit Enterprise in Health Care* (Washington, D.C.: National Academy Press, 1986), p. 101.

Note: Columns and rows may not add to totals because of rounding.

a. Annual number of admissions projected from data for a two-week period in January 1981. The data were collected by the Office of Civil Rights, Department of Health and Human Services, Washington, D.C.

*Table 5.2.* Average uncompensated and Medicaid discharges by type of hospital ownership, 1979–1984 (%)

| Type of ownership | Uncompensated care | Medicaid | Total |
|---|---|---|---|
| For-profit | 3.82 | 7.09 | 10.91 |
| Church-affiliated | 5.90 | 7.76 | 13.66 |
| Other nonprofit | 5.71 | 9.42 | 15.13 |
| Public | 10.91 | 12.93 | 23.90 |

Source: Data are means of the six years of data reported in Richard G. Frank, David S. Salkever, and Fitzhugh Mullan, "Hospital Ownership and the Care of Uninsured and Medicaid Patients: Findings from the National Hospital Discharge Survey, 1979–1984," *Health Policy* 14 (1990): 1–11.

ence of public hospitals and the adequacy of Medicaid programs—conditions vary widely from state to state. This means that the number of poor, uninsured people who potentially depend for care on the willingness of private hospitals (whether for-profit or nonprofit) to serve them also varies from state to state. The national data about nonprofit hospitals are influenced by the fact that in many states where they are located (and where there are few if any for-profit hospitals), the overall level of uncompensated care is very low because of state mechanisms that in effect compensate hospitals for providing charity care (as in Maryland, Massachusetts, New Jersey, and New York). In many other states where nonprofits are plentiful but for-profits are not, the Medicaid program covers a comparatively high percentage of the poverty population (as in Indiana, Michigan, and Pennsylvania). Thus, the national figures on uncompensated care are substantially influenced by the nonprofit hospitals' disproportionate presence in states where there is a comparatively heavy governmental presence and where the need for uncompensated care is, accordingly, comparatively low.[43]

It should be noted that this pattern is not due to nonprofit hospitals' having selected such states as places to locate. In most instances the hospitals predated the state programs. The operative factor seems to be that investor-owned hospitals tend *not* to locate in states with a heavy regulatory environment; those states have done disproportionately more to finance care for people who lack the means to pay.

Because of these state-to-state variations, the comparative behavior of for-profit and nonprofit hospitals can best be understood by comparing the two types within states where they are both present in reasonably large numbers. In many such states (for example, Florida, North Carolina, Tennessee, Texas, and Virginia), the state's Medicaid program covers a comparatively small percentage of the population with incomes below the poverty line. In these states, therefore, the potential uncompensated care burden for private hospitals is high. In California, however, the Medicaid (Medi-Cal) program offers comparatively high coverage, and a large number of public hospitals exist. Table 5.3 compares amounts of uncompensated care provided by hospitals in several states, using data from state commissions. In Florida, Tennessee, Texas, and Virginia—but not in California—the dif-

*Table 5.3.* Hospital uncompensated care as percentage of gross patient revenues, various states, 1981–1985

| Type of ownership | California | | Florida | | Tennessee | | Texas | Virginia | |
|---|---|---|---|---|---|---|---|---|---|
| | 1981–82 | 1985 | 1982 | 1985 | 1983 | 1985 | 1983 | 1982 | 1985 |
| Public | 7 | | 12.1 | | 18.7 | | 32.4 | | 21.5 |
| Nonprofit chain | 2 | | 6.6 | | 9.0 | | 6.5 | 5.5 | |
| Nonprofit independent | | 3.1 | | 7.6 | | 10.5 | | | 7.0 |
| Investor-owned chain | 2 | 2.7 | 3.8 | 4.9 | 8.7 | 4.8 | 3.5 | 3.5 | 3.7 |
| | | | | | 3.4 | | | | |
| Proprietary (independent) | 3 | | | | 4.6 | | | | |

Sources: Robert V. Pattison, "Response to Financial Incentives among Investor-Owned and Not-for-Profit Hospitals: An Analysis Based on California Data, 1978–1982," in Bradford H. Gray, ed., *For-Profit Enterprise in Health Care* (Washington, D.C.: National Academy Press, 1986), pp. 290–302. State of Florida Hospital Cost Containment Board, *1983–1984 Annual Report* (Tallahassee, 1984). State of Tennessee, Department of Health and Environment, Nashville. Unpublished data. Texas Hospital Association, Survey of Uncompensated Care in Hospitals, in "THA Statement of Fair Share Formula for Financing Care for the Medically Indigent, 1985" (Austin, 1985). Virginia Health Services Cost Review Commission, Richmond. Unpublished data. All in Gray, *For-Profit Enterprise in Health Care*, p. 103. 1985 data are from the same state sources and were reported in Lawrence S. Lewin, Timothy J. Eckles, and Dale Roenigk, "Setting the Record Straight: The Provision of Uncompensated Care by Not-for-Profit Hospitals," *New England Journal of Medicine*, May 5, 1988, pp. 1212–15. The Lewin data for nonprofit hospitals include both chains and independents.

ferences between for-profits and nonprofits are much more substantial than they are nationally. (Public hospitals provide consistently more than either nonprofits or for-profits, although in Florida and Tennessee the nonprofits occupy a more intermediate position between public and for-profit hospitals.)

Yet even these differences might not seem as large as expected when we consider that taxes were equivalent to perhaps 4 or 5 percent of the for-profits' revenues. This point has become relevant to debates about whether nonprofit hospitals are doing enough to justify their tax benefits. Nevertheless, the nonprofits appear to be more responsive than the for-profits to state-to-state differences in the need for uncompensated care.

This interpretation is strengthened by data in Table 5.4, which shows that as the overall levels of uncompensated care increased in Florida in the 1980s, a much larger increase took place among nonprofit hospitals than among investor-owned facilities. In 1980 the level was 26 percent higher in nonprofit hospitals than in investor-owned hospitals, but by 1985 the nonprofits were providing 44 percent more uncompensated care.[44]

Further evidence of a difference between for-profit and nonprofit hospitals comes from a 1984 American Medical Association (AMA) survey of a random sample of four thousand physicians, who were asked whether the hospital with which they were principally affiliated had policies meant to "discourage admissions" of uninsured, Medicare, or Medicaid patients (see

*Table 5.4.* Uncompensated care as a percentage of gross revenue in Florida acute care hospitals, 1980–1985

| Type of control | Year | | | | | | % increase, 1980–1985 |
|---|---|---|---|---|---|---|---|
| | 1980 | 1981 | 1982 | 1983 | 1984 | 1985 | |
| Government | 12.2 | 12.8 | 12.9 | 13.5 | 15.1 | 16.9 | 39 |
| Nonprofit | 5.3 | 5.7 | 7.2 | 7.0 | 7.9 | 8.3 | 57 |
| Investor-owned | 4.2 | 4.0 | 3.9 | 3.9 | 4.8 | 5.4 | 29 |

Source: State of Florida Hospital Cost Containment Board, hospital financial data, 1980–1985. Data provided by Kerry E. Kilpatrick, Director, Center for Health Policy Research, University of Florida.

Note: Exclusion of teaching hospitals slightly reduces the uncompensated care levels for government and nonprofit hospitals (e.g., to 16.0 and 7.8 percent, respectively, in 1985).

*Table 5.5.*  Percentage of physicians reporting that their hospital discouraged
admissions of various types of patient, by type of hospital in which they
practice, 1984

|  | Public | | Nonprofit | | For-profit | |
|---|---|---|---|---|---|---|
| Type of patient | Independent | System | Independent | System | Independent | System |
| Uninsured | 14 | 9 | 20 | 19 | 43 | 52 |
| Medicaid | 3 | 3 | 5 | 6 | 15 | 16 |
| Medicare | 2 | 1 | 1 | 1 | 4 | 5 |

Source: American Medical Association, SMS Survey, 1984; uninsured and Medicaid data
reported in Mark Schlesinger et al., "The Privatization of Health Care and Physicians'
Perceptions of Access to Hospital Services," *Milbank Quarterly* 65:1 (1987): 33. The final line
of the table comes from a prepublication version of this paper.

Table 5.5).[45] Physicians practicing in for-profit hospitals were two
to four times more likely to report such policies than were physicians who practiced in nonprofit hospitals. The differences were
more pronounced for hospitals in multihospital systems than for
independent hospitals. Whether or not these physicians' perceptions accurately reflect actual institutional policies, they suggest
that physicians may make fewer efforts to admit uninsured or
Medicaid patients at for-profit hospitals than at nonprofit hospitals.

The original publication of the state-level data shown in Table
5.3 prompted an objection from the Federation of American
Health Systems, the trade association of the for-profit hospitals,
which argued that nonprofit data are undoubtedly heavily influenced by a relatively small number of large urban teaching hospitals.[46] If the comparison were limited to like hospitals in suburban areas and small cities, they argued, the differences between
the for-profits and nonprofits would be small. Although it is
undoubtedly true that a hospital's location and educational
activities influence the extent of its uncompensated care, this
interpretation of the data concedes a major difference between
sectors—the range of types and locales of hospitals—that is
directly relevant to the point that the nonprofit sector is more
responsive than for-profits to local needs that cannot be met
profitably.

Several other differences between for-profit and nonprofit hospitals show the latter to be more involved in activities that do not provide an economic return. Even though the investor-owned companies started becoming active in medical education and research in the early 1980s, the examples either were isolated or were part of a strategy to build a regional patient care network that would provide marketing advantages. Except for a handful of examples, major teaching hospitals remain either nonprofit or public in ownership; the number of investor-owned hospitals with teaching programs remains very small.[47]

In addition, nonprofit hospitals tend to offer a wider range of services than do investor-owned hospitals of similar size.[48] Although there are no direct data regarding the profitability of specific services at particular hospitals, the services that are less common in investor-owned hospitals include many that are often unprofitable: intensive-care nurseries, outpatient departments, family planning services, and many others. Nonprofit hospitals are more likely than investor-owned hospitals to offer outpatient services that they report to be unprofitable.[49]

## For-Profit versus Nonprofit: A Broader View

As important as the hospital experience has been in the transformation of health care, it does not typify all types of health care organizations. Additional insights about the behavior of for-profit or nonprofit health care organizations can be gained by taking a longer historical view and considering evidence about organizations that provide different types of services.

Much of this literature has been summarized in two articles by Mark Schlesinger, Theodore Marmor, and Richard Smithey.[50] The empirical literature is strongest for hospitals and nursing homes; for other types of health care organizations the evidence is drawn from a small number of studies. The literature that they review can be summarized as follows.

First, whereas the literature on hospitals has found only slight ownership-related differences in the *costs of care* (expenses incurred), a different pattern exists among some other types of organizations. Studies have shown that costs tend to be lower in for-profit than in nonprofit nursing homes,[51] organizations that provide laboratory services, and health insurers.[52] Nonprofits appear to have equal or lower costs for renal dialysis and in health maintenance organizations.

Second, in terms of *quality of care* evidence is much more limited. Only nursing home data are available to compare with hospitals, and there were no clear-cut differences in quality. The literature review done by Catherine Hawes and Charles D. Phillips for the Institute of Medicine study of for-profit enterprise in health care concluded that it was not clear whether *average* quality of care differed in for-profit and nonprofit facilities, but that the "truly wretched ones are almost always proprietary."[53]

Finally, in the matter of *access to care,* for-profit providers avoid unprofitable patients or services by means of three different strategies about which Schlesinger, Marmor, and Smithey found at least some evidence. One is location away from low-income areas where reimbursement levels are low, a tactic that at least some evidence suggests has been used by for-profit hospitals, psychiatric hospitals, and home health agencies. A second strategy is not offering services that are not well reimbursed or that are used disproportionately by patients who are uninsured or covered by Medicaid. Mark Schlesinger and Robert Dorwart found that for-profit psychiatric hospitals were much less likely than nonprofits to offer emergency telephone and suicide prevention services (where the client is often unidentified and thus cannot be billed) or to offer home care and day care, programs that "tend, for historical reasons, to be under reimbursed by insurers."[54] In addition, several studies mentioned earlier in this chapter or cited by Schlesinger, Marmor, and Smithey provide evidence that for-profit hospitals are less likely than nonprofits to offer services that are heavily used by uninsured patients, a difference that is less pronounced among hospitals that are part of multihospital systems.

The third strategy is the use of admissions policies that tend to screen out the uninsured or those covered by Medicaid. I noted earlier that a 1984 survey found that physicians practicing in for-profit hospitals were much more likely than those who practiced in nonprofit hospitals to report that their hospital had a policy of discouraging admission of uninsured or Medicaid patients.[55] Another survey found that proprietary long-term care facilities (including nursing homes, psychiatric hospitals, and institutions for the mentally handicapped) were much less likely than their nonprofit counterparts to offer services at reduced charges.[56] For-profit nursing homes, however, serve larger numbers of Medicaid patients than do nonprofits, apparently because the latter are more attractive to patients who have the ability to pay.[57]

On the basis of this evidence and an examination of historical patterns, Schlesinger, Marmor, and Smithey offer several intriguing, if somewhat speculative, empirical generalizations. First, the type of service makes a difference in the consequences of type of ownership, in part because of the role of physicians:

> For health services in which physicians play an important role, facility ownership has little effect on quality or cost, although under some circumstances for-profit ownership may increase costs of care.
>
> In services in which professionals have a smaller role, proprietary services are less costly than those offered in nonprofit settings. For such services, however, investor-owned facilities are also disproportionately represented among the institutions offering very low quality treatment. Thus, where professional norms do not mediate the influence of ownership, there appears to be a trade-off between less costly services and a greater risk of exploitation of patients by providers interested in short-term profits.[58]

In addition, there is some evidence to suggest that the for-profit–nonprofit composition of an area of service delivery often goes through several stages. At first, services are offered in predominantly nonprofit settings (in part because reimbursement is limited or unavailable). Then demand grows and exceeds the capacity of nonprofit organizations because their ambition for expansion or their access to capital is limited. In this stage, for-profit facilities may play a leading role in expanding access to services. In later stages, as demand stabilizes, the ability of for-profits to attract capital becomes less of a factor in providing access to services, and the growing competitive situation begins to influence the behavior of nonprofits—perhaps leading them to introduce additional restrictions on access.

This analysis suggests that public policy should take account of the stage of development of a field, perhaps encouraging for-profits during the stage when demand is growing but favoring nonprofits when demand is stable.

The comparative behavior of for-profit and nonprofit health care organizations is not carved in stone. Expectations for nonprofit health care organizations should rest on more than assumptions about their behavior. By the same token, criticisms should be based on a realistic assessment of their resources. Though unsatisfactory to people who want a simple, unambiguous conclusion, the evidence examined in this chapter suggests that both for-profit and nonprofit forms of ownership may serve legitimate purposes in health care.

For-profits play a particularly important role in periods of rapid increases in demand, while nonprofits do so where there are serious flaws in the operation of market mechanisms, as when adequate payment is lacking or when the market has difficulty detecting differences in quality. As I suggested in earlier chapters, the comparative immobility of nonprofits' capital and their ability to draw on community support are sources of stability.

On economic measures, the relative performance of for-profit and nonprofit health care organizations appears to depend on a number of circumstances—the type of service that is involved, incentives built into payment systems, the role of physicians in making decisions that affect expenditures, and market niche. There are circumstances in which nonprofit organizations clearly provide care in a more economical fashion from the payer's standpoint. Whether because of their conception of mission or the fact that they must expend surplus revenues for the purposes for which they are chartered, it appears that nonprofits behave differently from for-profits at the margin. In nursing homes, for example, they appear more likely to spend money on enhanced quality than on expansion. In hospitals they seem more inclined to respond to needs that cannot necessarily be met profitably and to forgo opportunities to increase prices.

# External Accountability and Problems of Fraud and Abuse

Health care organizations are subject to oversight by a variety of external parties through an assortment of mechanisms. Two such mechanisms—malpractice suits and hospital accreditation procedures—were touched on in Chapter 5, as I noted that studies pertaining to quality have shown little difference between investor-owned and nonprofit hospitals. But what about the activities of government in its role as both regulator and purchaser of medical services?

To acquire greater understanding of the implications of the organizational and economic changes with which this book is concerned, I sought information about how institutions of different ownership types have fared with regard to these regulatory mechanisms. Such information is difficult to come by, but I was able to assemble various pieces and fragments about two areas—detection of Medicare and Medicaid fraud and abuse, and compliance with Medicare's conditions of participation. (I have chosen not to delve into nursing homes, where the history of fraud and abuse is all too familiar, but that situation is generally supportive of many of the points that are made in this chapter.)[1]

The available evidence suggests that hospitals owned by investor-owned companies and other multi-institutional systems have not often run afoul of the regulatory mechanisms. Even so, the evidence suggests that a variety of types of difficult-to-detect malfeasance can result from excessive zeal in the pursuit of economic goals, and that the corporate transformation of health care and the growing presence of profit-oriented providers have created new challenges and complexities for the parties with oversight responsibility.


## External Accountability Mechanisms

It is not difficult to understand why government mechanisms of accountability have prominence in health care. Recipients of medical services are often limited in their ability to evaluate those services in terms of necessity, quality, and reasonableness of price, and the purchasers and recipients of services are often different parties. Because matters of life and death as well as large amounts of money are involved, a strong rationale exists for government action to protect the interests of the public and for government and private payers to monitor hospital behavior to protect their own interests.[2]

Therefore, notwithstanding the private (for-profit or nonprofit) ownership of most U.S. hospitals, they are subject to a significant degree of accountability exercised in the public interest.[3] As I mentioned in Chapter 1, the Hospital Association of New York State in the mid-1970s claimed that its members had to deal with 174 regulatory bodies—including 96 state agencies, 40 federal agencies, 18 city and county agencies, and 10 voluntary or quasi-public bodies.[4] Another indication of the regulatory web surrounding hospitals comes from a small 1980 study by the General Accounting Office.[5] To illuminate the extent to which regulatory requirements might be contributing to the hospital cost problem, the GAO focused on inspections, reports, and Life Safety Code enforcement at two small samples of hospitals. Among the three hospitals in one sample a total of 101 different inspections were reported. (One of the three alone reported 65.) The four hospitals studied in the other sample had been requested to comply with 202 reports and forms—the highest number at any single hospital was 85—from 10 federal agencies and 49 "state and local government or private organizations." About half of the 202 were annual reports and forms; 126 were unique to hospitals; and the other 76 applied to all businesses. Even so, the GAO concluded that overlap and duplication were not serious problems.

Government regulation of hospitals follows two main avenues: state licensure procedures and the various mechanisms relating to payment for services. Licensure regulations include many detailed requirements regarding such matters as fire safety and qualifications of personnel. The main value of licensure, however, is as a threshold, not as an ongoing mechanism of accountability, for, as Tom Christoffel notes, "most states have many hospitals, detailed licensing requirements, and only a handful of inspectors to check on compliance."[6]

Most government mechanisms of accountability have been tied to the government's role as financier of health care. Indeed, in many states hospitals were subject to virtually no regulation before the late 1940s, when the federal Hill-Burton program required states to adopt a comprehensive system of licensure for hospitals as a condition of eligibility to receive construction funds under the program.[7] Medicare and Medicaid brought about major increases in regulatory activity in health care, initially through the adoption in 1966 of Medicare's conditions of participation for hospitals, which included many specific provisions regarding the organization and operation of hospitals and their medical staffs, and later through health planning programs, utilization review requirements, and so forth. The requirements attached to provider eligibility for participation in Medicare and Medicaid include not only state licensure but also accreditation by the Joint Commission for Accreditation of Health Care Organizations (or the equivalent of such accreditation) as well as review activities by peer review organizations (PROs), fiscal intermediaries, and agencies investigating fraud and abuse.

Payers have systems for monitoring and auditing to ensure that services being billed for are in fact provided and are necessary. Mechanisms to ensure quality include regulatory requirements built into conditions of participation, certification and accreditation requirements, and some activities of peer review organizations. These all have significant shortcomings, but at least some mechanisms are in place.

By contrast, procedures for monitoring access to care are much more rudimentary. Rather than imposing requirements on providers, the government's primary approach to ensuring access to care has been to give certain categories of patients the financial means to purchase care. Mechanisms by which the government has held providers accountable for caring for patients who lack the means to pay are quite limited.

One such mechanism stems from the so-called community service and free care obligations that hospitals accepted as a condition of receiving construction funds under the Hill-Burton program. Because for-profit institutions are not eligible for such funds, they are not so constrained, except under some very limited conditions.[8] Although enforcement of Hill-Burton obligations was difficult and fitful,[9] the contractual obligations of the program did require some accountability from nonprofit hospitals and, thus, might make nonprofits preferable from a social point of view. This obligation, however, was time-limited and resulted from legislation rather than the inherent characteristics of for-profit and nonprofit organizations; it is not a sound basis on which to criticize for-profit ownership.

In some states hospitals can also be held accountable for failing to provide emergency services to patients.[10] Regulatory authority to enhance patient access has also been part of the negotiation process involved in the operation of health planning activities. Most important, perhaps, the Federal Consolidated Omnibus Budget Reconciliation Act of 1985 added to the Medicare conditions of participation new provisions that forbid "dumping" medically unstable patients (that is, sending them to another hospital) for financial reasons. By early 1988 the Health Care Financing Administration (HCFA) reported that there had been 126 complaints nationwide regarding patient dumping and 31 "confirmed violations" since the law was passed in August 1986.[11] Investigations have also been undertaken under state laws. At least two hospitals have been removed from the Medicare programs for violations of the patient-dumping law.[12]

In sum, the external accountability of hospitals pertains primarily to financial accountability, secondarily to quality, and only peripherally to access for patients who lack the means to pay. Low levels of enforcement activities have been commonplace, perhaps reflecting a tradition of trust in nonprofit organizations.

Despite the fact that hospitals are subject to scrutiny from a wide variety of sources, very little information has been published about patterns of compliance with regulatory requirements. Either the information obtained by regulatory authorities is never made public, or the format in which it is presented does not show whether there are associations between the incidence of problems and the characteristics of organizations. This chapter is based on unpublished information obtained from several regulatory sources, generally by means of requests under Freedom of Information statutes.

The picture that emerges is complex, suggesting that the organizational changes with which this book is concerned have created new problems of identifying improper behavior while probably curbing some of the more traditional forms of fraud and abuse. The problem of detection has become increasingly more difficult. Moreover, there are serious limitations on the power, ability, and willingness of investigative agencies to pursue possible fraud and abuse in complex corporate organizational structures.

## Fraud and Abuse in a Commercialized Health Care System

### The Nature of the Problem

In health care the disparity of knowledge between providers and patients, the practice of third-party payment, and the exchange of huge amounts of money combine to create a fertile environment for fraud and abuse. As defined by federal and state agencies under Medicare and Medicaid, these terms have specific and narrow legal meanings. Under the statute, *fraud* is defined as "an intentional deception or misrepresentation with the intent of receiving some unauthorized benefit for the individual engaged in the fraud."[13] Program *abuse* includes "activity wherein providers, practitioners, and suppliers of services operate in a manner inconsistent with accepted, sound medical or business practices resulting in excessive and unreasonable financial cost to either medicare or medicaid."[14]

Depending on interpretations, these definitions may prove broad or narrow. Most investigations have been concerned with issues in which the payers' interests are directly at stake—as they are when inducements are offered in exchange for referrals or when unnecessary services are billed for—rather than those that pertain more narrowly to patients (for example, misleadingly informing a patient that discharge is necessary because the hospitalization period allowed by the Medicare diagnosis-related group has expired). Most of this chapter is concerned with fraud and abuse as defined and pursued by agencies with oversight and enforcement authority. No attempt is made to identify issues that potentially fall into these categories but have not been treated as such by these agencies.

Since the extent of undetected fraud and abuse is unknown, it is impossible to determine whether the incidence has increased along with the growing for-profit orientation of health care. It is clear, however, that the problem has received much attention. Between 1965 and 1982 the General Accounting Office and Congress issued more than one hundred reports and hearings on fraud, waste, and abuse in the Medicaid program alone. The Senate Committee on Aging itself held more than fifty hearings on Medicaid fraud.[15]

A steady flow of new laws and regulatory changes over the years suggests that the difficulty of detecting and correcting the problem has been consistently underestimated. For example, amendments to the Social Security Act in 1972 broadened existing provisions to include activities such as soliciting, offering, or accepting kickbacks or bribes for patient referrals.[16] In 1975 testimony before the House Government Operations Committee revealed that the Department of Health, Education and Welfare had no centralized mechanism to investigate fraud in its 334 programs.[17] In 1976 the federal government's first statutory Office of the Inspector General (OIG) was established to "reduce the incidence of fraud, abuse, and waste in the Department of Health and Human Services and to promote economy and efficiency."[18] Although OIG began slowly, sanctions imposed on health care providers and suppliers increased from 39 in 1981 to 390 in 1985.[19]

In 1977 new anti–fraud and abuse amendments increased the severity of violations from misdemeanors to felonies, expanded the provisions to cover a broader range of providers and treatment settings, and established mechanisms to aid in the detection of violations.[20] Matching funds were also made available for the creation of state Medicaid fraud units,[21] and disclosure requirements to aid in auditing were added.[22] In 1981 the Civil Monetary Penalties Law was adopted as an additional means of penalizing providers as well as recouping money lost to fraud and abuse.[23]

Even a cursory review of legislative changes to address this problem in Medicaid and Medicare conveys something of the difficulty of establishing effective mechanisms of accountability. Still, there is no reason to believe that fraud and abuse have been typical of health care providers. This may be due in part to ethical traditions in the medical profession, to the fact that its members could earn high incomes by legitimate means, and to the accountability of nonprofit institutions to boards of unpaid local citizens. Although such interpretation is consistent with the data on fraud and abuse that are examined here, it remains to be seen whether the incidence of malfeasance will be affected as changes take place that make it more difficult for health care providers to make money.

*Corporate Change and Modern Malfeasance*
Has there been a rise in fraud and abuse problems associated with the rise of for-profit health care? Although attention to and concern about fraud and abuse have increased in parallel with the growth of investor-owned health care companies, it would be naive to assume that official agencies have been able to keep pace with the changes in the activities over which they have jurisdiction. The hypothesis that the rise of for-profit health care has exacerbated the problem of fraud and abuse seems reasonable because economic motivations underlie both activities.

As we have seen, however, health care organizations of all ownership types are under pressure to perform well economically. Furthermore, individuals in any type of organization through which money flows may have opportunities to engage in illegitimate behavior for their own profit. Prominent examples have come to light in recent years in both public hospitals, like those in the New York City Health and Hospitals Corporation, and nonprofit hospitals such as Hermann Hospital in Houston.[24] Thus, it is conceivable that the rise of big for-profit organizations has been largely irrelevant to the problem of fraud and abuse. It is even possible that opportunities for individuals to engage in fraudulent behavior do not arise as often in large-scale organizations that have systematic administrative and financial controls in place as in smaller organizations, particularly proprietary ones.

Data on the activities of agencies whose task it is to detect malfeasance can be used to explore these somewhat contradictory hypotheses. First, however, it is necessary to delineate three types of fraudulent or abusive activities, which I term corporate deviance, organizational deviance, and individual deviance.

*Corporate deviance* refers to illegitimate activities or practices that an organization adopts and builds into its operations in the pursuit of its objectives. An example is provided by the 1986 indictment in New York of a company called Professional Care, Inc.[25] Described in the indictment as the nation's largest publicly owned home health care company (and listed as the eighth largest in *Modern Healthcare*'s 1986 survey of multi-institutional home health care organizations), Professional Care was accused of stealing more than $1.8 million from the Medicaid program between 1981 and 1985 and of participating in a statewide conspiracy to fabricate company records to deceive auditors and conceal the impropriety. Professional Care allegedly billed for services rendered by employees who lacked the qualifications and training required by the state. The executive vice president was also alleged to have issued orders to managers and employees to falsify the records whenever necessary to conceal from auditors the use of unqualified employees. The allegedly fraudulent behavior was initiated high in the corporate office, communicated downward to managers and employees, and made a part of routine operations.

Identifying corporate deviance can be difficult because the boundary between a clever business practice and a fraudulent or abusive one is not always clear. An organization that repeatedly chooses to operate close to (but, it hopes, within) the boundaries that separate the legitimate from the illegitimate risks crossing that line on occasion. Legal interpretations can be complex, and the boundary may not become apparent until someone tests it by adopting a new strategy or practice. For example, it was not until some hospitals began to waive Medicare co-payment to attract patients and some hospitals developed plans whereby profits on Medicare patients were to be shared with the medical staff that government agencies took up the question of whether such prac-

tices violated fraud and abuse provisions against offering inducements to patients and physicians to use the hospital.

Where is corporate deviance most likely to occur? Sociologists
who have studied the issue emphasize the role of organizational
goals. The for-profit organization's aims and accountability
structure are heavily oriented toward growth and profitability. In
addition, for-profit organizations may be managed by individuals
who are also stockholders and who may be able to pocket some
of the proceeds from corporate deviance. Such factors make it
plausible that for-profit organizations would exhibit corporate
deviance to a larger extent than nonprofit organizations. Nonetheless, the amount of hybridization that has taken place among
nonprofit health care organizations, the accountability of many
nonprofits to private sources of capital, and the dependence of
most health care organizations on sales to generate revenues all
serve to orient nonprofit hospitals toward economic ends. Furthermore, powerful parties in nonprofit hospitals may have goals
that are advanced when an institution generates profits. Corporate deviance, therefore, may not be limited to for-profit organizations.

The second type of improper behavior, *organizational
deviance*, occurs when individuals engage in activities to further
the interests of the organization but without the knowledge of
upper management. It is difficult to know how common such
deviance is, but an example came to light in 1984 in an investor-
owned hospital that I visited as part of a case study for the
Institute of Medicine's Committee on For-Profit Enterprise in
Health Care. Among the responsibilities for which the parent
company held the hospital administrator to account was maintaining the hospital's accreditation by the Joint Commission on
Accreditation of Hospitals (JCAH). (In 1987 this organization
changed its name to the Joint Commission for the Accreditation
of Healthcare Organizations.) During the most recent accreditation visit by the JCAH, a staff physician had suggested that the
contents of a truck in the parking lot be inspected. There the
visitors found a large number of incomplete medical records that
had been removed from the records department on instructions
from the hospital administrator. Prior to the JCAH survey visit,
the administrator had feared that the hospital had so many

incomplete medical records that accreditation might be jeopardized. After an unsuccessful effort to persuade staff physicians to complete the medical records, he ordered the incomplete records moved to the truck for temporary storage. The discovery led to termination of the JCAH survey and the firing of the administrator. (Both actions were later reversed: the company's request for another JCAH survey was granted, and the administrator was reinstated after the medical staff interceded with the parent company.)

Organizational deviance presumably can arise in any setting in which employees are expected to achieve a certain outcome and have some latitude in so doing. Designing a set of incentives that does not reward undesired behavior while encouraging desired behavior is never easy, and it may be particularly difficult in health care, where both illegitimate and legitimate means are available for achieving such goals as increasing utilization, revenues, or profits and decreasing lengths of stay, expenses, or bad debts.

The line between corporate deviance and organizational deviance is not always clear in actual operations. Although illegitimate practices may occur at the direction of top officials within an organization (corporate deviance), they may also occur in the context of an implicit understanding between superiors and subordinates that there is more than one way to achieve a goal. In both cases, however, the behavior in question pertains to the structure and goals of the *organization*.

The third type of illegitimate behavior, *occupational deviance*, can be engaged in by individuals or small proprietary organizations such as a pharmacy or a professional's practice. Instead of being oriented toward achievement of *organizational* goals, however, such behavior has the simple purpose of putting money into the pocket of the perpetrator, and it involves exploiting opportunities that arise in an individual's daily occupational activities.[26] Some behavior may involve theft from or fraud against one's own organization, as when a bookkeeper embezzles funds; such activities are outside the scope of this inquiry, which is concerned with illegitimate behavior that is directed outward, toward patients, payers, or regulators. In health care, examples of occupational deviance include the physician or dentist who bills the third-party payer for a patient who was never seen or for services that were not provided, the physician who receives a kickback for making a referral or for using or recommending a particular drug or device, or the pharmacist who bills a third-party payer for a prescription that was never supplied or for a brand-name medication when a generic drug was given.

The acquisition of small proprietary facilities by large corporations may have reduced the likelihood of occurrence of these types of illegitimate behavior, since most large organizations use systems for handling money and paying bills that are designed to minimize the chance that employees will siphon off funds. Although large-scale organizations must worry about such possibilities, they may be able to institute means for detecting and preventing many kinds of illegitimate behavior by individuals within the organization. In a large organization that has highly developed internal systems of control, certain forms of illegitimate behavior would require the knowledge and cooperation of many people, making the kinds of abuses that could easily happen in a "mom-and-pop" operation much less likely to occur.

*Data on Fraud and Abuse*

The results of the activities of fraud and abuse agencies are consistent with the idea that the emergence and growth of profit-oriented corporate health care may possibly have stimulated some forms of illegitimate behavior and curbed others. Fraud and abuse and related problems have not, by and large, been associated with big multi-institutional systems, regardless of type of ownership. Instead, most problems uncovered by these agencies consist of the types of activities undertaken by individuals or small organizations for their own enrichment, which large, well-managed organizations have internal procedures to prevent.

None of the available studies of fraud and abuse among medical practitioners and beneficiaries of public programs examine associations between such problems and the type of ownership of health care facilities.[27] (There is, of course, a long history of fraud and abuse in nursing homes, a field that I have not attempted to examine.) At least until recent years, however, those problems generally appeared to be due to individual behavior—the activities of proprietors—rather than to corporate strategies.[28] Little information is readily available about the overall distribution of fraud and abuse.

To address this topic I sought information directly from the government agencies that investigate the problem. Although some information can be gleaned from published reports of these agencies, I found it necessary to use Freedom of Information laws to obtain most information. Even under such requests agencies generally will disclose only information about closed cases, not pending ones (which may remain "pending" for many years). For the present work I obtained data from the Health Care Financing Administration (HCFA), the Office of the Inspector General (OIG) of the Department of Health and Human Services, and from Medicaid fraud units in Texas and California.

Table 6.1 summarizes the data obtained from those agencies. Hospitals, although the locus of 36 percent of expenditures in the Medicaid program and 66 percent of expenditures in the Medicare program,[29] are identified in relatively few cases of fraud and abuse. The majority of cases involve individual professionals or small proprietary organizations. (Most providers listed as "other" facilities in Table 6.1 are proprietary nursing homes or physicians' practices that are incorporated as clinics.)[30] For example, of the 1,079 cases that resulted in sanctions by OIG between 1975 and 1986, a facility (rather than an individual) was the object of the sanction in only eight cases; in four of these cases the facility was a hospital. Although ownership type was not identified, this small number of hospitals obviously means that large multihospital systems could not have run afoul of the laws governing fraud and abuse with any frequency.

To examine fraud in hospitals in more detail, I obtained information about hospitals investigated by the Texas Medicaid Fraud Unit.[31] Texas was selected because its fraud unit was said to be active and because of the large number of investor-owned hospitals there. In 1984, 159 (approximately one-third) of the general hospitals in the state were investor owned. (Another 44 were independent proprietary hospitals.) Between 1979 and July 1986, the Texas Medicaid Fraud Unit completed investigations of 28 hospitals. Of the hospitals involved in the 28 cases, 2 were proprietary, 4 were members of investor-owned hospital systems, 12 were nonprofit, and 10 were public. Thus, the investor-owned hospitals were, if anything, underrepresented. The activities investigated included billing for services not provided, improper cost accounting, submitting claims for services not covered under Medicaid, unnecessary admissions, denial of services, and billing for services already compensated for by an intermediary. No criminal action was taken in any of the cases.

### Compliance with Medicare Conditions of Participation

Activities for which providers are held externally accountable necessarily go far beyond problems of fraud and abuse. To be eligible for Medicare payment, hospitals must meet statutory requirements established under Title XVIII of the Social Security Act and additional health and safety requirements established by the secretary of Health and Human Services. Hospitals that fail to comply with those requirements can be dropped from the Medicare program.

Although OIG took this action against only four hospitals between 1975 and 1986, HCFA terminated fifty-seven hospitals from the Medicare and/or Medicaid program between 1981 and 1986 for failing to comply with various provisions (see Table 6.2). Most of these were small hospitals that may have encountered problems because of either insufficient capital or lack of good management. In relation to their total numbers, nonfederal public hospitals and independent proprietary hospitals had the highest rates of termination by HCFA; nonprofit hospitals were clearly underrepresented; and hospitals from investor-owned chains were slightly underrepresented.[32]

HCFA also took action against hospitals that state health agencies, through "substantial allegation surveys," had found to violate Medicare conditions of participation.[33] During the period from January 1984 to July 1986 the Medicare contracts of twenty-seven hospitals were terminated. Fifty-five percent of these hospitals were public facilities. Thirty percent were nonprofit. Only four of the hospitals were for-profit, and only one of these was a member of an investor-owned chain, Westworld.

Thus, investor-owned hospitals have had only a small number of serious problems with Medicare conditions of participation. Problems have arisen disproportionately in public hospitals and the rapidly disappearing proprietary hospitals. Other informa-

Table 6.1. Summary of Medicare and Medicaid fraud and abuse cases, by provider type (%)

| Cases | Hospitals | Other health care facilities[a] | Physicians | Other practitioners[b] | Pharmacy | Laboratory | Durable Med. Equip./supplies | Other |
|---|---|---|---|---|---|---|---|---|
| Fraud/abuse cases pending before state Medicaid fraud units, January 1, 1981 (N = 2,082) | 6.9 | 29.4 | 24.4 | 9.7 | 19.8 | 2.6 | 1.3 | 5.8 |
| Fraud/abuse cases referred by OIG to Department of Justice in 1981 (N = 91) | 18.7 | 12.1 | 19.8 | 6.6 | — | 5.5 | 11.0 | 26.4 |
| Fraud/abuse cases pending before Texas Medicaid Fraud Unit, July 1, 1986 (N = 356) | 7.3 | 13.8 | 36.2 | 18.5 | 5.9 | c | — | 18.5 |
| Fraud/abuse cases opened by Bureau of Medi-Cal Fraud, July 1978–March 1985 (N = 2,302) | 4.6 | 11.0 | 42.1 | 14.7 | 10.2 | 3.3 | 4.6 | 9.5 |

| Fraud/abuse cases closed by Bureau of Medi-Cal Fraud, July 1978–March 1985 (N = 1,871)[d] | 4.2 | 9.8 | 43.2 | 15.0 | 10.3 | 3.3 | 4.6 | 9.5 |
|---|---|---|---|---|---|---|---|---|
| Providers administratively sanctioned by OIG, 1975–April 1986 (N = 1,079) | [c] | 6.7 | 23.1 | 22.8 | 19.8 | 1.9 | 5.1 | 20.2 |

Sources: U.S. Congress, House of Representatives, Select Committee on Aging, *Medicaid Fraud: A Case History in the Failure of State Enforcement*, 97th Cong., 2d sess. (Washington, D.C.: Government Printing Office, 1982), p. 50. Department of Health and Human Services, Office of Inspector General, *Annual Report, January 1, 1981–December 31, 1981* (Washington, D.C.: Government Printing Office), app. C. Conversation with Charles Yett, Director, Texas Medicaid Fraud Unit. Sanction data are based on a listing, obtained under the Freedom of Information Act, of sanctions in effect against "physicians/practitioners, providers, and/or other health care suppliers" as of April 30, 1986. Sanctions include "suspensions, exclusions, and terminations of Physicians, Practitioners, and Other Providers of Health Care Services" under Sections 1128, 1862[d], 1160, 1156, and 1866 of the Social Security Act.

a. Includes nursing homes, intermediate care facilities, and clinics.

b. Includes chiropractors, podiatrists, optometrists, nurses, osteopaths, psychologists, dentists, and therapists.

c. Less than one percent.

d. Cases were closed because of insufficient evidence to prosecute.

*Table 6.2.* Involuntary terminations of hospitals from Medicare and Medicaid, by ownership, 1981–November 1986 (%)

| Ownership status | Terminated hospitals (N = 57) | Total nonfederal hospitals, 1982 (N = 6,569)[a] |
|---|---|---|
| Proprietary | 19.3 | 6 |
| Investor-owned chain | 7.0 | 10 |
| Public (nonfederal) | 54.3 | 32 |
| Nonprofit | 19.3 | 54 |
| Total | 100 | 100 |

Source: Data obtained under the Freedom of Information Act from the Health Care Financing Administration, Baltimore.

Note: Percentages may not total 100 percent because of rounding.

a. Includes both short-term and long-term hospitals. The percentages are derived from the 1983 American Hospital Association's figures. The numerators for the percentages of for-profit hospitals are based on the 1983 figures of the Federation of American Hospitals. American Hospital Association data for 1982 show 14 percent of nonfederal hospitals to be "for-profit."

tion, however, suggests that the rise of multihospital systems has complicated certain aspects of monitoring the performance of institutions.

### Limitations of Available Data

The data from agencies investigating fraud and abuse and other oversight bodies provide only part of the overall picture. The true incidence of improper activities is unknown. The data are undoubtedly influenced by the relative ease with which certain types of cases can be identified and documented sufficiently to justify the imposition of sanctions.

The data are also affected by the jurisdictional boundaries created by the different laws and organizations involved in the detection and adjudication of fraud and abuse and related activities. Jurisdiction is fragmented because of the decentralization of oversight responsibilities among regional and state agencies and because some relevant laws apply only to particular types of providers, such as HMOs, hospitals, and nursing homes, and some vary by state. Analyses over time are complicated by changes in laws, regulations, tools, and organizational responsibilities. For example, OIG is responsible for administering the criminal aspect of fraud and abuse laws; the HCFA Bureau of Quality Control administers the civil and administrative component of Medicare; criminal proceedings under federal law are initiated by the Department of Justice; and state Medicaid fraud units are responsible for criminal actions under state law.[34] Jurisdictional limitations also mean that an agency may be able to carry a case only so far before it must be referred elsewhere. Thus, a Medicaid fraud unit may investigate a case and then refer it to the Inspector General, who, in turn, refers the case to the Department of Justice for criminal adjudication.

Thus it is difficult to assemble a reasonably complete picture of the problems that have come to the attention of regulatory authorities. Furthermore, because the agencies are not research organizations, they may not maintain data on cases that have been closed or shifted to another agency's jurisdiction. In addition, agencies generally do not disclose information about cases that are pending. Hence, the data provided by federal and state agencies are far from exhaustive.

A 1985 case involving the sale of state approval for health care projects illustrates a further limitation of the data. Edwin Edwards, the governor of Louisiana, was indicted on fifty-six counts of fraud and obstruction of justice involving an alleged conspiracy to acquire and sell certificates of need for health care projects through the Health Services Development Corporation. It was alleged that the governor bribed the supervisor of the state's certificate-of-need program to approve certificates for corporations set up by Edwards and his associates. The corporations were then bought by investor-owned companies, including Hospital Corporation of America and American Medical International. The governor received $2 million for "certificate brokering." Yet, the criminal case involving Edwards ended in a mistrial.[35] How should such a case be counted in a compilation of data on fraud and abuse in health care?

If the data on detected cases inevitably and substantially underestimate the true incidence of fraud and abuse, as seems certain, this is probably true above all in large-scale, profit-oriented health care organizations, because the problems that can occur there may be particularly difficult to detect and document.

## Investor Ownership and the Problem of External Accountability

The experiences of three companies illustrate many of the kinds of difficulties that payers and regulators face in dealing with complex, strongly profit-oriented health care organizations. The three cases demonstrate the complexities that increase the cost and difficulty of unraveling the activities of large multi-institutional systems. Although the cases do not appear to be typical, they present the types of problems with which today's accountability structures must deal. They also suggest that even if the web of accountability in health care does not prevent certain problems from occurring, it is difficult for a company to sustain a pattern of dubious behavior for long.

*Westworld Community Healthcare, Inc.,* of Lake Forest, California, a publicly traded, investor-owned health care company, owned thirty-three hospitals in thirteen states, according to the 1986 *Directory of the Federation of American Hospitals,* although its holdings have changed unusually rapidly, as we shall see. The hospitals were very small (averaging thirty-three beds), and a Westworld hospital was typically the only one in a community. The company also operated rural clinics trademarked as Intercept and Paintrol programs for alcoholism treatment and pain control, respectively, and subsidiaries offering rural HMOs and air ambulance services.

Westworld acted as a "white knight" to small community hospitals in trouble. The company bought such hospitals and kept them open, and it also made substantial investments in renovations. Rayburn Allen, director of the Arkansas health department's Health Facility Services Division, estimated that Westworld had spent $1 million in renovations on the twenty-eight-bed hospital it acquired in Gurdon, $600,000 on renovations at the forty-bed Delta Medical Center in Brinkley, and $400,000 on surgical, obstetric, and emergency departments at the twenty-five-bed Eureka Springs Hospital.[36] Such large investments by an investor-owned company in small rural hospitals are difficult to understand, but they created strong local support. James Lee, the Arkansas attorney general's press secretary, stated that a publicly announced investigation of the Gurdon hospital had produced an "inch-thick stack of letters" in support of Westworld.[37]

Westworld's strategies and modes of operation brought it to the attention of many agencies and organizations concerned with the functioning of hospitals. An energetic reporter for the *Fresno Bee* managed to compile information about the company, which owned several hospitals in the Fresno area, from a wide range of sources.[38] The list of investigations and punitive actions taken against Westworld and the various issues that are involved convey a vivid picture of the web of accountability within which hospitals operate.

In December 1985, the *Bee* reported that investigations of Westworld hospitals were under way in three federal agencies and four states. The company's billing practices were under investigation by the OIG, the attorney general's office in California, the South Dakota attorney general's office, the Oregon Health Planning and Development Agency, and the Curry County, Oregon, district attorney's office. In August 1986 the *Bee* reported that investigations were also being conducted in Texas and Idaho, and that the Missouri attorney general had filed two lawsuits against the company. Many of the actions were prompted by complaints about Westworld's practice of adjusting charges on patients' bills so that they would total a predetermined sum, reportedly $1,150 per day. (The company eventually dropped that billing approach in favor of one that uses Medicare diagnosis-related groups—DRGs—to categorize patients, charging about one-third higher per DRG than the Medicare rate.) One of the Missouri suits, however, charged that the company had misled patients into believing that their insurance would pay for the alcohol treatment programs and alleged, in addition, that some patients were being charged for services not rendered.[39] The *Bee* also reported that Blue Cross/Blue Shield plans in four states (Arkansas, Idaho, South Dakota, and Texas) had taken action because of Westworld's excessive charges. The actions ranged from canceling contracts with Westworld hospitals to sending beneficiaries letters warning them that they would not have full coverage for charges billed by Westworld hospitals.

In addition, the HCFA had barred three Westworld facilities in

Texas and South Dakota from participation in Medicare because of improper actions to maximize the hospitals' reimbursement. According to an HCFA official, the peer review organizations (PROs) in the two states had discovered a pattern of abuse of "swing beds" in several Westworld hospitals.[40] The use of swing beds is intended to allow hospitals to provide patients with skilled nursing care when they no longer need hospitalization, particularly in rural locales where skilled nursing facilities are not available. Medicare pays the hospital for such nursing care on a per diem basis, in addition to the fixed DRG payment for the hospital stay. The PROs believed, and a subsequent investigation by the Office of the Inspector General confirmed, that the Westworld hospitals were improperly maximizing reimbursement by transferring patients to skilled nursing care too early in an admission, in effect being paid twice for care provided to patients. The fact that there was a pattern of such inappropriate transfers suggested that the intent was to circumvent or abuse the reimbursement system, and termination actions were brought against the hospitals.

Finally, the *Bee* reported that the U.S. Food and Drug Administration (FDA) was investigating Westworld's practice (subsequently discontinued) of manufacturing and transporting across state lines the drug pilocarpine for use in alcohol treatment programs in Texas and Arkansas.

Westworld's Intercept alcohol treatment program was the focal point of additional, separate investigations by the Arkansas State Department of Health and the Arkansas attorney general's office.

According to telephone interviews and accounts in the *Arkansas Gazette*,[41] the state health department became involved when it received a "resolution" in which fourteen staff physicians at the Central Ozarks Medical Center in Yellville said that they wanted no responsibility for the "widely advertised" alcohol treatment program using fourteen beds at the Westworld-owned fifty-nine-bed hospital there.[42] Westworld's Intercept program was offered at many of its hospitals, including three of its four Arkansas hospitals. The physicians for the program were often brought to communities by Westworld. The program involved two weeks of hospitalization and aversion therapy. The fourteen Yellville physicians (who were not part of the program) objected to the use of FDA-approved drugs for the unapproved purpose of inducing vomiting in patients after they had been offered their favorite alcoholic beverage. (Pilocarpine, which was administered along with the other drugs by injection, is licensed as an eyedrop for the treatment of glaucoma, but FDA regulations do not prohibit other uses. The importing of pilocarpine in injectable form from Oklahoma in apparent violation of Arkansas law was halted after the state health department notified Westworld of the violation; thereafter the compounding into injectable form was done at the hospital.)

In response to the physicians' action Westworld contended that the real issue was staff disgruntlement over loss of control of the hospital to the California company and that the physicians had violated the hospital's bylaws, which, according to the *Arkansas Gazette*, prevented the staff from disapproving of a hospital program without studying the issue and providing documentation to support their allegation. The hospital withdrew the staff privileges of the physician who was seen as the leading author of the resolution.

At a meeting three weeks later the hospital board agreed to drop aversion therapy from the Intercept program in Yellville. The health department's investigation was then closed the day before a scheduled public hearing. (The Intercept program continued at two other Westworld hospitals in the state.)

The Arkansas attorney general's investigation dealt with different but related concerns about consumer protection. The investigation arose from complaints about the Intercept program from three patients. The first case was concerned primarily with charges of $19,854 for a fifteen-day course of detoxification and treatment at the twenty-eight-bed Gurdon Municipal Hospital. The second complaint was also about charges. The third, concerning the details of the program, was summarized in the *Arkansas Gazette*.

> The person was watching television and saw a commercial about the Intercept Program, which mentions a telephone number. The person called and a woman who answered insisted on coming to talk with the caller. "I was drinking at the time and after reluctantly consenting to see her, continued to drink," the complainant said. About an hour later, the woman and a man arrived, talked with the complainant "for hours, packed up my belongings and got some beer from my refrigerator so I could drink on the way down

there. I remember vaguely being driven to Gurdon and signing papers. I also came to my senses somewhat and became enraged and troublesome to them, since I had no intention of being taken there," the complainant said.

"You do not walk around in the woods with street clothes on as the commercial implies. My wallet and clothes were locked up and no one is allowed outside. They gave me gin to drink as well as Serax and Haldol injections, which effectively kept me very calm."

Serax is an antidepressant and Haldol is a tranquilizer, according to the Physicians' Desk Reference. The person said when the hospital found that the person's insurance would not cover treatment, the person was discharged "still drunk, confused and with a bill for $3,885." The person said an attorney advised against paying the bill.[43]

Although Westworld's corporate counsel confirmed to me that the patient-recruitment methods described in this example are indeed used by the company, she contended that complaints of this sort are to be expected in substance abuse treatment programs because patients are often difficult and resistant and because high costs and high failure rates can easily lead to disgruntlement.[44]

Several caveats must be attached to the Westworld example. The company tells its own story about many of the charges, attributing some of its problems to the difficulty of trying to operate small rural hospitals profitably and others to misunderstandings about billing practices that ran afoul of the rules. Not all of the issues summarized here involve allegations of illegal conduct, and few have actually been adjudicated. Still, the variety of issues, organizations, and locales involved in the company's legal problems suggests at the very least a pattern of operating close to the line between legitimate and illegitimate innovation in the provision of services.

By late 1986 Westworld was exhibiting many symptoms of a company in trouble. Actions to restructure the organization included the appointment of a new president and a reduction of almost 50 percent in the number of facilities it operated.[45] By early 1987 there were real doubts about whether the company would survive at all after 1986 losses of $124.6 million ($15.33 per share) were announced. In mid-1987 Westworld filed for reorganization under Chapter 11 of the Federal Bankruptcy Code. Some of its former hospitals found ways of staying open, in some cases by reverting to local control.[46]

*International Medical Centers, Inc.* (IMC), provides a second example of an investor-owned health care company that violated numerous regulatory requirements and criminal laws. In only five years IMC became Florida's largest HMO and the nation's leading enroller of Medicare beneficiaries. Along the way it generated numerous complaints from patients and from the independent providers, such as hospitals and physicians, with which it had contracted to provide services. By 1986 complaints about various IMC practices had led to congressional hearings, a barrage of adverse publicity, and investigations by the Office of the Inspector General, the FBI, the Florida Department of Insurance, the General Accounting Office, and HCFA. The issues under investigation ranged from compliance with state and federal HMO regulations regarding financial solvency and quality of care to criminal investigations of alleged fraud.

IMC, which began its involvement with Medicare as a demonstration project in 1982, converted to a risk contract in 1985.[47] As a federally qualified HMO with Medicare contracts, IMC was subject to various federal and state regulations that are designed to ensure fiscal integrity and quality of care.[48] Those regulations include standards for financial solvency, enrollment requirements, marketing practices, beneficiary grievance procedures, and quality assurance.[49]

From the beginning IMC had persistent problems in complying with state and federal solvency requirements.[50] Between 1982 and 1986 several audits found serious problems, ranging from a lack of insurance against insolvency to the listing as assets of unsecured loans to company officials and related organizations.[51] Various corrective actions taken during those years successfully averted threats of takeover by the Florida Department of Insurance and the cancellation of IMC's Medicare contract.

Other problems grew out of IMC's structure as a service-delivery network contracting with other organizations that actually provided physician services and institutional care for IMC's enrollees in exchange for capitation payments from IMC. GAO found that this arrangement transferred the financial risks associated with providing care from IMC to the affiliated providers, which then became "entities that function in many respects as independent HMOs with little or no federal or state oversight."[52] A 1986 HCFA examination of IMC's compliance with the Public Health Service Act found that IMC did not have adequate personnel or systems to oversee the health services provided through its network.[53]

Federal and state agencies also received many complaints about IMC's processing of claims.[54] The company's slowness in paying its bills aroused concern about the potential adverse effects on enrollees' access to service should providers refuse to render services because of past delays in receiving payment. That problem had supposedly been resolved when HCFA established for IMC guidelines for paying bills, but the guidelines were not adhered to.[55]

Another persistent problem concerned the percentage of Medicare beneficiaries among IMC enrollees. HCFA granted IMC a three-year waiver from the congressionally established enrollment requirement that no more than 50 percent of a health plan's members be Medicare beneficiaries, on the understanding that IMC would make genuine efforts to meet this requirement within three years. (The 50 percent requirement was a quality-assurance feature designed to make sure that the HMOs in which Medicare beneficiaries enrolled would also have significant membership from employed groups, which in turn would ensure that the HMO would have to satisfy multiple payers, including some local ones.) Although failure to meet the 50 percent requirement was supposed to result in such sanctions as a moratorium on further Medicare beneficiary enrollment or termination of the Medicare contract, IMC never met it. Throughout its existence, 70 to 80 percent of IMC's enrollees were Medicare beneficiaries. Eventually, under pressure from HCFA to alter its enrollment mix, IMC announced in June 1986 a voluntary cap on the number of Medicare beneficiaries it would serve. Still, lack of compliance was the primary issue cited by HCFA administrator William L. Roper when he announced that IMC's $360-million-a-year contract would be terminated on May 1, 1987.[56]

In addition, IMC's legal and regulatory problems, as reported in Florida newspaper accounts compiled by Congressman Daniel Mica's office, included the following:

· A requirement that IMC pay a $5,000 fine for falsely listing two hospitals as members of its network in advertisements.[57]

· Investigations by the Office of the Inspector General and the FBI into allegations that IMC destroyed between 5,000 and 50,000 computer claims that recorded payments owed to doctors and hospitals that treated IMC patients on referral.[58]

· FBI and OIG investigations of allegations that IMC fraudulently billed for services and refused to accept people with serious health problems.[59]

· A federal investigation of possible criminal actions involved in IMC's purchase of liability insurance coverage from a related organization located in the Cayman Islands.[60]

· The targeting of Miami General Hospital, an organization related to IMC, as the subject of several investigations. (In 1980 Miami General allegedly did not refund money from patient overpayments. The hospital was assessed $121,977 in back taxes and penalties. The hospital was also investigated in 1980 by a federal grand jury for Medicare abuse. No criminal charges were filed. In 1982 the Department of Health and Human Services ordered the hospital to return $1.3 million in Medicare overpayments.)[61]

A frequent IMC practice was to hire or contract with former federal and state officials. These included nine former officials of the Department of Health and Human Services (DHHS), among them the former deputy director of the Health Care Financing Administration, a former DHHS general counsel, and the former head of DHHS's HMO program; the consulting firm of former White House aide Lyn Nofziger; the law firm of John Sears, a former campaign manager for President Ronald Reagan; a son of then Vice President George Bush; and various former state officials.[62]

By July 1986 IMC had submitted a detailed plan, approved by HCFA, by which it proposed to correct many of its quality and management problems. Rumors of a takeover of IMC by one of the major hospital companies gave rise to hopes of an infusion of managerial expertise and capital.

Nonetheless, the problems continued. IMC lost almost $20 million in 1986. It was later found that IMC had paid millions of dollars to other companies controlled by its president, Miguel Recarey.[63] The amount of such payments increased by $6 million in 1986, at a time when the company was going bankrupt. At this point IMC owed Medicare nearly $12 million in overpayments.[64] In 1987 IMC finally lost its Medicare contract, went bankrupt, and was taken over by the State of Florida, which sold it to Humana, Inc. Humana was able to continue services to enrollees. That acquisition took IMC out of the headlines, except for criminal charges lodged against Recarey, who was reported to have left the country.

The IMC affair left a legacy of suspicion and distrust that will take other HMOs that serve Medicare beneficiaries a long time to erase. As one knowledgeable observer put it, the experience taught HCFA that Medicare contracts with alternative delivery systems (such as HMOs) need close monitoring. "Without adequate safeguards to protect Medicare beneficiaries from the rougher edges of a competitive market, the bipartisan congressional support this innovative approach has enjoyed will soon wither."[65]

*Paracelsus Health Corporation*, a privately held investor-owned hospital company, became the subject of an investigation by the Office of the Inspector General because of an incentive system it established for its medical staff in 1985. Under that system staff physicians at fourteen of its hospitals were offered a share of hospital profits on Medicare patients as an incentive to practice in a way that controlled the hospital's costs for patients covered by Medicare's per–DRG-case payment system. "In each hospital, total hospital charges for Medicare patients admitted by each physician are compared on a month-by-month basis to Medicare prospective payments for those patients. If Medicare payments for a physician's patients for a month are above a set percentage of hospital charges for that month (70 to 75 percent in those we examined), the physician is paid a percentage of the difference."[66]

The Paracelsus plan was a rational approach to pursuing economic objectives within a particular payment system. Indeed, various approaches to aligning physician and hospital incentives had previously been suggested by hospital consultants.[67] Yet, questions about legality, ethics, and possible jeopardy to non-profit hospitals' tax-exempt status made many institutions hesitant. When the Paracelsus plan became known, the American Medical Association, among others, questioned whether this was a legitimate way of seeking to influence physician behavior or whether it put physicians in an untenable conflict of interest.[68] The issue went to OIG.

The primary question facing OIG was not about the facts of the Paracelsus plan, which had been publicly announced. Instead the issue was whether the plan technically violated the fraud and abuse statute's proscription against offering inducements to encourage the use of services covered by Medicare. During OIG's investigation Congress passed legislation prohibiting physician incentive plans, and Paracelsus announced that it would end its incentive plan.

Nonetheless, the OIG's investigation of Paracelsus' financial management practices found that the company had inflated its Medicare reimbursement in its 1982 and 1983 annual cost reports.[69] Paracelsus had charged the Medicare program for expenses that were unrelated to health care and had failed to disclose transactions with related organizations.[70] Some of the unallowable expenses that had been charged to Medicare were the cost of golf tournaments, country club dues and expenses, gifts to physicians, limousines and charter jets, political contributions, and expenses for foreign and domestic acquisitions.[71] In late 1986, under a negotiated settlement, Paracelsus pleaded guilty to one count of mail fraud and agreed to pay $4.5 million in reimbursements, fines, and interest to the government for the unallowable expenses reimbursed by Medicare.[72]

The examples of these three companies illustrate the difficulty in assessing the extent of malfeasance among health care organizations. Of the cases discussed here that involve investor-owned hospital companies (Westworld and Paracelsus), only a single Westworld hospital (in Texas) turned up in the data I obtained from agencies investigating fraud and abuse. This may be because cases had not been adjudicated (as in the case of Westworld), because a case was prosecuted under criminal laws rather than under the Medicare and Medicaid statute (as in the case of Paracelsus), or because no conviction was obtained.

## The Complexities Introduced by Corporate Change

Major organizational changes among providers always create new challenges for the payers and regulators who are concerned with accountability. This is true even for innovations that are generally regarded as positive.[73] The rise of investor ownership and of multi-institutional arrangements in health care introduced many stresses and strains into the mechanisms by which health care institutions are held accountable. The new organizations differ from previous types in the way they raise capital and make decisions. They have much more complicated organizational structures, and in many cases they are much more strongly oriented toward maximizing revenues and pursuing economic goals.

Under cost-based reimbursement methods long used by Medicare and some other payers, providers were reimbursed for allowable costs incurred in caring for beneficiaries. Such payment methods provided hospitals with incentives to inflate to the maximum (or disguise the nature of) certain reported costs. It is the job of auditors to detect improper accounting manipulations, uncover kickback arrangements with vendors, and verify and determine the reasonableness of reported costs. The growing complexity of organizational structures and interorganizational relationships created new, difficult-to-detect possibilities for exploiting weaknesses in payment and auditing systems.

Although cost-based reimbursement methods have now for the most part been abandoned, all payment systems have weaknesses that providers who are so inclined can try to exploit. A change in payment systems may reduce certain opportunities, but it does not change the underlying orientation of an organization that was willing to exploit the old system. And it is the *orientation*, not the weaknesses of a particular payment method, that I am seeking to document in this chapter.

Examples uncovered in various investigations by the General Accounting Office, the Office of the Inspector General, and state agencies reveal the endless provider creativity with which auditing organizations must contend. Bruce Vladeck's characterization of government–nursing home relations as a game of cops and robbers could be applied more broadly.[74] A more apt analogy may be found, however, in the relationship between taxing authorities and sophisticated taxpayers because paper transactions and accounting manipulations play such an important role.

The traditional problems of occupational deviance, such as billing for services that were not provided, are simple to detect and document compared to the problems that arise in the provision of and payment for services in the context of complex multi-institutional systems operating under cost-based reimbursement, a payment system that is still used for psychiatric care. Organizational complexities within those systems often exceed the capacity of accountability mechanisms to monitor certain types of activities effectively.

Three areas in which multi-institutional organizations present problems of accountability that are difficult to monitor are (1) providers doing business with related organizations; (2) determining the reasonableness of costs; and (3) allocating home office expenses. These three areas clearly illustrate the challenges to cost-based reimbursement that were raised by the introduction of complex health care organizations, particularly those that sought to exploit the weaknesses of auditing and payment systems. Although the cost-based reimbursement system that led to these particular problems has largely been replaced, an examination of these three problems demonstrates the proclivity of some health care providers toward exploiting the vulnerabilities that payment systems—all payment systems—have.

## Problems of Relatedness

Health care organizations that are to some degree vertically integrated encompass different organizational entities that are under a degree of common ownership and control and that do business with one another. Such arrangements appear to be common, particularly in multi-institutional systems and in individual institutions that have undergone corporate restructuring. For example, the California Health Facilities Commission reported that 707 of the 1,130 long-term care facilities in California had disclosed dealings with related organizations.[75] In another example, after Humana acquired American Medicorp, its organizational chart featured 37 different organizational entities in addition to the 111 hospitals that had been owned or managed by the two companies.[76] Many of the entities did business with one another. But not all the complex interrelationships of ownership and control that characterize many health care organizations appear on organizational charts available for public inspection.

Interrelationships of ownership and control among organizational entities that do business with one another may serve legitimate purposes regarding managerial incentives, efficiency, limitation of liability, and protection of markets or sources of supply. In health care, however, such arrangements also create significant possibilities for abuse because third-party payment and the vulnerability of patients long insulated providers from price competition and because interorganizational complexities can tax or exceed the monitoring ability of state and federal agencies.

The common ownership of two organizations that do business with each other results in transactions that are less than arm's length. The seller's income is a cost to the buyer. Under cost-based reimbursement, if the buyer were a hospital and the seller a supplier of goods or services, the transaction could be used illegitimately to increase the organization's income by inflating the expenses for which the third-party payer reimburses the hospital. With the move away from cost-based reimbursement, other types of potential abuse have presented themselves. For example, under payment systems that pay separately for different levels of care, such as acute hospital care and home care or skilled nursing care, common ownership of organizations that provide different levels of care creates the possibility that patients will be inappropriately shifted from one to another to maximize reimbursement, as with Westworld's use of swing beds.

Under Medicare law it is not illegal for hospitals to deal with related organizations as long as the relationship is disclosed and profits are not reaped. Medicare regulations require health care providers to identify persons or parties with an ownership or controlling interest in the provider organization. Subcontractors or suppliers with whom the provider has an ownership interest of 5 percent or more must also be disclosed. Failure to report such information can result in the termination of existing federal contracts. Such terminations have been rare, but this may be in part because violations can be difficult to detect and document.

A clue that this is true comes from a 1978 OIG investigation of chain-operated health care organizations. OIG concluded that Medicare costs and income of providers were being inflated as the result of "numerous cases" of providers' pyramiding expenses in transactions between related organizations.[77] Among the methods cited were lucrative lease arrangements and unreasonably high payroll costs for suppliers.

Perhaps the most notorious example of abuses perpetrated through the vehicle of related organizations was in the Medicaid experiment with prepaid health plans in California in the mid-1970s. It resulted, ironically, from an attempt by the state to screen out "bad apples" by requiring the participating HMOs to be nonprofit organizations. A General Accounting Office investigation eventually revealed complex interrelationships among the ostensibly nonprofit health plans and related for-profit corporations, which in most cases actually provided the health services. Four out of five prepaid plans basically served as fronts for related for-profit organizations by contracting their services to them. (This case illustrates that "nonprofit" ownership may in some instances not be genuine, a point that was also made about nursing homes during the mid-1970s.)[78]

The president of HMO International, one of the for-profit management companies that was associated with a prepaid plan, likened the convoluted organizational arrangements to a "pretzel palace." He said in congressional testimony that HMO International's "organizational structure [of different corporations and partnerships] is almost incomprehensible, onerous to manage, duplicative of expense, and in a word, it is wrong."[79] Much of the money intended for health services was converted into profits. A California auditor general's investigation of fifteen health plan contractors in 1974 showed that of the $56.5 million in Medi-Cal funds going to those plans, only $27.1 million, or 48 percent, was actually spent on health care services. The remaining funds went to administrative costs and profit.[80] Although state law required that prepaid health plans submit information on subcontractors to the state for approval, the GAO found that formal approval of the subcontractor arrangements had not been given by the state.[81] The entire Medi-Cal prepaid health care experiment was subsequently discontinued and is now widely cited as an example of abuses resulting from the profit motive. Another legacy of the California experience was a revision and strengthening of the antifraud provisions of the Social Security Act, particularly regarding disclosure requirements for health care providers.

The few attempts to document the prevalence of abuses in the operation of related organizations have foundered on the size and complexity of the task. An example was a project undertaken by the controller's office in California in cooperation with OIG in 1981 to examine whether corporate structures were artificially inflating medical costs through contracting procedures that allowed the improper disbursement of funds. The basic question was whether complex organizational arrangements were being used to generate and conceal profits that were illegitimate under cost-based reimbursement methods. The project began by screening data from 555 California hospitals to identify those with corporate structures that appeared to have potential for abuse on the basis of high costs coupled with a high dependence on service contracts. Seventy-two hospitals (13 percent of the total) were identified as potential subjects of investigation. It was soon recognized, however, that detailed auditing would be required to determine whether those hospitals were actually abusing the payment system. The project set out to examine the corporate structures of all seventy-two hospitals, but available funds were sufficient only for the examination of a single hospital—the thirty-six-bed, nonprofit Community Hospital of the Valleys.[82]

The investigation revealed several related corporations that were owned by a small group of individuals who controlled a large portion of the hospital's cash flow. The hospital contracted for ancillary services through one related organization, Perris Valley Scientific, which in turn provided or arranged for services through six other related organizations. As a result, the hospital did not use comparative shopping and bidding to minimize expenses, dramatically increasing the payments received from Medicare under the cost-reimbursement system.[83] From 1977 to 1980 Medicare paid $8.7 million to Community Hospital, of which $4.3 million was derived from organizations contracting with Perris Valley.[84] To conceal the hospital's relationship to those organizations, the minutes of hospital meetings were modified. Community Hospital was eventually closed in 1981 after an investigation of twenty-four deaths prompted a review and suspension of the hospital's operating license.[85]

The Community Hospital study was not the only one to produce evidence of abuses resulting from transactions among related organizations. A General Accounting Office study in 1982 of five hospitals in California and Nevada concluded that through dealings with related organizations the hospitals inflated their costs and, thus, government payments under Medicare and Medicaid.[86] The hospitals were selected for the study because of their large volume of federal business and because they were suspected of being engaged in less-than-arm's-length transactions. The hospitals chosen were *not* members of large multi-institutional systems (although four were for-profit) because GAO was not in a position to make the much more substantial investment of time and resources that an investigation of such organizations would have required. Even so, the report's conclusions emphasized the inability of fiscal intermediaries to identify transactions of less than arm's length without considerable effort. Furthermore, in some cases hospital costs were so intertwined with other organizations' costs that reimbursement could be based only on an arbitrary allocation of expenses among the organizations.

Problems of relatedness can also result from more subtle linkages among organizations. An OIG study of providers dealing with one Medicare fiscal intermediary, Mutual of Omaha, found instances in which companies that did business with a hospital chain, although not owned by the chain itself, were owned or controlled by the officers or directors of the chain.[87] OIG discovered many of the relationships only after doing extensive research on the organizations' structure and intercompany relationships in financial reports and publications, such as Dun & Bradstreet reports, Standard & Poor's reports, the *Wall Street Journal, Barron's,* and Moody's industrial manuals. In many instances the Medicare fiscal intermediary was unaware of the relationships between the hospital chain and its suppliers.

Relatedness also created problems with regard to the compensation of top officials. The difficulty of establishing relatedness between organizations and officers within a multi-institutional system made it possible for executives to receive large salaries from several organizations within the system. The combined salaries could exceed the costs that Medicare defined as reasonable for reimbursement purposes. An OIG review of health care chains found several instances in which individuals were listed as officers in different corporations within the same chain.[88] In one case an individual was receiving salaries as an administrator of one organization and as the chief executive of another, was being paid as a consultant to yet another chain, and was working full time in a non–health-related job. The questions of whether persons with multiple positions are performing services necessary to patient care and whether the costs incurred are reasonable can be addressed only if the auditor is clever enough (and has sufficient time) to unravel the organizational interrelationships.

*Reasonableness of Costs*

Medicare's cost-based reimbursement methods included provisions requiring that reimbursable costs be "reasonable."[89] Complex multi-institutional arrangements presented difficulties in determining the reasonableness of many costs, and abuses may have been common. For example, five of eight nursing home chains audited in a GAO study were found to have billed Medicare for excessive management fees charged to individual units by the home office,[90] for excessive interest on loans between the home office and individual units, and on property transactions between the chain and related parties.

Management contracts, so widely used among hospitals, presented several opportunities for abuse: incentives for overutilization of services created by management contracts in which fees were based on a percentage of the gross revenues; documentation problems regarding services that were billed for; and the failure of intermediaries to review the fees charged before approving payment.[91] Audits found that there was not always a reasonable relationship between the services provided and charges under a contract.[92] To reduce that type of abuse, the Tax Equity and Fiscal Responsibility Act of 1982 prohibited reimbursement under contracts in which the amount is based on a percentage of the provider's charges, revenue, or claims, on account of the cost-inflating incentives created by such contracts.

Yet even fixed-price management contracts contain potential for abuses that are not easy to detect. Insofar as the management contract allows the hospital administrator (a management company employee) to buy supplies or services from the parent company, it is possible that too high a price will be paid. A grand jury investigation in Habersham County, Georgia, of a management contract between the local hospital and the Hospital Corporation of America found that although the hospital was supposedly benefiting from HCA's purchasing power, the costs to the hospital (and, therefore, to cost-based payers) of supplies purchased by the administrator through HCA were in many cases higher than they would have been if the hospital had bought them through a consortium of nonprofit hospitals in the state.[93]

### Allocation of Corporate Office Expenses

The corporate or home office of a multi-institutional system was not directly reimbursable under Medicare's cost-based reimbursement rules. Medicare deemed the relationship of the home office to the hospital to be that of an organization related to a provider. When the home office provided patient–care-related services to hospitals, its reasonable costs could be included on the hospitals' cost reports. If the home office provided no services that were related to patient care, neither its operating costs nor the equity capital costs was recognized as allowable.[94]

The Office of the Inspector General concluded that health care chains had a "large potential for passing on unsupported or inflated home office expenses or other fees to health care providers," and that such potential greatly increased if the chain included large numbers of providers that were geographically dispersed and involved in both Medicare and Medicaid programs.[95] An illustration comes from a GAO study of a large nursing home chain.[96] The headquarters provided accounting services, liability and malpractice insurance coverage, and administrative services to its nursing homes. It assessed each home 4.5 percent of its gross revenue plus 1 percent of its salaries for those services. An audit found, however, that the fees so charged to the nursing homes exceeded the home office's actual costs of $3 million by nearly $817,000. In seeking reimbursement for costs, the nursing homes claimed their portion of the $3.8 million rather than the actual headquarters cost of $3 million. This resulted in the overpayment of $215,000 by four Medicaid programs.

In recent years several cases brought to Medicare's Provider Reimbursement Review Board have involved the allocation by home offices of pooled equity capital in multi-institutional systems. Once the amount of such pooled equity capital is determined by headquarters, it must be allocated by accountants to the institutions in the chain. The process is similar to the allocation of home office costs in that assets or liabilities attributed to a specific provider must be allocated to that provider. For example, capital costs involved in the purchase of a piece of equipment for a specific institution must be allocated to that facility. Reimbursement guidelines state that the basis for the allocation of home office equity capital must be the same ratio used in the allocation of other costs, such as patient days or total cost. Attempts by chains to allocate home equity capital using a different ratio could lead to a misallocation of funds.[97]

## Limitations of Investigatory Agencies

A large discrepancy undoubtedly exists between the number of cases reported by fraud and abuse agencies and the likely size of the problem presented by the proliferation of large-scale profit-oriented health care organizations. It is likely that instances of fraud and abuse have often not been identified because of shortcomings and constraints that hinder the operations of the organizations and agencies that have oversight responsibility. Several limitations can be identified.

First, there are *shortcomings of expertise.* The kinds of fraud and abuse that can arise in large, multi-institutional health care systems are very complex. At the time of the creation of the Office of the Inspector General in the Department of Health, Education and Welfare in 1976, oversight consisted almost entirely of financial auditing by fiscal intermediaries and was aimed at recovering overpayments.[98] OIG began with no experience at all in conducting investigations of hospitals, and such investigations remain only a small part of its activities.[99]

An additional problem for auditing and monitoring organizations, particularly in periods of rapid change, is that they are unable to adapt as quickly as the organizations they are monitoring. As providers innovate in various ways, lags inevitably develop while reimbursement, regulatory, auditing, and legal systems adjust to the changes. Years can pass as such systems go through the processes of recognizing developments that may affect a regulatory structure or procedure, determining what types of changes should be made in response, writing and promulgating whatever new policies and regulations may be needed, training personnel to implement those policies and regulations, and establishing judicial interpretations and precedents. In light of the rapid changes that have occurred in the health care industry in recent years, Sanford Tepliztky and Eugene Tillman's observation that "fraud and abuse structures have not experienced the same evolutionary changes as have the industry and reimbursement systems" is hardly surprising.[100]

When Medicare abandoned its cost-based reimbursement methods in favor of the prospective payment system, the activities of its medical care review organizations had to be refocused in recognition that the incentives faced by providers had been reversed and, consequently, the menu of types of possible mischief had been radically altered. The professional standards review organization (PSRO) program in the 1970s and early 1980s had been preoccupied with the problem of unnecessarily long hospital stays. This concern was swept away with the change from cost-based reimbursement to prospective payment. The analogous preoccupation of the current peer review organizations (PROs) is the opposite one of premature discharge. The methodological and logistical problems of determining whether a patient who is no longer in the hospital was discharged too soon are quite different from determining whether a hospitalized patient should be (or should already have been) discharged.

Second, there are *limitations of power and resources*. In 1982 a congressional committee found inadequacies regarding staff allocations to OIG to combat fraud, waste, and abuse.[101] The state-level agencies that pursue fraud in the Medicaid program also have some notable limitations. A 1980 investigation by the House Select Committee on Aging found that half of all state Medicaid fraud and abuse agencies did not have subpoena power, and some units did not have legal authority to initiate fraud investigations but had to wait for complaints or referrals.[102] Furthermore, serious problems of cost and legal authority can arise when the subject of an investigation is a multi-institutional company whose regional or corporate headquarters are out of state.[103] Coordination among the states has been limited.

Problems of jurisdiction and coordination also exist in the Medicare program because geographically dispersed facilities in a multi-institutional system deal with many different fiscal intermediaries. Although only one fiscal intermediary assumes responsibility for dealing with a chain's home office and the costs allocated thereto by individual institutions, the fact that many intermediaries might be involved in the company's business is a complicating and limiting factor. Medicare regulations also direct intermediaries not to spend audit funds on routine "attempts to locate situations where a provider may have failed to act prudently in its business operations."[104]

A third problem is *quality versus quantity* in the output of investigatory agencies. It is likely that the way in which investigatory agencies allocate their resources is affected by *their own* accountability to the organizations from which they obtain their resources. The pursuit of large and complicated cases, such as those involving multi-institutional systems, is risky. Because of the complexity of those cases and the technical nature of the violations that may be investigated, the process of developing and untangling evidence can consume many resources. The same factors may also make it difficult to obtain a conviction because the large stakes mean that a significant amount of legal talent may be arrayed in opposition. Even if a conviction is obtained, it may be viewed as only one case when the agency's accomplishments are being evaluated.

The so-called Spectro-Rubin case, the largest Medi-Cal fraud case of its kind in California, illustrates this difficulty. Spectro Health Services was a health care organization consisting of several hospitals and medical clinics owned and operated by a physician, Edward Rubin. A criminal investigation of Spectro Health Services was initiated in 1978 at the request of the California Department of Health Services. Audits by the Department of Health Services in 1978 revealed that Spectro Health Services and its subsidiary hospitals had been overpaid approximately $5 million by Medi-Cal. The overpayment was allegedly the result of overutilization of medical services, excessive diagnostic and lab tests, failure to disclose Spectro's relationship with related labs and pharmacies, and the use of false bills from attorneys and accountants to increase reimbursable costs.[105] In 1980 a thirty-two-count indictment was filed against Spectro Health Services. The case against the organization was dropped when charges were filed against individuals within the organization. The volume of financial transactions involved in the case required a lengthy investigation. In addition, Medi-Cal had to combat several petitions for injunctions to halt the investigation.[106] In 1981, two and one-half years after the California attorney general's office was informed of the case, a complaint was filed in municipal court, the first step of the superior court process.[107] By the time the case was heard by the superior court in 1984, charges against Rubin and others had to be dismissed because the statute of limitations had expired. Moreover, because funds drained from Spectro Health Services led to its bankruptcy, the Department of Human Services was unable to recoup any of the $7.5 million allegedly due from Spectro.[108] An analyst in Medi-Cal commented that the outcome of the Spectro case might have made Medi-Cal more cautious with regard to taking on large health care organizations.[109]

A safer course for investigatory agencies is to pursue relatively uncomplicated cases, such as those involving individual deviance (kickbacks, improper billing). These help build a record when the agency reports on the number of cases it has pursued and the number of successful outcomes (convictions or recoveries of money). The OIG concentrates its "limited resources on the areas of greatest vulnerability and highest possible return."[110] Even though the cumulative effect of cases of individual deviance may be relatively minor when compared to the scale of possible abuses by large organizations, agencies may consider it too risky to commit scarce resources to investigating the latter.

Both legitimate and illegitimate opportunities are available for deriving an income from the almost 12 percent of the nation's gross national product that passes through the health care system. Payers and regulators thus find it necessary to establish systems for detecting malfeasance. Much of the focus has been on problems that are variants of simple consumer fraud (did the consumer get what was paid for?), complicated by the fact that in health care the purchaser is often not present in the transaction between the provider and recipient of a service.

Most agencies pursuing fraud and abuse have targeted malfeasance by individuals or small proprietary organizations seeking to exploit the vulnerabilities of patients or the payment process. The movement toward larger, professionally managed health care organizations—whether they be group practices or multihospital systems—reduces the number of circumstances in which a single individual can charge for a service and pocket the payment. Accordingly, payers' problems with individual or occupational fraud and abuse may diminish as a result of the corporate transformation of health care.

At the same time, the creation of large, economically driven health care organizations greatly increases the likelihood that two other types of problems will arise. The first is deviance by employees who find themselves unable to achieve their assigned goals or responsibilities by legitimate means. The second resides in illegitimate strategies used by organizations themselves in pursuit of their economic goals. Although the latter problem could presumably arise in any type of organization that is driven by such goals, it may be a particular problem in an investor-owned company because of the pressure to increase earnings. Although relatively few cases of fraud and abuse have been detected among health care companies, the major examples that have been brought to light all involve for-profit firms.

This discussion has been much more illustrative than exhaustive regarding the potential for abuse presented by complex interorganizational relationships under cost-based reimbursement. Under that system economic goals emphasized maximization of reimbursement. The line between legitimate and illegitimate methods was not always clear, although some of the practices described in this chapter obviously crossed that line. An almost endless array of illegitimate opportunities existed for profiting from a system in which providers were supposedly being reimbursed only for their costs incurred in caring for patients.[111] It seems likely that organizations that were creative, determined, and willing to take some risks to maximize reimbursement under cost-based methods could often outstrip the ability of auditing and investigating agencies to keep up with them. Those difficulties are a largely unrecognized consequence of the corporate transformation of health care and are among the weaknesses that led to the demise of cost-based reimbursement methods.

Recognition of the cost-increasing incentives that were built into cost-based reimbursement—if not complete recognition of the auditing difficulties that it presented—led Medicare (and some other payers) to adopt alternative methods, most notably the so-called prospective payment system. Although prospective payment methods vastly reduce the incentives to find creative ways of building artificial but reimbursable costs into the care of patients, they produce their own set of incentives. Seen positively, they reward efficiency and eliminate such abuses as providing unnecessary services to hospitalized patients, pyramiding costs through transactions between related organizations, and juggling the allocation of home office costs. Yet, the incentives may reward unnecessary hospital admissions, premature discharges, manipulations in reporting diagnoses (since payment amounts vary according to reported diagnosis), and inappropriate transfers of patients between different levels of care for which separate payments are made.

It now appears that the difficulties of monitoring fraud and abuse in complex health care organizations are less severe in a prospective payment system than were the problems under cost-based reimbursement. Nonetheless, the same pressures that led to unnecessary services and fraud and abuse under cost-based reimbursement may now create a different set of problems relating to quality of care, since the incentives under prospective payment and capitation encourage the provision of fewer services. The potential problems that this raises clearly go far beyond the means of traditional fraud and abuse agencies to control. More sophisticated data systems for monitoring are needed and, as we shall see in Chapters 10 and 11, are already coming into use by large purchasers of medical care.

# 7

# Provider Efforts to Shape
# the Reimbursement
# and Regulatory Environment

At the end of *The Social Transformation of American Medicine,*
Paul Starr wrote, "No less important than its effect on the culture of medical care institutions is the likely political impact of
the growth of corporate enterprise. As an interest group, the new
health care conglomerates will obviously be a powerful
force . . . and will also [resist] public accountability and participation."[1] Despite the concern of critics of for-profit health
care about the ability of large investor-owned health care companies to influence health care policy and regulation, the
aggressiveness and effectiveness of those companies' efforts to
influence their environment have not been studied empirically.

To shed some light on the pursuit of influence over the reimbursement and regulatory environment in which health care
institutions operate, I examined three very different sets of records, which pertained to (1) appeals to an administrative agency,
(2) the use of the courts, and (3) the lobbying of legislative bodies.
What I found provides some support for the concern about the
aggressiveness of the investor-owned health care companies.
There are also indications, however, that the payoff may be small
in proportion to the effort.

## Appeals to the Provider Reimbursement Review Board

Hospitals vary widely in their approach to third-party payers and
the fiscal intermediaries that administer claims for payment

under the Medicare program. Some are averse to submitting claims that may be rejected and are hesitant to bill for costs that may be disallowed. Others persistently test the limits of payment systems. The investor-owned hospitals have been characterized by officials of their own trade association as having "pioneered the art of maximizing reimbursement."[2] So-called reimbursement maximization, however, is undoubtedly not a goal whose pursuit is limited only to one sector. The question is how aggressively it is done.

One indicator of aggressiveness vis-à-vis the reimbursement system is in the use of Medicare's Provider Reimbursement Review Board (PRRB). A provider organization that disagrees with a Medicare fiscal intermediary's determination of what costs are allowable for payment has 180 days to appeal. Appeals for amounts greater than $10,000 are heard by the PRRB. (Amounts disputed by *groups* of providers must exceed $50,000.) The provider and the fiscal intermediary present evidence to the board, which can affirm, reverse, or modify the decision of the intermediary. The board then submits its written decisions to the deputy administrator of the Health Care Financing Administration (HCFA), who can affirm or reverse the decision.

The PRRB was established in 1972 to give due process to providers who had objections to determinations of allowable costs for reimbursement purposes.[3] Although the board originally reviewed issues that arose in the cost-based reimbursement system, new matters continue to be referred to it.

The PRRB has examined a wide range of issues that involve the costs allowed for reimbursement purposes.[4] The most basic issues can arise in any type of hospital, such as the costs of special care units or the treatment of interest expenses and income in bond financing. Some issues pertain primarily to nonprofits, for example, how charitable contributions will affect reimbursement. Other issues primarily concern for-profit providers, such as stock maintenance costs, return on equity, and tax matters. The growth of multi-institutional systems also raised specific questions, such as how home office costs or the costs of centrally raised capital should be allocated to individual institutions.

The PRRB has thus been a key arbiter of many practical questions arising from the corporate transformation of American medicine. Some cases have been resolved only after substantial amounts of money and time have been spent.

To assess differences in how hospitals use the PRRB to influence their economic environment, I compiled information from the Commerce Clearing House volumes on cases decided by the PRRB from 1980 to 1986. The information included the type of provider that brought each appeal, the kinds of issues that were raised, and the outcome of the decision. Of the 807 cases decided during that period, 652 involved hospitals.[5] My analysis focused on those.

The investor-owned sector seems to have been notably active. Although investor-owned hospital companies owned about 13 percent of U.S. hospitals during the period studied, 28 percent of the cases brought to the PRRB came from investor-owned hospitals, and another 4 percent were from independent proprietary hospitals.[6] (The remaining 68 percent of the hospital cases involved public or private nonprofit institutions.) The issues raised by the investor-owned sector illustrate the challenge that its rise posed for the Medicare payment system.

Humana, Inc., brought to the PRRB a series of cases seeking reimbursement for costs incurred from 1973 to 1977 in attracting private investment capital for thirty-five of its hospitals. Humana maintained that these costs, which included stock maintenance expenses, income taxes, liability in calculating equity capital, and return-on-equity capital, were necessary to the delivery of health services. The PRRB denied the claim, and Humana took the decision to the courts. A federal appeals court ruled that the costs in question were not necessary to the delivery of needed health services. Humana appealed the 1985 appeals court ruling to the Supreme Court, which declined to review it.[7]

Other cases of major significance for investor-owned companies dealt with depreciation expenses after acquisitions or mergers. Prior to a change in the law, the purchase price of an asset such as a hospital established the value on which the Medicare payments for depreciation expenses were based. The question then arose whether the purchase of a company's stock could be considered the purchase of its facilities. If so, the provider could obtain Medicare reimbursement for depreciation expenses, as well as interest costs and return-on-equity costs associated with those facilities.[8] The PRRB upheld an intermediary's decision that a transfer of stock was not reimbursable as an acquisition of assets.

This ruling involved high stakes and considerable complexity. For example, in 1978 Humana acquired 54 percent of American Medicorp's outstanding stock in a hostile takeover. Several months later a merger occurred, followed by a liquidation of American Medicorp's remaining assets. The PRRB eventually decided that Humana had gained control of American Medicorp when it acquired a majority interest in the latter's stock and that the subsequent merger and liquidation of assets amounted to a transaction between related parties for which revaluation of transferred assets would not be permitted.[9]

An examination of the *outcomes* of cases brought to the PRRB (see Table 7.1) shows evidence of both the aggressiveness of the investor-owned companies and their relative lack of success. Although the PRRB did not often reverse the decisions of the fiscal intermediaries (only on an average of 14.5 percent of the time), investor-owned hospitals were particularly unsuccessful in

*Table 7.1.* Outcome of decisions by Medicare's Provider Reimbursement Review Board (PRRB), by ownership of hospitals, 1980–1986

| PRRB ruling on intermediary's determination[a] | Cases from nonprofit and public hospitals (N = 420) | Cases from proprietary hospitals (N = 29) | Cases from investor-owned company (N = 172) | Total cases (621) |
|---|---|---|---|---|
| Affirmed | 37.1% | 51.7% | 14.5% | 196 |
| Reversed | 19.7 | 3.4 | 7.5 | 97 |
| Mixed | 20.0 | 31.0 | 30.9 | 146 |
| Appealed | 14.5 | 13.8 | 43.1 | 139 |
| Other | 8.6 | — | 4.0 | 43 |
| Total | 100 | 100 | 100 | 100% |

Ownership determined by reference to the American Hospital Association's *Guide to the Health Care Field* and the Federation of American Hospitals' *Directory of Investor-Owned Hospitals.*

Source: "PRRB Decisions," in *Medicare and Medicaid Guide* (Chicago: Commerce Clearing House, 1986).

a. For an explanation of the categories, see note 10 of this chapter.

gaining reversals, winning only 7.5 percent of their cases.[10] Investor-owned hospitals were much more likely to appeal PRRB decisions (43.1 percent of their cases) than were nonprofit and public hospitals. (The large percentage of nonprofit hospital cases shown as affirmed reflects the fact that they were much less likely than for-profit hospitals to appeal a PRRB affirmation of an intermediary's payment decision.)

There are several possible reasons for the investor-owned chains' comparatively greater use of the PRRB. It may be more economical for organizations that own multiple facilities to make appeals. There may also be greater returns for a favorable decision. Or, in a dynamic delivery system the actions of an investor-owned hospital chain may be particularly likely to outpace the rules being used by Medicare intermediaries. Whatever the reasons, the investor-owned sector has been notably active in using the PRRB to shape the reimbursement system in ways that serve its own interests.

### Lawsuits Involving Health Planning Agencies

Another area in which hospitals challenged or sought to influence the regulatory environment involved certificate-of-need decisions by health planning agencies. Operating under the National Health Planning and Resources Development Act of 1974, health planning agencies were responsible for reviewing the need for capital expenditures by providers under Medicare and Medicaid (section 1122 of the 1972 Social Security amendments) and under state certificate-of-need (CON) laws. Such reviews were based on statewide plans and priorities for allocating capital expenditures.

Health care providers viewed the certificate-of-need system negatively or positively depending on their circumstances. For providers seeking to make capital expenditures above a certain threshold—by constructing a new facility, by adding beds, or by purchasing a major piece of capital equipment—local and state health planning agencies were an obstacle to be overcome, particularly if excess capacity already existed or the proposed expenditure would duplicate existing facilities. For other providers the health planning agencies in effect protected their franchise by restricting entry of competitors into the market. Always controversial and unpopular with many providers, the federal health planning program was ended in 1986, although CON laws remain in many states.

Because the decisions of health planning agencies could have considerable economic impact on health care providers, they were often the subject of litigation. Over a twenty-year period the number of suits involving CON/1122 decisions increased, as did the likelihood that a health planning agency would win (see Table 7.2).[11]

During the period 1975–1986, for-profit hospitals were plaintiffs in a disproportionately large number of lawsuits against health planning agencies (see Table 7.3).[12] They were plaintiffs in 46.4 percent (26 of 56) of the cases brought by acute care general hospitals in the eleven states where they make up at least 10 percent of such hospitals (for-profit hospitals account for 30 percent of all types of hospitals in those states).[13] For-profit hospitals were plaintiffs in 17.1 percent (14 of 82) of the acute care cases in

*Table 7.2.*  Disposition of CON/1122 court decisions,[a]
             1965–1985

|  | Health planning agency upheld[b] | Health planning agency reversed/not upheld |
|---|---|---|
| 1965–1968 | 1 | 0 |
| 1969–1972 | 3 | 1 |
| 1973–1976 | 9 | 8 |
| 1977–1980 | 26 | 33 |
| 1981–1985 | 81 | 39 |

Source: James B. Simpson, Western Consortium for the Health Professions, Inc., Berkeley, California, and Simpson and Ted Bogue, *The Guide to Health Planning Law: A Topical Digest of Health Planning and Certificate of Need Case Law,* 4th ed. (San Francisco: Western Center for Health Planning, 1986), and cases slated for inclusion in the next edition.

a. The court actions in this table pertain to decisions made by state agencies under two types of health planning authorities—state certificate-of-need (CON) statutes or section 1122 of the Social Security Act. These programs were intended to assure the necessity of significant capital expenditures for health care facilities.

b. Those cases in "which a state health planning agency administering a CON program or 1122 program was a party litigant and was upheld, was not a party litigant but the state health planning agency's position was upheld, or the state CON statute, state 1122 program, or federal 1122 program was upheld."

*Table 7.3.*   Analysis of hospital litigants in health planning cases, 1975–1986 (%)

| Type of case | Hospitals in states with more than 10% for-profit hospitals, 1980 (N = 85 cases)[a] | Hospitals in other states (N = 149 cases) |
|---|---|---|
| Percent of cases in which plaintiff was an acute care general hospital | 67.1 | 55.0 |
| Percent of cases brought by acute care hospitals in which a for-profit hospital was plaintiff | 46.4 | 17.1 |
| Percent of cases in which a for-profit hospital was plaintiff, which the plaintiff won | 46.1 | 25.0 |
| Percent of cases in which an "other" hospital was plaintiff, which the plaintiff won | 50.0 | 44.1 |
| Percent of cases in which a hospital was protecting its franchise | 44.7 | 25.6 |
| Percent of franchise-protecting cases in which a hospital was protecting its market from a for-profit hospital | 23.5 | 19.0 |
| Percent of cases in which plaintiff was not an acute care general hospital ("other providers")[b] | 32.9 | 45.0 |
| Percent of "other provider" cases which the plaintiff won | 39.3 | 35.1 |

Source: Data in James Simpson and Ted Bogue, *The Guide to Health Planning Law: A Topical Digest of Health Planning and Certificate of Need Case Law,* 4th ed. (San Francisco: Western Center for Health Planning, 1986).

a. Includes 11 independent for-profit hospitals and 29 investor-owned company hospitals.

b. It was not possible to identify reliably the type of ownership of many of these providers, because so many different types are involved—most notably nursing homes—and because no directories identify ownership type.

the other states, where they made up 5.8 percent of such hospitals. Over this period the frequency of certificate-of-need lawsuits in which for-profit hospitals were the plaintiffs (4.35 suits per 1,000 hospitals) was significantly higher than the rate for nonprofit and public hospitals (1.6 suits per 1,000 hospitals).[14]

Thus, for-profit hospitals were proportionately involved in 2.75 as many cases as nonprofit and public hospitals.

Although for-profit hospitals were more willing to sue, they were slightly less likely than other hospitals to *win* their lawsuits. As shown in Table 7.4, for-profit hospitals won 38.8 percent of the cases in which they were the plaintiffs, compared with a rate of 46 percent for other hospitals. In the states with high concentrations of for-profit hospitals, they won 46.1 percent of their cases, compared to 50 percent for other hospitals (see Table 7.3). In other states for-profit hospitals won just 25 percent of their cases, while other hospitals won 44.1 percent of theirs. This raises the possibility that lack of success with health planning agencies in the states where there are few for-profit hospitals may partially explain their scarcity in those states.

Health care organizations also used health planning laws to protect their market position. This was true of 44 percent of the cases involving hospitals in the high investor-ownership states and only 25 percent of cases in other states. Of the cases that involved hospitals seeking to protect their market, investor-owned hospitals were the encroaching party in 23.5 percent of the cases in the eleven high investor-ownership states and in 19 percent of the cases in other states.[15]

In sum, for-profit hospitals have brought substantially more than their share of lawsuits involving health planning agencies. No doubt this reflects the fact that these companies were seeking to grow in an environment in which there was a broad consensus

*Table 7.4.*   Disposition of certificate-of-need lawsuits brought by hospitals, 1975–1986 (%)

| Disposition of suits by hospitals | Suits by for-profit hospitals (N = 40) | Suits by other hospitals (N = 98) | Total |
|---|---|---|---|
| Won (N = 60.5) | 38.8 | 45.9 | 43.8 |
| Lost (N = 77.5) | 61.2 | 54.1 | 56.2 |

Source: Data in James Simpson and Ted Bogue, *The Guide to Health Planning Law: A Topical Digest of Health Planning and Certificate of Need Case Law,* 4th ed. (San Francisco: Western Center for Health Planning, 1986).

Note: Suits in which hospitals won a partial victory were counted as one-half a win and one-half a loss.

among health policy analysts that the nation had too many hospital beds. Nonetheless, their legal activities against health planning agencies provide a second confirmation that the investor-owned institutions have been more aggressive than nonprofit institutions in seeking to shape their regulatory environment. The fact that they lost almost two-thirds of the time (a greater percentage than for other hospitals) indicates that their success in this regard was relatively modest.

## Political Activities

Political activities furnish a third arena in which to examine providers' efforts to shape the regulatory and reimbursement environment. Lobbying activities and political contributions (financial and otherwise) are a basic part of the political process in the United States. Because the federal government plays a major role as a regulator and as the largest purchaser of health care, health care providers have long been very active in trying to influence government policies. During the 1977–1978 election cycle, for example, 112 health-related political action committees (PACs) contributed funds to political candidates.[16]

The political activities of the American Medical Association have far exceeded the activities of the hospital industry,[17] but corporate changes in health care have introduced new participants seeking to advance their own interests. I examined information on two aspects of the political activities of the hospital organizations: 1985 lobbying expenditures of hospital-related organizations and political action committee contributions to candidates in three election cycles. In both areas federal reporting requirements compel the filing of reports that, though imperfect in many ways, provide some basis for comparing the political activity of different sectors. Although the data reported here are limited, they provide some insight into the comparative political activities of different sectors of the hospital industry.

Political involvement occurs either through providers themselves, through organizations they create to represent them for that purpose, or through trade associations. Trade associations include those representing nonprofit hospitals only (Volunteer Trustees of Nonprofit Hospitals, American Protestant Health

Association, the National Council of Community Hospitals);[18] the American Hospital Association, which is the largest trade association and represents both the for-profit and nonprofit sectors; and the Federation of American Health Systems (formerly the Federation of American Hospitals), which represents for-profit hospitals.[19]

Table 7.5 compares lobbying expenditures of hospital organizations during 1985 by sector. Not surprisingly, the largest organization, the American Hospital Association, representing all hospitals regardless of ownership type, far outspent all the other groups. For-profit hospital organizations accounted for 36 percent of total hospital lobbying expenditures, considerably more than nonprofit hospital organizations. This is particularly striking when one considers the overall percentage of for-profit and nonprofit hospitals (approximately 15 percent and 85 percent of private hospitals, respectively).[20]

*Table 7.5.*   Lobbying expenditures[a] filed with the Clerk of the House of Representatives, by hospital sector, 1985

| Sector | Expenditure ($) |
| --- | --- |
| *For-profit* | |
| Federation of American Health Care Systems | 98,270 |
| Hospital Corporation of America | 66,309[b] |
| National Medical Enterprises, Inc. | 9,675 |
| Total | 174,254 |
| *Nonprofit* | |
| Volunteer Trustees of Nonprofit Hospitals | 39,437 |
| American Protestant Health Association | 14,599 |
| National Council of Community Hospitals | 10,363 |
| Total | 64,399 |
| *Mixed[c]* | |
| American Hospital Association | 214,320 |
| Alabama Hospital Association | 21,680 |
| American Osteopathic Hospital Association | 10,485 |
| Total | 246,485 |
| Total | 485,138 |

Source: Data in "Report-Pursuant to Federal Regulations of Lobbying Act," filed with the Clerk of the House of Representatives, 1985.

a. Includes organizations' and individual lobbyists' funds.

b. Rounded to nearest dollar.

c. Membership includes for-profit and nonprofit hospitals.

The for-profit and nonprofit sectors also differed in the size of contributions made by political action committees to candidates. Table 7.6 summarizes PAC contributions during three election cycles by for-profit and nonprofit hospital organizations and by organizations whose membership includes both types of hospitals. Two facts are notable. First, for-profit hospitals contributed substantially more money to candidates than nonprofit hospitals and organizations that represent both types of hospitals. This is true not only in relative terms but in absolute terms as well. Second, for-profit multi-institutional systems made sizable contributions, particularly in 1984 and 1986, funding 29 percent and 24 percent, respectively, of total PAC contributions by hospitals.

During this period two investor-owned systems were involved in incidents that drew negative attention to their political activities. The first case concerned National Medical Enter-

Table 7.6.  PAC contributions[a] to political candidates reported to the Federal Election Commission, by hospital sector, 1981–1986 ($)

| Sector | 1981–1982 | 1983–1984 | 1985–1986 |
|---|---|---|---|
| *For-profit* | | | |
| Universal Health Services | — | 7,500 | 2,654 |
| National Medical Enterprises, Inc. | 29,460 | 56,026 | 81,150 |
| Humana, Inc. | 3,800 | 16,500 | 8,300 |
| Charter Medical Corporation | 9,570 | 27,050 | 10,450 |
| American Medical International | 3,000 | 15,000 | 53,500 |
| Hospital Corporation of America | 8,150 | 25,075 | 35,034 |
| Subtotal of multi-institutional systems | 53,980 | 147,151 | 191,088 |
| National Association of Private Psychiatric Hospitals | 19,300 | 31,600 | 25,800 |
| Federation of American Health Systems | 201,625 | 201,500 | 135,517 |
| Total for-profit | 274,905 | 380,251 | 352,405 |
| *Nonprofit* | | | |
| Voluntary Hospitals of America | — | — | 17,500 |
| *Mixed*[b] | | | |
| American Hospital Association | 182,925 | 228,141 | 279,896 |
| Total | 457,830 | 608,392 | 649,801 |

Source: Data in Federal Election Commission, Index D, 1982–1986.
a. Total contributions during the election cycle.
b. Membership includes for-profit and nonprofit hospitals.

prises, Inc. (NME), one of the largest investor-owned health care companies. In 1985 a $50 million lawsuit was filed alleging that NME had bribed state officials to approve its application for the construction of a $23.8 million hospital that it had submitted to the state Health Planning and Development Bureau. NME donated $10,000 to the New Mexico Democratic party two days after the state decided to reconsider NME's application, which had originally been turned down. The FBI investigated donations made by NME as part of a larger investigation into state corruption.[21]

In the second case, International Medical Centers (IMC), as part of its growth strategy, cultivated political connections at both the state and federal levels as well as the expedient use of state and federal campaign contributions. IMC hired individuals who had been employed in the Department of Health and Human Services and others with ties to the administration of President Ronald Reagan. One IMC employee, a former adviser in Reagan's 1980 campaign, was instrumental in gaining approval for IMC's participation in a government demonstration project.[22] Between 1982 and 1986 IMC made contributions to federal and state campaigns totaling $87,150.[23] In Florida IMC officials and associates contributed $30,150 to Senator Paula Hawkins' campaign and $20,000 to Congressman Claude Pepper's campaign.[24] Both Hawkins and Pepper had opposed a proposal requiring IMC to sign a non-Medicare patient for every Medicare patient it enrolled.[25] (See Chapter 6 for more details about the IMC case.)

Although the activities discussed in this chapter—appeals to the Provider Reimbursement Review Board, lawsuits against health planning agencies, and lobbying activities and political contributions—are not limited to the for-profit health care sector, this sector has been more active than the nonprofit sector in all three areas, particularly in the political arena.

Lobbying and other political activity by health care organizations will continue as long as government plays a major role in regulating and purchasing health care, but even here there are changes that have implications for the for-profit and nonprofit sectors. Many of the issues that were uniquely or primarily of interest to for-profit hospitals—such as revaluation of acquired assets for the purposes of calculating depreciation expenses for reimbursement—have been resolved. And despite the Federation of American Health Systems' reputation as a highly effective lobbying organization, its major accomplishment in these areas has been to delay, not to alter, the eventual outcomes. (Nevertheless, the economic benefit of such delays can far outweigh the costs of the lobbying activities that brought them about.)

As policy issues that concerned the investor-owned sector have been resolved in ways that diminish that sector's comparative advantages, the reasons for the for-profit sector's trade association to speak with a different voice from that of the American Hospital Association have lessened. Although the most significant legislation supported by the Federation of American Hospitals—Medicare's prospective payment system—was adopted, the change was also supported by other hospital groups, including the American Hospital Association. Furthermore, the law was not designed to convey advantages to any particular sector; in its role as purchaser the federal government no longer seemed to see any reason to treat the for-profit and nonprofit sectors differently. The Federation of American Hospitals responded to the question of what it can offer its members that the broader trade association cannot by expanding its concerns and membership to include for-profit HMOs, changing its name to the Federation of American Health Systems along the way.

Although the narrowing of differences between sectors may lessen the for-profit sector's need for separate political activities, such a conclusion may be premature. Issues in which the interests of for-profit and nonprofit hospitals diverge still exist. The continuation of capital payments that include return on equity is one example. Also, both the pace of the transition to prospective payment and adjustments to the prospective payment formulas involve elements that have an incidental, differential effect on the two sectors. New payment issues may emerge. Furthermore, in its role as a taxing authority the government continues to treat for-profit and nonprofit hospitals differently.

The for-profit sector's more aggressive efforts to shape the reimbursement and regulatory environment may still have important implications for the future. We have seen that the investor-owned health care organizations make disproportionate use of the tools that are available to shape the political system. But they have been less likely than the nonprofit sector to prevail in these conflicts, although this conclusion may understate the impact of aggressive companies on their own environment.

Something that is less tangible but nevertheless very real may be at stake when health care providers actively pursue their economic interests. An atmosphere of mutual distrust of motives may develop among providers, regulators, and payers and become a pernicious legacy. This lesson, which can be drawn from the American Medical Association's half-century-long battle against government programs for the purchase of medical care,[26] may also apply to the corporate influence in health care.[27]

# 8

# For-Profit Health Care and the Accountability of Physicians

This book has thus far concentrated on two important aspects of the traditional accountability structure of health care: the predominantly *nonprofit* and *locally controlled* nature of the organizations in which health services are provided. In the next three chapters I focus on a third element: medical *professionalism* and presumptions about what it entails. Three significant changes have been occurring in the conditions of physicians' work: the growth of physician involvement in entrepreneurial activities (Chapter 8), the growing dependency of physicians on organizations that are driven by strong economic incentives (Chapter 9), and the rise of new cost-containment methods that shift some responsibility for patient care decisions to third parties (Chapters 10 and 11). These changes have broad implications for the two elements that have been hallmarks of medical professionalism: the fiduciary ethic and physician autonomy.

## The Fiduciary Ethic

Physicians are the key decision makers in the health care system in regard to the needs of individual patients. Approximately 75 percent of the ongoing expenditures in health care are attributable to decisions made by physicians.[1] For patients, the physician's advice can obviously have great consequences. Accordingly, societal expectations for the medical profession have been very high. Physicians are expected not only to maintain considerable technical competence but also to be faithful to the interests of their patients.

Doctors are often in a position of making recommendations to patients about the need for services that they will themselves provide and from which they derive income. The vulnerability of patients and the wide disparity in knowledge that commonly exists between doctor and patient create tremendous potential for exploitation and distrust. In response, ethical and legal norms and expectations have developed that define the doctor's first responsibility as to act in the interests of the patient. As Robert M. Veatch notes, "Historically, all of medical ethics in the Hippocratic tradition, including that of Anglo-American medical ethics, affirms as the basic principle the idea that the physician should use his or her judgment to do what he or she thinks will benefit the patient."[2] An example comes from the American Medical Association's Council on Ethical and Judicial Affairs:

> Under no circumstances may the physician place his own financial interest above the welfare of his patients. The prime objective of the medical profession is to render service to humanity; reward or financial gain is a subordinate consideration. For a physician to unnecessarily hospitalize a patient or prolong a patient's stay in the health facility for the physician's financial benefit would be unethical.
>
> If a conflict develops between the physician's financial interest and the physician's responsibilities to the patient, the conflict must be resolved to the patient's benefit.[3]

Terms such as *agent, advocate, trustee,* and *fiduciary* are often used to describe the physician's responsibilities to patients. Even though the body of case law that would define the physician's fiduciary obligations is not very extensive, Frances Miller argues that doctors "owe a duty of loyalty to their patients' interests that requires them to elevate their conduct above that of commercial actors."[4] Yet, most lawsuits in which fiduciary obligations have been invoked have arisen *not* from economic conflicts of interest or exploitation of patients' vulnerabilities but from such problems as the failure to obtain informed consent or to maintain confidentiality.[5] Whether the infrequency of lawsuits alleging self-interested behavior by physicians reflects their general adherence to fiduciary principles or is due to patients' inability to assess this matter is a question for speculation.

In the past the fiduciary ethic of the medical profession was reinforced by commonplace organizational arrangements. In traditional solo practices the physician's accountability to the patient was relatively unambiguous. A continuing flow of patients depended on the physician's reputation and ability to satisfy his or her patients, or, in the case of specialists who received patients on referral, to satisfy the patient's primary physician. Moreover, the physician of a hospitalized patient was not ordinarily an employee of the hospital but was the patient's own physician.

Despite rapid changes in the organization of health care, the ethical statements of professional associations continue to emphasize fiduciary principles. No one knows, however, how much the fiduciary ethic has actually guided the behavior of physicians and how often it has been abused or used to disguise other motivations. Nonetheless, patients and policy makers have by and large behaved as if the fiduciary ethic were operable. This has facilitated the trust that is widely deemed necessary to the doctor-patient relationship, and it has made self-regulatory mechanisms credible. These values are at stake when economic and organizational changes reduce the perceived reality of the fiduciary ethic.

*Trust in the Doctor-Patient Relationship*

The degree of trust that patients place in the skills and advice of physicians is remarkable in view of the potentially high stakes—even the patient's life—and the knowledge disparities between doctors and patients. Patients are often unable to make informed decisions about their own well-being without relying on the information and advice provided by a physician. Such circumstances could create grounds for suspicion.

The legal doctrine of informed consent obliges physicians to provide patients with all information that they could reasonably be expected to want to know about proposed treatments.[6] But because physicians who wish to do so can often manipulate patients' decision making, the effect of the law of informed consent lies more in clarifying the rights of patients than in protecting patients from physicians who do not deserve their trust. Thus, in spite of the views of some physicians, the doctrine of informed consent is not a denial of the fiduciary aspects of the physician's role. Instead, it recognizes the patient's dependence on information provided by the doctor, defines the doctor's fiduciary obligations, and helps to distinguish the doctor-patient relationship from commercial relationships in which the ethic of caveat emptor applies.

The patient's need to trust the physician anchors many analyses of the dynamics of the doctor-patient relationship. The physician Eric Cassell describes the need for trust as follows:

> Uncertainty is intolerable at all times but more so in the ill because their existence seems threatened, and yet they are required to make decisions about themselves . . . But decisions and actions that are seen as having to do with one's very life require levels of certainty that are not available to the sick person—they simply do not have enough information, as does no one in such circumstances. Trust in others is one of the central human solutions to the paralysis of unbearable uncertainty. It is for these reasons that the sick put the kind of trust in doctors that they do.
> Sick people, then, are people who are forced to trust.[7]

The patient's willingness to trust reflects a degree of confidence not only in the training and regulatory processes that determine who can practice medicine and who has hospital privileges but also in the integrity of the particular doctor whose skills and advice will be relied on.[8] The plausibility of the fiduciary aspect may thus be central to trust in the doctor-patient relationship.

### Trust and Professional Autonomy

Autonomy—"the right to control their own destinies, to set educational standards, regulate admission to practice, prescribe ethical codes, and discipline deviant practitioners"[9]—is the central characteristic defining a profession. Trust in the fiduciary ethic is a key factor underlying the status of the medical profession and its ability to "exercise its powerful knowledge with a minimum of external control."[10] As the physician and sociologist Jeffrey Berlant has observed:

> In a general way, trust inducement increases the market value of medical services and helps covert them into commodities. It also creates a paternalistic relationship toward the patient, which may

undermine consumer organization for mutual self-protection, thereby maintaining consumer atomization. Essentially, it persuades the patient that he need not protect his own interests, either by himself or by organized action. Through atomization of the public into vulnerable patients, paternalism results in the profession's dealing with fragmented individuals instead of bargaining groups.[11]

Although individual practitioners have long enjoyed and prized a considerable degree of freedom from supervision (particularly by laymen) in their work, many aspects of professional autonomy operate not at the level of the individual practitioner but at the level of the organized occupation.[12]

The medical profession's combination of autonomy and responsibility for making life-or-death decisions has long fascinated sociologists. How can such important decisions be left in the hands of individuals who operate with such minimal supervision? One aspect of the answer has been the practical difficulty of supervising physicians' work. Another may lie in societal acceptance of the medical profession's claim of ethicality with regard to patients.

Not so many years ago leading theorists in England and the United States saw an element of altruism and a special ethical orientation toward one's clientele as characteristics that distinguished professions from other occupations. In his classic formulation of the physician's role, Talcott Parsons emphasized *affective neutrality* (that is, like or dislike of a patient should not affect the care provided) and *disinterestedness* (putting the welfare of the patient above the physician's personal interests) as elements that made medicine a profession.[13] Since the 1960s, however, sociological analysts have been more likely to see *monopolistic institutions* and *high status* as the critical factors that distinguish professions and to view knowledge, skill, and special ethical orientations not as objective characteristics of professions but rather as ideological claims by which professions seek to gain or preserve status and privilege.[14]

In short, an altruistic or fiduciary orientation is not a fixed characteristic of the professions but a variable that determines the extent to which an occupation can properly be seen as a profession and, therefore, entitled to the prestige and autonomy that are the hallmarks of professions. Bernard Barber, for example, argues that "a group's behavior is the more professional the more the group actually displays, and not just claims to possess, . . . powerful knowledge, considerable autonomy, and a high level of fiduciary obligation and responsibility both to the individual clients and to the public welfare."[15] David Mechanic has noted that the characteristics identified by Parsons have less value in actually predicting the behavior of physicians than in predicting "those elements of the physician's behavior that the public will criticize and those the doctor will be defensive about."[16]

In sum, a profession's ability to win and retain a high degree of autonomy depends on more than political power (a function of numbers, money, and prestige) and the esoteric nature of the knowledge that is involved. It also rests on the plausibility of the claim that individual practitioners act primarily in the client's interest and that the organized profession acts primarily in the public interest.

## Changes Affecting the Fiduciary Ethic

Today the medical profession's claims of devotion to the patient's welfare and of trustworthiness are met with increasing skepticism. Such claims are redolent of a paternalistic ethic that has fallen out of fashion, which denies the ability of laymen to participate meaningfully in decisions concerning their own health. Moreover, because developments and proposed policies that might affect the autonomy or income of physicians have often been attacked by the profession on the grounds that they would jeopardize patients' interests and the ability of physicians to protect those interests, the suspicion arises that claims of fidelity to the patient disguise self-interest.

The plausibility of the fiduciary ethic is also affected by major changes that are occurring in the conditions of medical practice—particularly the growing extent of for-profit and entrepreneurial activities by both investor-owned companies and physicians themselves (a topic examined later in this chapter) and the growing economic dependency of physicians on organizations that are strongly driven by economic incentives (see Chapter 9).

In discussing such disturbances of the status quo, I am not

suggesting that we are moving from an era in which the matter of physician accountability to patients was handled well into one in which it is not. Because of the low levels of enforcement that have characterized both the self-regulatory and state-regulatory mechanisms of health care, and because of the norms of privacy in the doctor-patient relationship, the question of accountability has been a chronic one in the profession. I do not believe it to be either possible or desirable to return to an era in which physicians were essentially accountable only to their patients.

Nevertheless, trends toward greater entrepreneurship and organizational dependence are significantly changing the structure of accountability within which physicians operate. Pressures on the physician to consider interests other than the patient's are increasing. Qualitative financial and organizational changes are taking place that may affect whether physicians will behave as if responsible first and foremost to meeting the needs of their patients. Is the fiduciary ethic plausible in the face of changing conditions? What are the alternatives to leaving oversight in the hands of the physician and patient?

## Entrepreneurial Trends and the Fiduciary Ethic

The rise of investor-owned health care companies and the emergence of new forms of physician entrepreneurship both have potential implications for the medical profession's fiduciary ethic. I believe that physicians' adherence to this ethic may be affected more by their own entrepreneurship than by investor ownership of facilities. Both developments, however, evoke conflicts with deeply held views in medicine about how the ethic of the profession differs from the ethic of business.

### The Traditional Ethic: Medicine Is Not a Business

The fiduciary ethic of the medical profession is often discussed in terms of how it differs from the business ethic.[17] Arnold Relman, editor of the *New England Journal of Medicine* and a strong proponent of traditional concepts of medical professionalism, argues that because patients must depend on doctors, doctors must act under legal and ethical constraints that do not apply to businessmen.[18] Observers outside the medical profession also point to the incompatibility of medicine's fiduciary ethic and the ethic of business. For example, the sociologist Paul Starr contends that

> the conflict between professionalism and the rule of the market is long-standing and unavoidable. Medicine and other professions have historically distinguished themselves from business and trade by claiming to be above the market and pure commercialism. In justifying the public's trust, professionals have set higher standards for themselves than the minimal rules governing the marketplace and maintained that they can be judged under those standards by each other, not by laymen. The ideal of the market presumes the "sovereignty" of consumer choices; the ideal of a profession calls for the sovereignty of its members' independent, authoritative judgment. A professional who yields too much to the demands of clients violates an essential article of the professional code: Quacks, as Everett Hughes once defined them, are practitioners who continue to please their customers but not their colleagues. This shift from clients to colleagues in the orientation of work, which professionalism demands, represents a clear departure from the normal role of the market.[19]

The incompatibility of the ethic of business and the professional fiduciary ethic raises questions, then, about the significance of entrepreneurial trends in health care, both in the activities of investor-owned companies and in the investments of physicians themselves.[20]

## Investor-Owned Companies

The potential conflicts between the fiduciary ethic and the obligation to generate a return for investors has been a source of concern about the rise of investor-owned health care companies.. Might investor ownership of hospitals erode physicians' adherence to the fiduciary ethic? This could happen if the institutional atmosphere were changed, or if physicians' power and influence were reduced or new constraints were placed on their decision-making power. These possibilities deserve examination.

*Institutional Atmosphere*

Might the entrepreneurial atmosphere of an investor-owned institution produce subtle changes in the thinking and decision making of its staff physicians? A suggestion of differences in institutional culture comes from the research finding that physicians who practice in for-profit hospitals are more likely than physicians in nonprofit hospitals to perceive that their hospital discourages the admission of uninsured or Medicaid patients.[21] This finding does not necessarily mean, however, that for-profit hospitals actually encourage staff physicians to depart from the fiduciary ethic in caring for their *own* patients. Moreover, because nonprofit hospitals have themselves become increasingly entrepreneurial, better documentation is needed before sweeping conclusions can be drawn about differences in the organizational cultures.[22]

If one were to look for evidence that physicians' adherence to the fiduciary ethic is affected by investor ownership of the facility in which they practice, it might be sought in patient care patterns that are influenced by physicians' decisions and that have financial implications for the hospital. The limited available evidence is both inferential and contradictory. Robert Pattison and Hallie Katz found substantially higher rates of use of ancillary services (presumably ordered by physicians) in for-profit than in nonprofit hospitals.[23] Because hospitals billed for ancillary services separately and priced them to be profitable, the thought arises that the for-profit hospitals were perhaps encouraging physicians to do some unnecessary testing. Unfortunately, no evidence was available about the necessity of the services, and the higher rates could have been the result of other factors.[24]

Other evidence does not fit with the hypothesis that investor-owned hospitals influence medical decision making to increase profitable services. Studies conducted when hospitals were paid more if patients stayed longer generally revealed shorter lengths of stay in for-profit hospitals than in nonprofits.

In sum, although the idea that the culture of an investor-owned hospital may affect the adherence to the fiduciary ethic of its staff physicians is provocative, there is little evidence that it is true. But, of course, the evidence itself is very sketchy.

*Physician Influence*

Investor ownership of hospitals might also affect the impact of the fiduciary ethic by reducing the influence of physicians within hospitals, supplanting the professional ethic with a business ethic. Physicians have traditionally had a great deal of influence in hospitals, not because of their formal place of power in the administrative structure but because of their prestige and technical expertise. There was also an important economic factor: "The institutional providers of health services—the most powerful of which have been the private, voluntary hospitals— have traditionally had their policies determined by their professional staffs. The financial consequences that would result from the desertion by the leading members of the medical staff have usually . . . prevented the board of trustees or the administration of the voluntary hospitals from expressing attitudes that differ significantly from those held by that conservative profession."[25]

"The coming of the corporation," as Starr dubbed the rise of the hospital companies, has been seen by some as a threat to the hegemony of physicians and, by extension, to the fiduciary ethic.[26] Investor ownership of hospitals does not appear to have had this effect, however. For one thing, few physicians (14 percent, according to a 1983 AMA survey) admit their patients primarily to for-profit hospitals,[27] and these hospitals actually employ very few physicians.[28] In addition, physicians at investor-owned hospitals have privileges at more hospitals than do physicians at other types of hospitals.[29] This is important because, notwithstanding the size and power of large hospital companies, hospitals attract patients in local markets. The ability of physicians with multiple hospital appointments to shift patients elsewhere puts them in a strong position to influence hospital policies and to resist control.

Moreover, compared to nonprofit hospitals, investor-owned hospitals have been more oriented toward pleasing the physicians who make up their medical staffs and less oriented toward controlling them. The attitude of investor-owned hospitals to physicians on their staffs can be seen in hospital governance. Compared with nonprofit hospitals, investor-owned hospitals have a larger number of physicians on their boards, are more likely to have physicians as voting members, and are much more likely to have a physician as chairman of the hospital board (43 percent of the time, compared with 5 percent at hospitals generally).[30] Perhaps for that reason those who practice in investor-owned hospitals are particularly likely to report that their hospital administrator is "responsive" to the concerns of physicians, according to a 1984 AMA survey.[31]

It is, of course, possible that hospitals that were solicitous of physicians and facilitated their ordering services for which the hospital could bill may have changed their behavior since the advent of fixed, per-case reimbursement methods by Medicare. This gave hospitals strong incentives to save money and, thus, to find ways of encouraging physicians to order fewer services for hospitalized patients and to discharge them more quickly.[32]

Available evidence regarding whether investor-owned institutions put greater constraints on physicians is mixed and inconclusive. A 1984 AMA survey found that 28 percent of physicians believed that doctors had less clinical discretion at for-profit hospitals than at nonprofit hospitals, while only 9 percent believed the opposite (the rest believed there was no difference or had no opinion).[33] Another 1984 AMA survey, however, produced contradictory evidence. It asked physicians about hospitals' efforts to influence the practice of medicine by setting guidelines to reduce lengths of stay, doing retrospective reviews of lengths of stay, and formally reviewing clinical decisions. The majority of physicians in both for-profit and nonprofit hospitals reported that their hospitals were doing these things, but the percentage was slightly lower among physicians in for-profit hospitals.[34]

Although there is little evidence that the rise of investor ownership of hospitals has made it more difficult for physicians to act in a fiduciary capacity, the changed incentives that affect hospitals, the growing involvement of for-profit and nonprofit multihospital systems in financing as well as providing care, and the willingness of some companies to enter into contractual relationships with physicians that are virtually the equivalent of an employment relationship (but skirt legal restrictions against the corporate practice of medicine) are all matters for concern. Although rapid changes occurred in patterns of patient care decisions by physicians in the 1980s (most dramatically in the decline of hospital admissions and lengths of stay), there is little evidence that the investor-owned companies are placing more constraints on physician decision making than are nonprofit hospitals. At this point it appears that a more serious threat to the fiduciary ethic comes from another trend: the growth in entrepreneurial activities by physicians themselves.

## Physician Entrepreneurship and the Fiduciary Ethic

In a speech about ethical issues in medical practice, the lawyer Alexander Capron considered the contradictory responses that the term *physician-businessman* provokes.[35] Some see this term as an oxymoron and adhere to the view that the medical profession has special ethical responsibilities, quite different from the ordinary ethics of the business or commercial world, to act in the patient's best interests. Other observers see redundancy in the term, since a private physician's office practice copes with all of the problems that any business faces—raising capital, generating new business, collecting debts, meeting payroll, and so forth.

Bridging those divergent views is the economist Robert Evans' notion that a physician's practice can be thought of as a "not-only-for-profit" organization.[36] That is, although a successful practice does generate profits, the physician is expected to behave in ways that depart from the norms of business.

### Tensions between Business and Professional Sides of Practice

Physicians who wish to enter practice (whether by establishing a new practice or joining an ongoing one) clearly must make a substantial investment, as any entrepreneur must. Indeed, researchers at the AMA attribute the rise in employment among younger physicians in part to "the costs of purchasing or establishing a new practice [which] may exceed their ability to borrow through capital markets, particularly in the presence of debts from medical education."[37] The income of most physicians is derived from the difference between their practice's revenues and its expenses. The average professional expenses of self-employed physicians in 1987 were $123,700, according to an AMA survey, an amount that was equivalent to about 48 percent of the revenues of the typical practice ($256,000).[38] The average self-employed physician's net income before taxes was thus $132,300 (ranging from general and family practitioners' $91,500 up to surgeons' $187,900). That income could be characterized as the practice's profits.[39]

The dual role of the physician as entrepreneur and medical professional causes tensions and contradictions for the individual and the profession. By tradition, and in some cases by law, there are circumstances under which physicians are expected to provide services for which they may not be compensated.[40] The Medicare and Medicaid programs greatly reduced the number of people dependent on physicians' willingness to act charitably.[41] Approximately 10 percent of the population remains uninsured, however, and many others have inadequate coverage. A national survey in 1982 found that about 15 percent of families who lacked insurance had experienced an unmet need for health care in the previous year; 3.6 percent of uninsured families reported having been refused care for financial reasons.[42] There are indications that physicians have helped deal with the problem of uninsured patients. Uninsured people reported an average of 4.4 physician visits in 1981—less than the average of 5 visits for insured people but substantially more than zero.[43] Although many uninsured people pay for the care they receive, some must at times rely on the charity of the providers. Seventy-seven percent of physicians responding to an AMA survey reported that they had provided some free or reduced-fee care in 1982.[44] Such care averaged about 9 percent of total billings, or an amount equivalent to $16,000.

Yet, many physicians apparently take a colder economic view in evaluating such issues as whether to accept Medicaid patients when Medicaid payment rates are substantially lower than their usual fees. Physician refusal to participate in the Medicaid program has been a persistent problem and is strongly related to the level of state reimbursement for doctors' services under the program.[45]

Criticism of physicians unwilling to treat uninsured and Medicaid patients is often couched in terms of the difference between the professional ethic and the business ethic, as in this excerpt from a doctor's letter to the *New England Journal of Medicine:* "Physicians who limit their office practice to insured and paying patients declare themselves openly to be merchants rather than professionals . . . It fosters the myth that physicians as a group are greedy and self-serving rather than dedicated and altruistic, [and] it deprives a large segment of our fellow humans of care. Physicians who value their professionalism should treat office patients on the basis of need, not remuneration. Physicians who do not do so deserve the contempt and censure of their colleagues."[46]

Tensions between the physician as professional and as businessman are perhaps as old as the practice of medicine. Professional associations have sought to define and proclaim the characteristics that distinguish their members from businesspeople.

The original 1847 AMA code of ethics included flat prohibitions on certain entrepreneurial or commercial activities— advertising (including "boast[ing] of cures or remedies"), holding patents, and dispensing "secret nostrums."[47] Through much of the twentieth century the AMA urged physicians to avoid selling drugs to patients when "ethical pharmacies" were available locally to meet their needs. Continuing prohibitions against rebates and fee splitting are in this tradition. The American Medical Association's ethical standards long required eliminating certain conflicts of interest, particularly those in which a physician might derive secondary income from patient care decisions. Such approaches are found in ethical codes of the nineteenth and twentieth centuries in Britain and the United States.[48]

Such prohibitions were most effectively imposed by professional associations on individual practitioners in an environment where solo practices predominated. Here physicians were in effect accountable only to themselves and their patients for the care that was provided, and to the local medical society, which enforced strictures against breaches of ethics. Indeed, organizational forms that involved payment methods other than fee-for-service were viewed as unethical, as were physicians who had dealings with them. For many physicians, maintaining good standing in the medical society was essential to receiving referrals and gaining or maintaining hospital admitting privileges. For much of the first half of this century, the American Medical Association and its constituent state and local medical societies controlled hospital privileges and, thus, had considerable power with which to bring individual practitioners to heel. How this power was used was a matter of dispute, with the AMA contending that it sought to protect the interests of patients, and critics seeing monopolistic self-interest as the operative principle.

In any case, organized medicine's power to impose ethical standards on individual doctors has declined substantially. The growth of specialization, the proliferation of professional associations (such as specialty societies), and the increased diversity of practice arrangements and settings have reduced the ability of organized medicine to speak with one voice. Each of the various professional organizations represents a decreasing proportion of all physicians (only about half are now members of the AMA). In addition, it is difficult for a membership organization to take uncompromising stands without alienating and perhaps losing an economically and politically significant number of members.

Organized medicine's power over the ethics of individual practitioners has also declined for external reasons. Despite being couched in terms of serving the public interest, many ethical restrictions imposed by professional associations on their members came to be viewed by the public, the courts, and policy makers as self-interested. Particularly noteworthy have been the lawsuits finding professional societies in violation of antitrust laws, beginning with the 1943 Supreme Court decision upholding the AMA's conviction for violating the Sherman Antitrust Act in its attempts (made in the name of ethics) to destroy one of the early prepaid group practices—Group Health Association of Washington, D.C. Until the mid-1970s, however, the learned professions were by and large seen as exempt from antitrust laws. "Although the courts had never squarely so held, it was thought that physicians, lawyers, and perhaps some other professionals were not engaged in 'trade or commerce' and that professional activities, undertaken in the name of professional ethics and the quality of professional services, were fundamentally different from similar concerned activities carried out by industrial groups."[49]

That position was firmly rejected by the Supreme Court in a 1975 decision (*Goldfarb v. Virginia State Bar*), which held that the self-regulatory activities of the "learned professions" (in this case attorneys) were not exempt from scrutiny under the antitrust laws. This was followed by a successful Federal Trade Commission (FTC) action against the American Medical and American Dental associations establishing that the codes of ethics of such organizations were subject to the jurisdiction of the FTC because such codes could be used to restrain trade and competition. Subsequently there has been a series of cases regarding restraint of trade resulting from the concerted action of members of professional associations, even though those actions were undertaken in the name of moderating health care costs (as in the maximum fee schedule that was found to be illegal in *Arizona v. Maricopa County Medical Society,* 1982) or of protecting quality of care (*FTC v. Indiana Federation of Dentists,* 1986). Professional societies' restrictions concerning truthful advertising were also successfully attacked in a Supreme Court First Amendment decision (*Bates v. Arizona State Bar,* 1977) and in a 1980 FTC order against the American Medical Association on grounds of unfair competition.[50] Throughout the 1980s the FTC continued its active opposition to anticompetitive practices in health care, defeating a concerted effort by organized medicine to get legislation enacted that would have removed its jurisdiction.

Today's ethical standards of professional associations have become much more flexible than the old blanket prohibitions against certain arrangements.[51] Nevertheless, major professional societies in medicine continue to be concerned with distinguishing the professional ethos of medicine from that of business and with the more specific problem of making credible the claim that physicians are oriented first and foremost toward the needs and interests of patients.

## Is the Fiduciary Ethic Necessary to the Doctor-Patient Relationship?

Commercial and entrepreneurial aspects of medicine do not necessarily entail serious conflict with the fiduciary ethic,[52] as many critics seem to believe. Even some developments that depart from past ethical guidelines in the medical profession and that undoubtedly appear unseemly to leaders who worry about the profession's dignity do not necessarily conflict with the ostensible purpose of the fiduciary ethic: to protect the interests of vulnerable patients. Two such activities are engaging in marketing and advertising, and offering services to meet patient-defined needs.

## Marketing and Advertising

Long prohibited by professional codes of ethics, advertising and other marketing activities have become increasingly common in health care in the wake of the court decisions mentioned earlier. In 1982 an AMA survey found that 40 percent of physicians had used some marketing strategy or technique in the previous five years.[53] Advertising by physicians and medical organizations has become increasingly common in the traditional outlets of broadcasting, print, and the Yellow Pages, and through approaches that are more specific to medical care, such as telephone referral services.

Much advertising seeks to bring the name of a practitioner, institution, or alternative delivery system before the public in a favorable way by stressing convenience, amenities, cost, and quality. Although the use of advertising for such purposes is still relatively new, efforts by institutions and practitioners to present themselves favorably are not. A more significant break with tradition occurs in advertising designed to encourage the use of particular procedures (such as ophthalmological or plastic surgery) or services (such as treatment of substance abuse).

Although the idea of marketing and advertising produces negative reactions from some leaders of the profession, only the most rigid defender of tradition would object to marketing in the form of providers' efforts to assess their patients' satisfaction with various aspects of the care they have received or to assess and respond to unmet needs in their community; their opening a new facility in an area where demand appears to exist; or their making known the availability of a service. Marketing raises two concerns that merit discussion, however.

The first is the potential for abuse in situations where risks might be underplayed and the benefits overplayed.[54] This danger, though real and worth monitoring, is mitigated by several factors. As with advertising generally, the demand for truthfulness applies to health care. In addition to the legal requirements that are enforced by government agencies such as the Federal Trade Commission, professional associations are active in enforcing ethical strictures against misleading advertising.[55] Furthermore, advertising by its nature is a public activity, and there are plenty of competing practitioners and institutions to scrutinize competitors' advertising and to make an issue of anything that seems misleading.[56]

Nevertheless, the tendency to exaggerate benefits no doubt occurs in health care advertising as elsewhere. In health care, however, such exaggerations seem most likely to occur in advertising for services that pose little risk to the consumer, such as health status evaluations based on hair analysis, or weight-loss programs. To exaggerate the benefits (or conceal or fail to disclose the risks) of a treatment that could have serious negative effects might make the advertiser liable under informed consent doctrines. The desire to avoid liability will thus provide some deterrence against misleading advertising, at least when real risk is present. When there is no real risk, advertising in health care appears to raise no special problems or policy issues beyond those that exist in all advertising. (There are, however, some areas of health care where malfeasance is difficult to prove and where patients, competitors, *and* payers have difficulty monitoring performance. Psychiatric and substance abuse treatment are examples of areas in which misleading advertising could have serious consequences for patients while posing relatively little risk for the organizations that advertise.)

How consumers respond to advertising by the health professions is not entirely clear, but they may well be more adept at distinguishing valid from false claims than was assumed when professional strictures against advertising were adopted. This may partially explain why articles about failed advertising and marketing efforts have become fairly common in the trade press.

A second concern about increased advertising by medical professionals is what it suggests about the doctor's orientation toward the patient. The devices of the salesman seem inconsistent with the fiduciary ethic. Seeking to create demand is quite different from seeking to evaluate need objectively. Even though sales personnel are ethically and legally obligated to be truthful about certain matters, they have no ethical obligation to ascertain and act in their customers' best interests, and only the most naive consumers are unwary. The doctor-patient relationship, by contrast, is supposedly one of comparative trust.

### Services to Meet Patient-Defined Needs

Frequently overlooked in sociological and ethical analyses that emphasize the fiduciary aspects of the physician's role are areas of medical care in which it is largely up to *patients* to decide whether they want a service (or what services they want), and where the physician's main role is to provide the service in a technically competent way. In such areas the fiduciary ethic and its restrictions may be irrelevant.

An instructive example comes from one of the few sociological studies of the entrepreneurial side of medical practice—Michael Goldstein's study of physicians whose practices consisted largely of abortion services in Los Angeles in 1967–1972.[57] He described a subgroup of physician-entrepreneurs "who actively seek out opportunities to maximize their income through the ownership of businesses that employ other physicians and who, in general, model their behavior on that of business people as opposed to medical professionals." Among the patterns that emerged in his interviews with such physicians were frank admissions that money was a motivating factor, that health care was a commodity to be marketed, and that they were responding to needs defined *by* clients rather than defining needs *for* patients, as the traditional professional ideology sees the physician's role. The entrepreneurial orientation of a small number of physicians in the wake of court decisions that legalized abortion "shaped the transition of legal abortions as a procedure controlled by physicians and performed in hospitals to one controlled by clients and performed in freestanding outpatient clinics." Along the way the price came down, and patients' access to the service was enhanced.[58]

Goldstein's study documented how physician entrepreneurship can transform the way a specialized service is provided. A similar entrepreneurial orientation may well characterize the physicians who have established hemodialysis centers, ambulatory surgery centers, urgent care centers, pathology laboratories, imaging centers, sports medicine centers, substance abuse clinics, and obesity centers. Goldstein's respondents at the time realized that their entrepreneurial ideology "was deviant and stigmatized among their colleagues."[59] In the ensuing years it seems likely that the commercial trends sweeping health care have produced changes in how physicians view themselves. Entrepreneurial physicians may no longer see themselves as deviant. If physicians increasingly consider themselves businessmen or entrepreneurs as well as professionals, the effect on the operation of the fiduciary ethic is worth studying.

I have described Goldstein's physician-entrepreneurs not to argue that the fiduciary ethic is no longer of relevance to medical practice, but to show that its applicability is not universal. An entrepreneurial orientation may be quite appropriate for physicians whose services meet needs that are defined by patients. A distinction can be drawn between those areas of medicine in which patients typically make their own determinations about whether they want or need a service before approaching a physician and those areas in which patients rely on physicians' advice about whether the service itself is needed. "Physicians [ordinarily] do not sell injections of antibiotics or surgical incisions, but rather the judgment of whether an antibiotic or incision would be in the best interest of the patient . . . After liberalization [of abortions], abortion became elective surgery. Women wanted abortions, not the judgment of a physician about whether they needed one."[60] From the standpoint of the fiduciary ethic, the orientation of entrepreneur to customer rather than professional to patient is much less troublesome in areas where patients are typically able and willing to define for themselves whether or not they want a particular service. Here the ethics and legal accountability of business may be sufficient to protect the interests of patients.[61]

## Entrepreneurship in Conflict with the Fiduciary Ethic

The entrepreneurial and commercial aspects of business are most problematic in those areas of medical practice where the physician's role is to assess patients' needs and to make recommendations and take actions based on that assessment. Conflicts of interest in such situations threaten the credibility of the fiduciary ethic and may put patients in the position of having to follow the advice of someone they have reason to mistrust. Particularly noteworthy is the trend toward physicians' making investments that create opportunities to derive secondary income from the services they order for or recommend to patients.

Although a complete catalog of such developments is beyond the scope of this chapter—and is probably impossible, given the rapidity of change in this area—several examples illustrate the direction in which commercial and entrepreneurial values are taking medical practice. I will focus on in-office testing by physicians, direct sales of pharmaceuticals and other products, and ownership of (or economic relationships with) facilities to which doctors make referrals, including joint ventures.

*In-Office Testing*

Physicians have long done some laboratory and X-ray work in their offices. In less urbanized areas the absence of local laboratories often led physicians to develop testing capabilities of their own. In-office testing has increased markedly in recent years, however, and has become a significant source of revenue for a growing number of physicians. Table 8.1 shows the results of a 1985 survey of in-office testing by primary care physicians. Thirty-one percent reported that they had increased the amount of in-office testing in the previous year, and 38 percent anticipated a further increase in the following year.[62] One analyst estimated that Medicare payments for physicians' in-office testing would increase by 200 percent between 1984 and 1986, while payments for hospital outpatient testing would increase by 31 percent and payments for independent lab testing would decline by 9 percent.[63]

The growth of in-office testing is a result of several factors, including development of new technologies (such as desktop analyzers), convenience for patients, and, undoubtedly, the income opportunities for physicians. A 1985 Medicare rules change about billing practices for work referred to outside labs also contributed. Whereas previously a physician who referred work to a lab could be billed by the lab and then, in turn, bill Medicare (after a markup), the rules were changed to require the tester to bill the government directly. Although the rules change was

*Table 8.1.* Tests performed in doctors' offices, 1985[a]

| Test | % of doctors performing test | Test | % of doctors performing test |
|---|---|---|---|
| Urinalysis | 87 | PT/PTT | 18 |
| Occult blood | 73 | AST | 15 |
| Blood glucose | 65 | Electrolytes | 14 |
| Hemoglobin | 62 | ALT | 12 |
| Hematocrit | 52 | CK | 11 |
| Pregnancy | 48 | LDH | 11 |
| Strep | 43 | RPR | 8 |
| WBC | 41 | TDM | 6 |
| WBC differential | 32 | Rubella | 5 |
| Gonorrhea | 27 | Fibrinogen | 2 |
| BUN | 26 | Other | 19 |
| Bilirubin | 20 | | |

Source: *Medical Laboratory Observer* 17 (October 1985): 9.

a. Percentages based on responses of 304 (of 1,000 sampled) family practitioners, general practitioners, and internists in solo, partnership, and group practices.

stimulated by the cost increases that had resulted from the markups and by the incentive for unnecessary testing that came from the physician's deriving income from it, the effect was to encourage physicians to develop an in-house capacity to do more testing, for which they could then bill directly and profitably.[64]

One concern raised by in-office testing is whether quality standards are the same as in commercial laboratories. Physicians' offices escape most of the regulatory controls that affect hospital and commercial labs.[65] Testing in physicians' offices is often done not by specialized personnel but by people with various other types of training and duties.[66] There is also evidence of lower levels of accuracy and higher levels of operational and analytical deficiencies in physicians' office labs.[67]

Physicians' investments in laboratory equipment and personnel provide additional incentives for unnecessary testing. The cost of an expensive piece of technology must be recovered. (A desktop analyzer can cost $60,000 or more.) Several studies of laboratory and X-ray use show a direct relationship between physician ownership and rates of testing.[68] Although most of the studies are small and subject to various interpretations (for example, physicians who order many tests may tend to invest in equipment), it seems likely that physicians' investments in testing equipment and facilities do affect their patient care decisions. Although it is hard to know how often these are contrary to the medical interests of patients, unnecessary testing is clearly contrary to the economic interests of purchasers of care (whether patients or third-party payers).

### Direct Sales of Devices, Drugs, and Services

Physicians can also generate secondary income by having a financial interest in whatever they recommend patients purchase. This practice sometimes violates both law and ethics, as was demonstrated in congressional hearings in the early 1980s into the apparently widespread use of kickbacks by manufacturers of intraocular lenses (IOL) as a way to encourage ophthalmologists and surgeons to use their products.[69] The practices in the IOL industry were identical to practices described in an earlier congressional staff investigation of the cardiac pacemaker industry.[70]

Both congressional investigations also contained strong allegations and some evidence of unnecessary or inappropriate surgery. Arrangements by which physicians are given an economic stake in recommending and using a particular manufacturer's product are clearly inconsistent with the physician's fiduciary responsibility to decide whether an implant is appropriate to the patient's needs and to select a particular device solely on the basis of quality.

Some physicians generate secondary income from their patient care decisions through the direct sale of prescription drugs. From its earliest days, organized medicine sought to restrict the sale of drugs and "nostrums" by physicians as a way to professionalize medicine, distinguishing the ethical practitioner from the quack. But in the mid-1980s new arrangements whereby physicians sell drugs directly to patients gained sufficient economic importance to merit a major story in the *Wall Street Journal*[71] and a congressional hearing.

Indeed, a new industry, known as pharmaceutical repackaging or prepackaging, has developed. Firms buy drugs from manufacturers, repackage them into dosages suitable for treatment of common illnesses, and market them to physicians in cabinets that are regularly restocked with the thirty or forty most commonly prescribed drugs.[72] Repackagers' advertisements to physicians stress the economic benefits of selling drugs directly to patients. "One direct mail piece carries a headline that advises: 'How to earn $52,000 this year with no investment.' Another asks: 'Why pass the buck? Every time you sign a prescription, it's like writing a check to a pharmacy.'"[73] The $52,000 figure may be more advertising hype than fact, but significant income opportunities are nevertheless present.[74]

The direct sale of drugs by physicians is still somewhat unusual. Although the president of one repackaging company says that at least 5 percent of primary care physicians dispense pharmaceuticals, the president of another believes that only 1 percent do so.[75] The repackaging industry's revenues were estimated in 1986 as less than $20 million of the pharmaceutical market's $20 billion. Nonetheless, physicians' interests in finding new sources of revenue and the broader trend toward commercialization of medical care suggest that direct sale of drugs could increase substantially. In 1986 projections from industry leaders (not an unbiased source, it should be noted) put the potential market above $3 billion over the next five years.[76]

Although sales of drugs by physicians are said to have cost and convenience benefits for patients, the practice raises questions. Might it become more likely that drugs that are not needed will be prescribed, purchased, and used? Is there a danger that physicians will tend to prescribe what they have in stock, even if it is not the most appropriate drug? Will patients' suspicions about such matters reduce their confidence in their physician and their compliance with the drug regime? Does elimination of pharmacists from the process by which prescription drugs reach patients remove an important check against errors, as pharmacists contend?

Professional codes of ethics and state laws are in flux on this matter. A Texas physician was cited by the state board of pharmacy for "practicing pharmacy without a license" in 1985. Only in four states (including Texas), however, is direct dispensing of pharmaceuticals by physicians illegal. The AMA's Council on Ethical and Judicial Affairs stated in 1986 that "reputable firms rely on quality and efficacy to sell their products . . . and do not appeal to physicians to have financial involvements with the firm in order to influence their prescribing."[77] In early 1987, though, physician sales of drugs were reportedly supported by the AMA, as well as the Federal Trade Commission.[78]

Another new form of physician entrepreneurship is the full-fledged "turnkey" operation that physicians can purchase and incorporate into their practices. An example is the "NOW" (nutrition and overweight) program developed and marketed to physicians and hospitals by Medical Nutrition, Inc., of Englewood, New Jersey.[79] Under the program, physicians can offer their patients a complete diet-control regimen that includes weekly counseling sessions, behavior modification, patient information and videotapes, and foods for special dietary use. Medical Nutrition provides everything from marketing to training of personnel to the foods that are sold to patients. "The company sells a week's worth of food to the physician for $27.50, and recommends that the physician double the price to the patient to $55. Then, the company says, the patient should come in each week to be weighed, to have a urinalysis and his blood pressure checked, and to be given his next week's supply of food. This office visit—which in most cases a nurse can handle—should cost the patient $25, the company suggests."[80] According to the company's founder, a physician who has an average of six patients per week in the program will generate additional revenues of $28,000 and net $15,000.[81]

### Ownership of Facilities to Which Referrals Are Made

In the 1980s awareness grew that some physicians had ownership or other economic interests in the facilities to which they were making referrals, and concern increased about the effects that this development might have. Although many examples (some of which are described herein) can be cited, I have found only one attempt to document the extent of such arrangements. In legislation passed in 1988, Congress directed the Office of the Inspector General in the Department of Health and Human Services to conduct a study. OIG did two surveys—one of physicians and one of independent clinical laboratories, independent physiological laboratories, and durable medical equipment manufacturers.[82] They also used Medicare data to assess utilization patterns of patients of physician-owners identified in the survey.

The study found that 12 percent of physicians who bill Medicare have ownership or investment interests in entities to which they make patient referrals—clinical and physiological laboratories, durable medical equipment suppliers, home health agencies, hospitals, nursing homes, ambulatory surgical centers, and HMOs. Eight percent of physicians had compensation arrangements with entities to which they made referrals. Regarding the ownership of the organizations that were surveyed, the OIG found that at least 25 percent of independent clinical labs, 27 percent of independent physiological labs, and 8 percent of durable medical equipment suppliers were owned in whole or in part by referring physicians.

The study of services provided by physicians who billed Medicare showed that patients of physicians who owned or invested in clinical laboratories received 45 percent more services (at a cost of $28 million) than did Medicare patients in general. Patients of physician-investors in physiological labs received 13 percent more services than did Medicare patients in general. No relationship between ownership and patient services was found for suppliers of durable medical equipment.

Obviously, laboratories and durable medical equipment suppliers are not the only areas where physician investments potentially affect patient care decisions. Home health agencies, ambulatory surgery centers, and diagnostic imaging centers come immediately to mind. Some employee benefits managers speak of the difficulty of controlling costs for inpatient psychiatric and substance abuse services when the professional who is advising patients and families about the need for and benefits of services is also the owner of the facility within which the services will be provided.

## Joint Ventures

A particularly visible form of physician investment in the 1980s was the joint venture involving physicians and hospitals or companies that develop specialized services such as laboratories or various types of ambulatory care centers for diagnosis, treatment, and rehabilitation. Some joint ventures were stimulated substantially by tax considerations and were adversely affected by the Tax Reform Act of 1986. Nonetheless, many joint ventures that give physicians an economic stake in services and facilities are designed, at least in part, to influence doctors to recommend particular procedures or services or to refer patients to a particular facility or institution. Again, the obvious danger is that considerations other than the patient's interest will come to influence physicians' decisions and recommendations.[83] In addition, as with the developments that are discussed in the next chapter, physicians' involvement in such joint ventures means that their patient care decisions have an economic impact on other organizations, which may then seek to influence the physician and, perhaps, to divide the physician's loyalty. Much empirical research will be required before we know what the consequences are for patients and payers.

Because of the diversity of joint ventures, data on them are fragmented. The frequency with which such ventures are discussed in the trade press (the entire April 1986 issue of the American Society of Internal Medicine's magazine, *The Internist*, was devoted to the topic) may give an exaggerated impression of the extent of such activities. It does appear, however, that the practice of physicians' investing in various types of ambulatory care facilities has become common.[84]

In 1984 the American Hospital Association found in a national survey that 12 percent of hospitals were engaged in some type of joint venture with physicians, most commonly a preferred provider organization or a medical office building.[85] A 1985 survey of four hundred hospital executives whose hospitals were already involved in or interested in joint ventures found that ambulatory care centers were the most common type (37 percent), followed by alternative delivery systems (16 percent), and that physicians were the most common joint venture partners (in 40 percent of the ventures).[86] A 1985 AMA report states that 1,200 joint ventures existed between hospitals and physicians.[87]

A substantial number of these ventures involve investor-owned health care companies and physicians. For example, in late 1986 Republic Health Corporation had more than fifty joint ventures involving more than four hundred physicians. The joint ventures included surgical suites, equipment, mental health units, one new hospital, and a variety of branded specialized services: Balance (for eating disorders), Reach (adolescent chemical dependency), ReNew (cocaine addiction), You're Becoming (cosmetic plastic surgery), Second Sense (hearing disorders), Miracle Moments (maternity), Step Lively (foot care), Impotency Solutions (male impotence), and View (comprehensive women's services).[88]

*How joint ventures work.* Because hospital-physician joint ventures are local, private arrangements, few details about them become public. Still, information about the logic of joint ventures is available from examples in which a public solicitation has been made or the companies involved are large enough to be written about in the trade press. From this a picture emerges of tensions with the fiduciary ethic and with laws against fraud and abuse.

In general, joint ventures are structured so that the physicians derive financial benefits—generally a share of the facility's profits—in addition to charging for their own services. Referring to the joint ventures for outpatient surgical operating rooms in ten Republic hospitals, Republic's CEO described the arrangement as follows: "We regard the surgical joint venture as a kind of a 'everybody wins' situation. The patient gets the surgery done in the safety of a hospital environment at competitive prices that Republic has established in order to attract volume. The physician gets the opportunity to share in the profits of the surgery room. And Republic gets the increased volume plus the other ancillary services that goes [sic] along with the surgery."[89]

Some joint ventures enable physicians to develop new capabilities in their own office practices, as in the following promotional information for prospective investors from Meris Laboratories, Ltd.:

Through the legal entity of a limited partnership, the MERIS concept allows physicians to invest in a clinical laboratory as owners and users of the laboratory's services. From a financial perspective, physicians can significantly increase their annual income level . . . by participating in profits generated by laboratory operations. *Returns are projected at an average annual return of approximately 70% of the original investment through each year of the partnership.* Physicians can also share in a potential capital gain when the laboratory is sold. From a professional perspective, *physicians can utilize improved laboratory services that are tailored to the physician's own practice.* (emphasis in original)

In another offering, physicians are told that they need only make referrals to enjoy increased revenues of "$15,000–$25,000 annually." The arrangement is described in a letter from "CP Rehab Corp West" that begins "Dear Doctor":

> If you have not already been approached, you probably soon will be with various offers to become involved in a free standing radiology imaging center. Most will be in the form of limited partnerships [and] will require some investment on your part . . . [However] *no person or organization will offer what CP Rehab Corp West provides.* With the right group of neurologists, neurosurgeons, internists, orthopedists, family practitioners and others our company will take *all* of the financial risks without any capital investment whatsoever by the physicians.
>
> Our company will design and provide the space, supply the equipment, stock the patient consumables, pay the utilities and employ the administrative and technical personnel. The physician group will receive revenues from the profits of the center based on stock ownership.
>
> Stated in its simplest form, we tell you without reservation that you can increase your income significantly by merely referring your radiology studies to your own facility *which has cost you nothing* . . .
>
> We are a public company with assets of fifty-four million dollars.[90]

Yet another example comes from the prospectus filed with the Securities and Exchange Commission in 1986 for a company called Physicians Clinical Services Limited Partnership, which "intends to engage in the business of providing quality and timely out-patient clinical laboratory testing." Its customers would be "patients of physicians, health care providers or facilities in . . . the Defined Service Area" (four states and the District of Columbia). Not coincidentally, the limited partnerships were to be offered "primarily to physicians, other health care providers and facilities located in the Defined Service Area." The prospectus makes it explicit that the customers would be the patients of the partners: "While the Partnership intends to market its services to the general health care community, the Partnership anticipates that a significant portion of its initial laboratory business may be derived from referrals from the Limited Partners. To the extent that the Limited Partners do not make such anticipated referrals, the Partnership's forecasted revenues and distributions will be adversely affected." The prospectus then describes the steps being taken to avoid violating fraud and abuse statutes and warns investors that the self-referral arrangements created a risk that the enterprise could nevertheless be found in violation.

The relationship of joint ventures to the fraud and abuse laws, and the agility required to stay on the right side of those laws, reveals much about the conflict-of-interest problems that joint ventures can entail.

*Legal and ethical issues posed by joint ventures.* Joint ventures and other cooperative arrangements between physicians and institutions raise both legal and ethical questions. Because the legal issues have greater immediate consequence for providers—the risk for nonprofit hospitals of losing tax exemptions or the possibility of fines and imprisonment—the legal ground is better mapped than the ethical ground.[91]

The legal issues posed by fraud and abuse statutes go to the heart of the conflict-of-interest problem posed by joint ventures. According to Richard Blacker and W. Bradley Tully, two attorneys with the law firm that acts as counsel to the Federation of American Health Systems (FAHS), the trade association of investor-owned hospital companies and alternate delivery systems, a primary motivation of many joint ventures is "the securing of a patient referral base": "Placing persons who are referral sources in an ownership position allows them to indirectly receive a return from the business they generate, thereby providing a strong incentive towards utilization of the venture's services."[92] Fraud and abuse provisions of the Medicare law (43 U.S.C. sec. 1395nn), however, forbid providers to pay for referrals of Medicare patients for treatment. (Similar prohibitions exist for Medicaid patients and in some state laws as well.)

The lawyers who advise joint venture principals seek ways to reconcile the intent of the joint venture with the fraud and abuse statutes. But it is not easy to reward physicians for making referrals while not appearing to do so. For example, as Blacker and Tully note, some arrangements have been "structured as purchases of services from referring professionals," but the courts have begun to "look behind the documentation of these kinds of transactions to determine whether payments which are ostensibly for services, are actually for referrals."[93] Similar legal difficulties may arise in lease arrangements between facilities and physicians when one refers business to the other. Depending on who is leasing from whom, payments that are substantially above or below the market rate can be viewed as compensation for referrals. Another court case (*U.S. v. Greber*) brought a conviction under fraud and abuse laws even though the referring physicians were being paid for services they actually performed for the provider of Holter monitoring equipment, to whom they were referring patients.[94]

Blacker and Tully's suggested route around such legal problems is joint ownership "because distributions based upon ownership are made out of profits and the reasonableness of the return is not generally subject to scrutiny."[95] This "solution" creates another problem, however: free riders. It enables physician-owners to profit even if they do not refer patients, which defeats the purpose of the whole enterprise. Nevertheless, there are ways to structure things so as to "maximize the likelihood that all investors will support the venture while avoiding arrangements that would be deemed to be payments for referrals."[96] These approaches, while minimizing the free-rider problem, raise the risk of violating fraud and abuse statutes and, though seldom mentioned, the fiduciary ethic.

Some joint ventures have been set up not to engage in substantial business activities but only as a front for channeling business to other providers. In an effort to make up for income they lost when prohibitions were established on billing for lab work referred to outside laboratories, some physicians set up and secured a license for a clinical laboratory to which they could refer work. Yet, as Blacker and Tully warn, if the "laboratory" has all its tests performed by another laboratory on a referral basis, "the venture could be criticized as being a mere conduit for referrals." They close by observing that "this sham business test is becoming an increasingly important one for cooperative ventures."[97]

Most patients rely on their physician for advice and guidance about services, treatment, and the hospital or facility to be used.[98] If physicians who have investments in joint ventures and patient care facilities recommend certain services or steer patients to those facilities when it is not in the patient's best interests, they clearly violate the fiduciary ethic.

Defenders of joint ventures sometimes assert that the involvement of referring physicians provides some assurance of quality. There is no evidence that this is true, however, and an organization that has secured a flow of patients by giving referral physicians an economic stake has less need to compete with other organizations on the basis of quality or efficiency. The possibility of unnecessary services and increased costs was no doubt the reason why in 1989 the Office of the Inspector General implemented a "Special Fraud Alert" regarding joint ventures and gave wide circulation to a pamphlet that described various types of "suspect" arrangements—primarily those in which "investors are chosen because they are in a position to make referrals"—and published a hotline number along with a plea to "Help Protect Your Tax Dollars."[99]

## "Solutions" to Conflicts of Interest

Among the regulatory bodies, standard-setting organizations, and third-party payers who deal with the medical profession, three general approaches have been developed for addressing the problem of conflict of interest in medical practice: prohibitions, disclosure requirements, and utilization review and management by parties external to the doctor-patient relationship. This last development is sufficiently significant in the accountability structure of health care to merit two separate chapters (10 and 11). In the remainder of this chapter, I will briefly examine the other two approaches.

### Prohibitions on "Unnecessary" Conflicts of Interest

Professional associations such as the American Medical Association have been urged to take firm positions against some of the conflicts of interest that have been described in this chapter. For example, Arnold Relman urged in 1983 that "the medical profession . . . should declare as an article of its ethical code that doctors should derive income in health care only from their professional services and not from any kind of entrepreneurial interest in the health care industry."[100] In similar fashion the Institute of Medicine Committee on For-Profit Enterprise in Health Care stated in 1986 that "it should be regarded as unethical and unacceptable for physicians to have ownership interests in health care facilities to which they make referrals or to receive payments for making referrals."[101]

Nonetheless, the medical profession seems unable to resolve the problem of conflicts of interest from economic arrangements that generate self-referrals and secondary income from patient care decisions. Organized medicine's commitment to fee-for-service practice is very deep, and the conflicts of interest that arise when a physician refers a patient for testing to a lab that he or she owns have similarities to situations that arise daily in fee-for-service practice when physicians recommend services that they will provide or suggest that the patient return for a follow-up visit.

Because the "new" conflicts of interest are so similar to the conflicts of interest that inhere in fee-for-service, criticisms of the new arrangements can be seen as criticisms of arrangements to which organized medicine is wedded. If the physician who invests in facilities to which he refers cannot be trusted to resist economic temptation and to put the patient's interest first, then why should fee-for-service physicians—who are faced with analogous decisions daily—be trusted? To accept the need for control over temptations to violate the fiduciary ethic in the one area implies the need for change in fee-for-service itself. This logic makes the profession reluctant to condemn any economic arrangement on the basis of the temptations to which it exposes physicians.

Relman and others have argued that the conflicts of interest that arise from economic relationships between physicians and facilities to which they make referrals are worse than traditional conflicts of interest because they are "unnecessary" (that is, not inherent in the fee-for-service arrangement) and because the older conflicts are well understood by the patient, who can switch physicians if mistrust develops. Such arguments generally fail to convince those who are predisposed to either of two opposing beliefs: that fee-for-service has given physicians so much experience in coping with economic conflicts of interest that they can handle any temptations that might arise from owning a piece of the surgicenter or referral lab, or that the incentives of fee-for-service have already hopelessly corrupted medical decision making, leaving patients with little choice but to accept the advice of someone whom they have objective reason to mistrust.

Also contributing to the profession's reluctance to adopt ethical standards that would restrict physicians' income to the fruits of their own professional services is the belief that if physicians do not become involved in the ownership of the facilities to which they make referrals, they will sacrifice control (and, presumably, income).[102] Also militating against taking a strong stand is the increasing fragmentation of the profession by specialization, type of practice setting, and many other internal distinctions. Finally, the profession's ability to enforce ethical standards is significantly limited by the antitrust considerations that were described earlier.

Thus, the trend in setting the ethical standards of professional associations in medicine has been away from blanket prohibitions on practices that are deemed to be unethical—advertising, ownership of patents, investments in facilities to which patients are referred—and toward standards against which compliance can be judged only on a case-by-case basis.[103] Perhaps the strongest statement by a major professional association is put forth by the American College of Physicians, which holds that "the physician should avoid any business arrangement that might, because of personal gain, influence his decisions in patient care"; but even this statement acknowledges that the "business aspects" of a physician's practice should be guided by the intent to offer "reasonable support of that practice and for the effective provision of quality care for patients."[104] Intent, obviously, is a difficult matter for independent parties to assess.

Indifferent or ineffectual responses from the medical profession are not the only impediment to addressing the problems raised by physician entrepreneurism. There are practical difficulties in defining just where conflict of interest begins. The assertion that physicians should not invest in laboratories to which they refer their patients is met with the question of whether it is acceptable for them to do lab testing in their own offices (where many tests can be done quickly and cheaply while the patient waits). The argument that physicians should not own a pharmacy is countered by examples of rural areas in which patients would not otherwise have access to prescription drugs. The issue then hinges on the difficult task of trying to distinguish necessary or acceptable conflicts of interest from unnecessary or unacceptable ones.

Nevertheless, it is possible to define some clear conflicts of interest and to move against them through either the medical practice laws under which physicians are licensed or the conditions of reimbursement established by third-party payers. Medicare, for example, has for years forbidden physicians who own more than a 5 percent interest in a home health agency to certify that a patient requires the services of that agency.

Legislation has addressed the issue in only tentative and limited ways. A survey by the Office of the Inspector General in 1989 found some pertinent licensure-related legislation at the state level, although only Michigan had an outright prohibition— against physicians' "directing or requiring an individual to purchase or secure a drug, device, treatment, procedure, or service from another person, place, facility or business in which the licensee has a financial interest."[105] Many states have laws that prohibit unnecessary referrals or referrals made only to benefit the physician financially. Such legislation does not provide clear lines between what is acceptable and unacceptable and faces obvious enforcement difficulties. OIG found that "the overwhelming majority of respondents responsible for enforcing applicable State statutes reported that they were unable to monitor for compliance of existing laws" because of lack of resources or vagueness in the law.[106]

The U.S. Congress has addressed the issue twice in the last several years. The first was in the Medicare Catastrophic Coverage Act of 1988, which directed the Office of the Inspector General to make the study, described earlier, of physician ownership and compensation. The second was in Congressman Fortney Stark's Ethics in Patient Referrals Act, which passed late in 1989 and is limited to Medicare.

That act demonstrates the difficulty of distinguishing acceptable from unacceptable situations. From the beginning, because of the need to define a "bright line" between what was covered and what was not, it was limited to investments that were *external* to the physician's practice. Thus, it would have been acceptable for a physician (or group of physicians) to invest in laboratory testing equipment for their offices but not to invest in an external organization to which they would make referrals. As the legislation was developed and considered, a series of exceptions was included—for labs in the physician's own building, for prepaid health plans, for investments in publicly traded companies, for rural areas. The legislation that was passed nevertheless introduces a prohibition on physicians' referring patients to a clinical laboratory for a Medicare-covered service if the physician or an immediate family member has an ownership or investment interest or other compensation arrangement with the laboratory, and it bars laboratories from submitting bills for reimbursement pursuant to a prohibited referral.

It seems unlikely that the problem of economic conflicts of interest can be dealt with effectively through prohibitions alone. Moreover, it is difficult to have confidence that new rules against certain conflicts of interest will not have unintended effects. As has been shown in this chapter (and also in Chapter 6), health care is full of examples demonstrating that where economic opportunities or pressures are present, great creativity will emerge from entrepreneurs, including the more entrepreneurial portion of the medical profession (people can argue about how large that portion is), in finding a means to an end. Recall that payment rule changes to discourage referrals for unnecessary testing helped to stimulate an increase in testing in physicians' offices, where monitoring and quality control are much more difficult to achieve. Documentation of increases in the number of services provided by physicians after fees were frozen furnishes another example.[107]

### Disclosure

An alternative to prohibitions on conflicts of interest is disclosure requirements. The AMA, for example, follows its statement that it is "not unethical" for physicians to own a "commercial venture with the potential for abuse" with the stipulation that "the physician has an affirmative ethical obligation to disclose to the patient or referring colleagues his or her ownership interest in the facility or therapy prior to utilization."[108] The Institute of Medicine report followed its statement about the ethical unacceptability of physicians' owning facilities to which they make referrals by calling for disclosure in the absence of prohibitions.[109] The Inspector General's survey of states found that eleven had laws or regulations requiring physicians to disclose conflicts of interest to patients, although "the stringency of this requirement varies."[110]

Although disclosure of conflicts of interest seems to be a minimal but essential requirement in fiduciary relationships, it presents several problems. First, the confidential nature of the doctor-patient relationship makes disclosure requirements difficult to enforce. Second, virtually nothing is known about patients' responses to disclosure by their physicians that they have an interest in the facility to which they are referring patients. Does it breed distrust and noncompliance with physicians' recommendations? Or does it increase the confidence with which patients approach the facility? Third, if the fears about conflict of interest are well founded, and physicians' patient care decisions are indeed biased by their having an economic stake in the services they recommend, there is no reason to believe, a priori, that disclosure would lessen the bias.

Less pessimistically, a requirement that economic conflicts of interest be disclosed to third-party payers (as well as to patients and referring physicians) would increase the possibility of addressing the problem of biased decision making.[111] Equipped with such knowledge of conflicts of interest, third-party payers could use claims data to identify providers whose utilization patterns appear to be influenced by physicians' financial interests and could act accordingly through utilization controls or selective contracting. In effect, the market could play a role in determining the acceptability of certain conflicts of interest in the physician-patient relationship.

The medical profession has long propounded ethical standards that distinguish the practice of medicine from commercial enterprise. Foremost among those standards is the fiduciary ethic, which holds that the physician's primary obligation is to serve the patient's interest ahead of any personal interest. Because of the vulnerability of patients, the plausibility of the fiduciary ethic has been instrumental in establishing a relationship of trust between patients and physicians and between the medical profession and society. Self-regulation has been characteristic of the medical profession, and individual practitioners have enjoyed a considerable degree of autonomy.

Because the fiduciary ethic is different from the ethic of business, the rise of for-profit health care appears to be inconsistent with the stance adopted by the profession in establishing relationships of trust with patients and in public policy negotiations over social accountability. The analysis in this chapter suggests, however, that the plausibility of the medical profession's fiduciary ethic is threatened less by the rise of the investor-owned hospital companies than by entrepreneurial activities among physicians themselves. Investments in diagnostic technologies, direct sales of prescription drugs, equipment, and products, and various types of joint ventures have become increasingly commonplace. Such entrepreneurial activities provide ways for physicians to generate secondary income from their patient care decisions, create pressure to recover invested capital, put physicians in a position where co-venturers have an economic stake in their patient care decisions, and raise ethical and legal issues that test the limits of fraud and abuse statutes. Although it is not known how large a percentage of physicians is involved in these arrangements, it is sufficient to bring into question the plausibility of the fiduciary ethic and the public policies that rest upon it.

For a variety of reasons it is difficult to prohibit these arrangements, although some steps have been taken in that direction. Disclosure of arrangements that create economic conflicts of interest for physicians seems to be a minimum ethical requirement. Among payers a new kind of solution—utilization review and management—has rapidly taken root and is changing traditional conceptions about physician autonomy. These approaches are examined in Chapters 10 and 11. First, however, another major trend that runs counter to the traditional structure of accountability must be examined: the rise of physicians' dependence on organizations for patients and income.

# 9

# Organizational Dependence
# and the Fiduciary Ethic

The conditions of medical professionalism have been altered in recent years by some striking changes in the autonomy of physicians. A considerable degree of autonomy has long characterized medical practice in the United States, as was noted in Chapter 8. Indeed, autonomy has been identified by the influential medical sociologist Eliot Freidson as the single most important feature that defines professionalism itself.[1] A decline in physician autonomy denotes much more than a major change in the occupation that is generally seen as the prototypic profession, however. It also involves a basic change in the accountability structure of health care.

This chapter is concerned with the independence of medical practice and the new forms of organizational dependency among physicians. Changes in their autonomy in making patient care decisions are discussed in the next chapter.

## Traditional Organization of Practice

Most physicians in the United States have traditionally been self-employed in solo practices or small partnerships and have been paid on a fee-for-service basis. The physician's autonomy was maximized by several basic elements, most notably self-employment, fee-for-service payment, and a passive orientation on the part of third-party payers regarding whom the patient chose as a physician and what services were provided. These elements were integral to the profession's concept of the ideal doctor-patient relationship and have been stoutly defended as essential to the physician's ability to carry out the fiduciary ethic by putting the patient's interest ahead of all other considerations.[2]

The idealized view of traditional private practice emphasizes the importance of the physician's unambiguous allegiance to the patient: "Those who wish to eliminate fee for service may overlook the fact that the physician-patient relationship is one of deep intimacy and trust. The patient's monetary power, large or small, is the symbol attesting to the fact that the physician is the agent of the patient. Surprisingly, 'unholy mammon' more adequately protects the fiduciary-covenant relationship of physician and patient than if the former is salaried by a company, the military, or the government."[3] In their activities and ethical codes, professional associations such as the American Medical Association long held that departures from fee-for-service practice would divide or dilute the physician's loyalty to the patient. Others have seen the independence of physicians as a buffer against the potential excesses of the for-profit health care organizations. Thus, the physician and health services researcher James Lo-Gerfo observed at a conference in the mid-1980s that, "given the relative independence of physicians from direct administrative control and their fiduciary obligations to patients, it is unlikely that cost reductions will be readily identifiable in decisions about the care of individual patients."[4]

Of course, not all observers have seen the doctor-patient relationship in traditional private practice as a pure agency relationship. Critics have faulted the lack of any real accountability since patients were seen as largely unable to evaluate the care provided by physicians, who were described by the health services researcher Milton Roemer, M.D., as "small entrepreneurs, with enormous freedom to mishandle and even cheat patients."[5]

The autonomy-maximizing structure of solo (or small single-specialty group) practices with fee-for-service as the mode of payment and with third-party payers confining their role to removing financial barriers to care is part of what the economist Alain Enthoven describes as the "guild free choice model."[6] The elements of this model are that the patient has free choice in selecting a doctor; the doctor is subject to no outside interference regarding choice of therapies; the doctor and patient negotiate fees without third-party intervention; payment is based on fee-for-service; practice is in solo (or small single-specialty group) settings; and licensure is under the control of the profession (the guild). Enthoven's analysis of this structure shows it to be inherently inflationary of physicians' incomes and, therefore, of health care costs.[7] This is one of the reasons why the guild free choice model has long been the object of the attention of reformers.[8]

The traditional organization of practice and third-party payment gave physicians considerable opportunity for income enhancement, particularly where doctors were in relatively short supply. I am not referring primarily to knowingly providing, and charging for, unnecessary services, although this undoubtedly occurred in some instances. Of more economic significance, I suspect, was the fiduciary ethic itself, which provided a rationale for (and therefore encouraged) increasingly service-intensive patterns of care.[9]

Under circumstances in which third-party payment eliminates cost to the patient as a factor, the question of whether an additional test or procedure or hospital day is worth the money becomes irrelevant to both doctor and patient. Indeed, the fiduciary ethic can be interpreted to make it illegitimate for the physician to weigh whether the benefit to the patient is worth the cost to a third party. This interpretation can justify or even require the provision of whatever services might benefit the patient, so long as the patient consents, no matter how marginal the benefit might be.

That this view of the requirements of the fiduciary ethic generally coincided with physicians' economic interests was a happy circumstance from their standpoint but a problem from the payer's, and it contributed significantly, I believe, to the continuous, rapid growth in the volume of services provided to patients.[10]

In short, both the traditional form of practice and the fiduciary ethic added to the cost inflation that has stimulated so much change in health care. The developments that are examined in this chapter and the following ones are radically altering the traditional accountability structure of medical practice. How the fiduciary ethic will be affected is not yet clear.

## Dependency of Physicians

The concept of accountability that has been used throughout this book is closely related to the concept of dependency because it is concerned with control of access to needed resources. In discussing the changing dependency of physicians, I will focus first on access to resources, including money, and next on access to a flow of patients.

### Access to Resources

Physicians have traditionally had a relationship of mutual dependency with hospitals, with physicians providing patients and the hospital providing facilities, technologies, and personnel needed for patient care. Although physicians traditionally held no formal role in the administrative structure of the hospitals in which they practiced, they nevertheless had tremendous influence, in part because of their control over which hospital their patients would use. Hospitals were thus seen as "doctors' workshops" by some analysts.[11] In theory, at least, the fiduciary ethic required physicians to use their power on behalf of their patients (that is, to select the hospital that would provide the best care). The extent to which this occurred is, unfortunately, not as well documented, nor is the use of this power for self-interested purposes.[12]

Competition among hospitals has reflected the degree of physicians' control over the flow of patients. Although the use of direct economic inducements ("paying for patients") has gained attention,[13] the traditional form of competition among hospitals has been through the purchase of new technologies; hospitals have tended to acquire a new technology that was being adopted by nearby hospitals.[14] By so doing, they could reduce the risk that physicians would take their patients elsewhere. This dynamic largely doomed government efforts (the regional-medical and health-planning programs) to regulate the adoption and diffusion of very expensive technologies. In the era of cost-based and charge-based reimbursement, it also meant that competition among hospitals had an unusual economic effect: costs tended to be higher in highly competitive locales than in areas where there were no competing hospitals.[15] Competition that resulted in multiple hospitals' doing the same complex procedures (such as open-heart surgery) had another negative effect: some hospitals did too few to do them well.[16]

Changes in the reimbursement environment have led hospitals to seek ways to alter the balance of power with physicians. Under past payment systems that reimbursed hospitals for costs incurred or for billed charges, the economic interests of both hospitals and physicians were served by the provision of additional services to patients. By contrast, under more recent payment methods—Medicare's prospective payment system and contractual arrangements with private payers—hospitals increasingly receive a fixed or limited amount of money for caring for particular patients. The hospital's costs, however, are still heavily influenced by physicians' patient care decisions (whether to admit the patient to the hospital, what tests and procedures to do, when to discharge the patient).

Hospitals began to develop their own agendas—not just to serve as doctors' workshops—and to seek ways to influence physicians' care decisions in the interests of those agendas. As I will discuss later in this chapter, some approaches are aimed directly at shaping those decisions. A less obvious set of approaches concerned the hospital's traditional dependent position vis-à-vis physicians. One way that change has been accomplished—whether intentionally or not has not always been clear—is by providing staff physicians with services that benefited their practices and, therefore, raised the consequences to physicians of shifting patients to other institutions. By tying physicians more closely to itself, a hospital could increase physicians' dependency and, therefore, its own power in relation to physicians. Many of the services thus provided had the added benefit—and even the primary purpose—of generating additional revenues for the hospital.

Some approaches, such as construction of a medical office building adjacent to the hospital, were not necessarily new but were effective ways to make the physician's use of that particular hospital much more convenient than the alternatives. Hospitals also began providing staff physicians with services to benefit their office practices, such as scheduling and computerized record keeping. Some hospitals began joining selected staff physicians in forming new organizations for marketing packages of physician and hospital services to large purchasers.

The logic underlying many of these developments was laid out by an influential health care consultant, Jeff Goldsmith, in the early 1980s. He wrote:

> Hospitals should consider making technical and financial resources available on a joint venture basis to selected members of their medical staffs to further their professional practices . . . The hospital should not be construed as offering its resources in exchange for physician business through formal contracts. It is far better to offer some types of assistance which, if withdrawn, pose some economic risk to the physician and to let the performance expected under terms of such an agreement remain implicit, though crystal clear . . . Hospitals do not need to own or operate their own feeder systems. Through joint ventures [with physicians] they can assure the same result—sustained hospital utilization.[17]

It hardly needs to be noted that competing by offering physicians the most attractive amenities and economic advantages is not the same thing as competing to provide the best quality of care to patients. In fact, arrangements that discourage physicians from admitting patients to another hospital may reduce the physician's ability to exercise leverage on behalf of patients. But whether or not that is true, hospitals have increased physicians' dependency by providing at least some of them with benefits that made admitting privileges increasingly valuable.

### Access to Money

The lengths to which some hospitals have gone to assure themselves of a flow of patients (in part by creating physician dependency) were described in a 1989 *Wall Street Journal* investigative report entitled "Warm Bodies: Hospitals That Need Patients Pay Bounties for Doctors' Referrals."[18] The article describes in some detail a number of different arrangements—some legal, some probably not—by which hospitals have made it financially rewarding for physicians to use their facilities.

These methods include: (1) paying a flat "consulting fee" ($70) per admission to the admitting physician; (2) providing and then forgiving a $75,000 loan to a clinic in exchange for a promise that

75 percent of the clinic's patients would be referred to the lending hospital; (3) direct kickbacks for referrals; (4) a $1 million "subsidy" to a medical group by an investor-owned hospital company whose officials were quoted as saying that it was an industrywide practice to help physicians build a patient base near a hospital; (5) payments (disguised as financing for office locations and for consulting fees) of $1.2 million to another medical group by the same company; (6) payments of $2.5 million by a prominent nonprofit Minneapolis hospital to a nationally known group practice (Park Nicollet) in exchange for 90 percent of Park Nicollet patients who require CT scans, home care, inpatient rehabilitation, and selected outpatient surgical procedures (Medicare and Medicaid patients were excluded, in deference to the federal fraud and abuse statute); (7) leasing hospital beds to physicians who can put their patients in them at a marked-up price (a medical consultant was quoted as saying that this practice was "on the cutting edge" but perhaps illegal); and (8) the purchase of physicians' practices.

The authors of the article quote the consultant Barry Moore as observing, "If you have locked in that supply of patients, then you have assured your future and you have significantly damaged your competing hospital," and they observe that "the word 'kickback' isn't fashionable among hospital administrators. They refer instead to 'physician practice enhancement' and 'physician bonding.'"[19] Echoes can be heard of Jeff Goldsmith's advice to hospitals in the early 1980s.

Arrangements between hospitals and *group* practices may also affect the flow of patients. Because they tend to distribute rather than accumulate profits, group practices often need outside capital for expansion or new ventures, and joint ventures with hospitals or other investors may result.[20] There have been numerous reports of the sale of group practices' assets to hospitals, which then take over the management of the practice. According to a leading consultant, the purchase agreements do not usually specify that the group's physicians will admit patients to that particular hospital, but "it's commonly understood that that's the expectation."[21]

Various of the developments described herein have attracted the attention of the Office of the Inspector General at the Department of Health and Human Services and of legislators. Regulations aimed at many of these arrangements were proposed in January 1988 and again in late 1989 under the 1987 Medicare and Medicaid Patient and Program Protection Act. The purpose of these regulations was to distinguish certain "safe harbors" from those arrangements that might subsequently be found to violate the fraud and abuse statutes. As was described in Chapter 8, limited legislation in the form of the Ethics in Patient Referrals Act was passed in 1989, which forbade certain economic arrangements between physicians and laboratories for services billed to the Medicare program.[22]

## Access to Patients

A third and, I believe, a much more significant form of organizational dependency involves access to *patients* and, therefore, to income. I have described how physicians' control over which hospital to admit their patients to gave them a powerful (if informal) role in the structure of accountability that hospitals traditionally faced. Eliot Freidson's analysis of how *physicians* obtain their patients provides a useful point of departure for a discussion of how the dependencies of physicians have changed.

*Client-dependent and colleague-dependent practices.* Writing in the late 1960s, Freidson noted that although the key defining characteristic of a profession is autonomy, and although medicine is the quintessential profession, physicians' practices are nonetheless subject to varying degrees of control by patients and colleagues.[23] He found that, depending on the type of specialty and organizational setting, patients came to physicians either via self-referral (or through the "lay referral system," as with the recommendation of a friend) or through referrals from doctors' colleagues. Freidson used the terms *client-dependent* and *colleague-dependent* to describe the two resulting types of practices.

Primary care physicians in solo or small-group practices had client-dependent practices in which a continuing flow of patients depended on the physician's ability to satisfy *lay* criteria of good care. To be chosen again or recommended to a friend, the physician had to "be prepared to provide services that honor the client's prejudices sufficiently to make him feel . . . treated properly."[24] Because practice in client-dependent settings was neither easily observed by nor dependent on colleagues, professional standards were likely to be comparatively low, assuming, as Freidson did, that patients' standards were not as high as professional standards. He saw this as more than a matter of the relative emphasis placed on, say, bedside manner as opposed to technical virtuosity. For example, patients might sometimes ask for medications or procedures that would not generally be approved of by physicians.[25] Doctors whose practices were heavily client dependent would be tempted to respond by practicing in ways that colleagues would not necessarily condone, and they would be economically rewarded for doing so.

By contrast, specialists in fields such as radiology or anesthesiology had colleague-dependent practices in that their patients were not attracted directly but were referred by other physicians. The economic health of such a practice depended on satisfying those physicians; this suggested that professional standards of ethical and technical performance would be honored more than the wishes of clients.

In practice, most physicians probably fell somewhere between the extremes of the quack, who is completely indifferent to professional standards, and the technician, who is completely indifferent to patients' evaluations. Freidson's key insight was that the behavior of a physician is subject to influence by the physician's relative dependence on one or another source of patients. His categories of dependence serve as a useful reference point from which to analyze fundamental changes that have taken place in the constraints faced by practicing physicians, for physicians have since become organization dependent, in the same sense that Freidson found them to be either client dependent or colleague dependent.

*Factors leading to change.* Certain organizations are coming to control the access of ever-larger numbers of physicians to a flow of patients. These organizations include hospitals and, more important, ambulatory care centers, HMOs, and preferred provider organizations. They have gained this control either by marketing to the public or by establishing contractual relationships with large purchasers of health care. Before I discuss the marketing approaches and types of organizations that are involved, it is worth noting several interrelated causal factors that lie behind this development.

A variety of legal changes have contributed. Federal legislation (the HMO Act of 1973) was among the key factors that stimulated the growth of HMOs; state laws to allow the selective contracting essential to preferred provider arrangements are another.[26] The increased marketing of medical care is in part due to Federal Trade Commission actions and court decisions against professional associations' prohibitions concerning truthful advertising, as was described in Chapter 8. Laws forbidding the corporate practice of medicine have fallen into disuse in most states.[27]

A second set of causal factors, described in more detail in Chapter 10, includes the search by payers for ways to control health care costs. Organizational arrangements whose incentives differ from fee-for-service practice have been particularly attractive, and the quest for cost containment created a market for organizations that contract directly with third-party purchasers for the provision of medical services.

The breakdown in physicians' unwillingness to enter into arrangements other than traditional solo or small fee-for-service practices also has economic roots. As we saw in Chapter 8, the increasing cost of becoming established in practice and the debts incurred in training make physicians more willing to accept salaried positions. But a more basic economic factor is also at work: the increasing number of physicians. (Interestingly, Freidson saw a threat to professional standards in too much client dependence, but, writing in the late 1960s, he saw the relative *scarcity* of physicians as a mitigating factor.)

Between the mid-1960s and the early 1980s, the number of physicians graduating annually from U.S. medical schools doubled.[28] Also, the number of foreign medical school graduates who practice in the United States has been growing. The result has been a 51 percent increase in the number of physicians per 100,000 population.[29]

The supply of physicians has produced innumerable ripple effects.[30] Physicians' services have become more accessible in terms of both time and location. Even so, the number of patient visits per physician per week has been declining (from 139 to 118 between 1975 and 1985).[31] This decline was due not only to the increased number of physicians but also, since 1982, to an absolute reduction in patient visits.[32] It is also worth noting that while patient visits were declining, physicians' incomes were increasing at a slower rate than the consumer price index.[33]

Given these changes, it should not be surprising that relations among physicians and between physicians and institutions have become more overtly competitive and commercialized. Patients, rather than physicians, are becoming the party in short supply, leading to an increased willingness on the part of physicians to enter into various types of relationships with organizations that promise access to a flow of patients.

Let us turn to the elements that have been integral to this situation: the marketing approaches that give organizations themselves access to patients, the creation and growth of new organizational types, and the increasing number of physicians who are employed by, or who have contractual relations with, such organizations.

### Marketing and Organizational Dependence

The growth of marketing in health care has enabled organizations to gain access to patients through channels other than the traditional one for hospitals—via their staff physicians. Advertising aimed at the public is the most visible form of marketing. After being resisted successfully as unethical by organized medicine for half a century, it developed rapidly after professionally erected barriers were knocked down as an unwarranted restraint of trade.

Although the primary objections to advertising had been that it was unprofessional and would often mislead the public, experience has shown that a more important aspect is that it lends itself to economies of scale.[34] That is, *organizations* are able to advertise more extensively and with more sophistication than can individual physicians. Whether the goal is to create patient preferences for certain institutions or demand for certain services, success brings a flow of patients that the organization can make available to affiliated physicians.

Advertised telephone referral services that are operated by hospitals and that steer callers to staff physicians are designed not only to increase admissions to the hospital but also to make privileges at that particular hospital more valuable to staff physicians. Some marketing approaches, such as the champagne dinners offered by hospital obstetric services, are directed at creating patient preferences for certain hospitals, taking advantage of obstetricians' client dependency.[35]

Consultants recommend advertising that has an educational element, addresses consumers' hopes and fears, and focuses on services in which physicians' influence over treatment decisions is relatively small.[36] In several such areas brand-name services have been developed and advertised to the public. Examples include CareUnit for substance abuse treatment; Share for occupational health; Medical Plus, a computer-based fitness assessment program; Reflections Breast Health Centers; and Easy Street, simulated environments for rehabilitation patients.[37]

In some instances the advertised service is staffed by physicians who are either employees or are under contract. In other instances the service is a variation on the telephone referral service approach. The way that such services create organizational dependency in physicians was described by James Buncher, CEO of Republic Health Corporation, which has a number of "branded" health care products that are advertised to the public:

> When we have a concept and start developing the advertising materials, the physicians help us develop the advertising materials so we are sure that what we say is medically correct. The program is designed entirely to generate referrals to the physicians. We have a telemarketing function in which telephone and mail inquiries come into our hospitals and we in turn pass them along to the qualified physicians in the appropriate specialty. The physician in turn gets in touch with the patient as a response to the inquiry. If the patient is interested, it usually will result in at least an office visit with the physician.
>
> For example, let's look at our plastic surgery program, You're Becoming. In the first step, the office visit, the patient describes his area of interest. The physician then determines if the patient is suitable. A lot of patients either are not suitable for plastic surgery or the risks would be too great. If plastic surgery is determined by the patient to be desirable, then the physician is free to use any hospital he desires. But since physicians are getting the referrals from us, they feel they have a joint relationship with us. We are helping them build their practice, and they in turn use our hospitals.[38]

Despite its visibility, advertising aimed at the public is less significant in terms of numbers and implications than is marketing by alternative delivery systems. The selection of physicians by thousands of patients is affected by the decision of a benefits manager to encourage beneficiaries to enroll in a particular alternative delivery system—an HMO, a preferred provider organization (PPO), or some other type of network of providers.

Perhaps the most significant development that has reshaped the health care system is the growth of the several types of organizations that provide purchasers and patients with an alternative to the traditional practice arrangements in which all of the incentives encouraged the provision of additional services. These organizations all have some type of cost-containing elements built in, but their nature varies among organizational types. Distinctions among these types have become fuzzy as they borrow elements from one another, but three prototypic models can still be identified: HMOs (two models) and PPOs.

HMOs provide subscribers with a comprehensive set of hospital and medical services for a set prepaid premium; they have generally been able to make their premiums lower than the cost of conventional health insurance.[39] Data for 1987 published by the HMO trade association, the Group Health Association of America (GHAA), showed days of hospitalization (352 per year per 1,000 enrollees) for HMO enrollees under age sixty-five to be about 60 percent of the national average; hospital use for enrollees above age sixty-five was about 55 percent of the national average for that age group.[40] (The fact that the differences in hospitalization are so much larger than the differences in premium may be partially due to the data's being collected at different times, their being based on different sources, or their being released by trade associations whose interests differ.)

Although there are several types of HMOs, the key distinction for present purposes is between prepaid group practices and individual practice associations.[41] In the prepaid group practice (PGP) model all of the patients for a group of physicians come from the HMO. These physicians may be employees of the HMO (as with the Group Health Association in Washington, D.C., or the Yale Health Plan), or they may be part of a group of physicians that has a contractual relationship with it (as with Kaiser-Permanente). In either case their degree of professional and economic identification with the HMO is very strong, as is the ability of the HMO to affect conditions of professional work via data systems and its control over resources and staffing levels. (As a practical matter, such issues are subject to negotiation.) The PGP model also lends itself to the development of internal policies governing clinical matters—the circumstances under which certain technologies will be used, the adoption of formularies for which drugs will be used, and so forth. As of July 1989 a slim majority of prepaid group practices were nonprofit organizations.[42]

The contrasting HMO model, the independent practice association (IPA), arose initially as a way for solo practitioners to compete with prepaid group practices while retaining their independent, office-based, fee-for-service practices.[43] Often started under the auspices of county medical societies in the 1970s, IPAs in the 1980s became the primary vehicle for the entry of investor-owned companies into the HMO field. In July 1989, 75 percent of IPAs were for-profit, and the average IPA was only five years old.[44]

As with a PGP, the IPA provides subscribers with a defined set of hospital and physician services for a set, prepaid premium. Unlike in the group model, however, the physicians in an IPA continue to practice in their own offices and to see patients who are not enrolled in the IPA in addition to patients who are. For services to the IPA's patients, the physicians are paid by the IPA. These compensation arrangements are varied and can be very complicated, but they range from fee-for-service to some type of capitation arrangement whereby the physician receives a set monthly fee per enrollee. The IPA has much less control over the conditions of practice than does a PGP, but nevertheless has a number of tools for trying to keep costs in line with collected premiums. These include incentives built into compensation arrangements with physicians, various types of utilization controls (described in Chapter 10), and selectivity regarding which physicians may join the network.

Preferred provider organizations or arrangements (PPOs or PPAs) bear some similarities to IPAs, but the organization does not accept the financial risk of agreeing to provide a full set of services for a set premium. Instead, the organization agrees that the providers in its network will give services to beneficiaries at negotiated fees or at a discount from ordinary charges. Although the details of these organizations are highly varied (the joke that "if you've seen one PPO, you've seen one PPO" became a staple of consultants' speeches in the 1980s), the essence is captured in this definition: "A PPA is a fee-for-service alternative to traditional health insurance under which those covered are given financial incentives to choose from a panel of preferred providers with whom the payer has contracted. Rather than a specific entity, a PPA is a series of contractual arrangements among an insurance plan (or a self-insured payer), those covered by insurance, and the preferred providers, with a third-party administrator or other broker sometimes serving as a middleman."[45] As with IPAs, cost containment in PPOs is sought through price negotiations with providers and utilization controls, and by excluding high-cost providers from the network.

In PPOs providers seek increased market share in exchange for price and autonomy concessions—increases that are possible only if the payer contracts with *selected* providers—and purchasers agree to give beneficiaries significant incentives to use providers that are part of the network. These incentives may include reduced cost sharing, coverage of additional services, or low premiums.

Although alternative delivery systems also market directly to the public, mainly through advertising aimed at employees of organizations that have agreed to offer the plan as part of their employee benefit package, a key threshold is decisions by employers and unions regarding which plans will be offered to beneficiaries. The organizations that market to benefit managers may stress location (national networks may have an advantage in marketing to large corporations whose employees are geographically dispersed), quality (prestigious hospitals are commonly part of the package), and, most important, price or cost containment. One 1987 estimate predicted that as many as 50 percent of employers would "direct employees to providers" in 1988, up from virtually none in 1983.[46]

### Employment and Contractual Relationships

The number of physicians who obtain patients through contractual or employment relations with an organization has grown rapidly. The most common relationship between physicians and organizations continues to be admitting privileges in hospitals. But employment of physicians (in hospitals and elsewhere) is growing and now involves more than one in four physicians.[47] The trend seems likely to continue, since the percentage of employed physicians is highest among the younger doctors.[48]

Other types of connections between physicians and organizations have also become more common. For example, the majority of physicians who have a "financial arrangement" with hospitals are not employees but have lease agreements and contractual relationships in which the physician provides patient care services and receives either fee-for-service payments or a percentage of department revenues.[49] These arrangements may be similar to an employer-employee relationship, but they are commonly structured as contracts in deference to laws against the corporate practice of medicine.

In addition to hospitals, a growing variety of organizations now employ or contract with physicians to provide patient care. An estimated 3,400 freestanding primary care or urgent care centers market directly to the public through advertising and commonly hire physicians on salary or contract.[50] Physicians also gain access to patients by way of relationships with firms that contract with hospitals to provide specific patient care services. Such services range from the traditional (emergency departments) to the relatively new (substance abuse treatment programs). Such firms' arrangements with hospitals usually include the provision of services of physicians who are hired under contract.

Nonetheless, the organizations that are by far the most instrumental in providing physicians access to patients are HMOs and PPOs. In some areas of the country individual physicians may have contracts with several HMOs or PPOs. Over 160,000 of the country's half-million physicians were under contract to a PPO by 1986 (this is a minimum number, arrived at by adding the numbers enrolled in the largest PPO in each state),[51] and an estimated 145,000 physicians had contracts with an HMO in 1987.[52]

The number of patients to whom physicians have access through participation in HMOs and PPOs has grown rapidly. Six million people were members of the nation's 175 HMOs in 1976. By 1988 more than 32 million people were members of 600 plans.[53] PPOs were an invention of the 1980s, but by late 1986 at least 535 were operational, and 28 to 30 million people had access to PPOs as an option in employee benefit plans (up from

5.8 million in mid-1985).[54] Actual enrollees in the ten largest PPOs increased from 2.9 million people in the spring of 1985 to 6.2 million in February 1986.[55]

A noteworthy aspect of this growth is that as enrollment in alternative delivery systems climbs, it will become increasingly difficult for physicians to make a living by providing care only to patients who are *not* members of such systems. Trends in population growth, the supply of physicians, and enrollment in HMOs make this graphically clear, as has been shown by Alvin Tarlov, who chaired the Graduate Medical Education National Advisory Committee (GMENAC), which in 1980 issued a landmark report on the nation's present and future supply of physicians.[56] Writing only a few years after the report was issued, Tarlov found that the picture had already been changed by the rapid growth of enrollment in HMOs.[57]

In 1978 there had been about 584 people per physician in the United States. Within HMOs there was one physician for every 875 people. Because only about 3 percent of the population was enrolled in an HMO, however, the HMOs' physician-to-population ratio had relatively little effect on the pool of patients available to other physicians. GMENAC concluded, on the basis of population and physician supply trends that were already in place, that by the year 2000 there would be about 430 people per physician in the United States. But because the physician-to-population ratios within HMOs will remain relatively constant, the more the enrollment in HMOs grows, the more seriously physicians who are *not* in HMOs will be affected.

In his 1986 examination of the issue, Tarlov assumed that 44 percent of the U.S. population would be enrolled in HMOs by the year 2000.[58] (This is not an outlandish figure, having been reached in the Twin Cities and approached in some parts of California.) If the same ratio of persons enrolled per physician in HMOs were to continue, this would leave an average of only 309 persons available as potential patients to each physician who is *not* in an HMO. That is obviously a very small number on which to try to base a practice, but such circumstances already exist in some areas. For large numbers of physicians, affiliation with an HMO or other alternative delivery systems will be essential if they are to have enough patients to make a living practicing medicine.

My intent in emphasizing the growth in enrollment in HMOs and PPOs is not to suggest that such organizations are necessarily problematic in terms of either costs to payers or quality of care. An exploration of those topics is beyond the scope of this chapter, but it should be noted that these systems are designed to correct well-understood shortcomings of traditional practice arrangements. As systems of health care delivery they have the potential for monitoring costs and patterns of care and for developing forms of accountability that did not exist in traditional practice. In addition, there is considerable evidence that HMOs are able to restrain costs (primarily by reducing hospitalization) in ways that do not have an unacceptable impact on quality.[59] (Virtually all of the evidence about quality, however, is based on studies of non-profit prepaid group practices and should not be generalized to the whole population of HMOs or to PPOs.)

Rather than attempting an overall evaluation of HMOs and PPOs, I am concerned here with only one aspect of these and other types of health care organizations: the creation of increased organizational dependency on the part of physicians and the implications of this change.

## Significance of Organizational Dependence

Organizational dependence creates a new source of power that has the potential to influence physicians' patient care decisions. Obviously this has implications both for patients and for payers.

I take it as axiomatic that this new source of power will be used for whatever purpose the organization adopts, within whatever constraints the organization faces via regulation, the market, employee relations, and so forth. It must be borne in mind, therefore, that the organizations involved range from patient cooperatives (such as the widely admired Group Health Association of Puget Sound) to investor-owned IPAs and proprietary ambulatory care centers. The internal accountability structures of such organizations were discussed in earlier chapters of this book.

It is also axiomatic that the organizations on which physicians are dependent have their own economic interests and constraints. The ambulatory care centers have fixed costs and generally have a profit-seeking orientation. Hospitals face economic constraints, either from fixed payment methods or from the need to compete economically for the business of large private payers and alternative delivery systems. For their part, alternative delivery systems that have agreed to provide beneficiaries with a package of physician and hospital services for a set amount of money are thereby put at economic risk and must, therefore, be more actively concerned about the costs of physician-ordered services than traditional third-party payers have been.

Broadly speaking, health care organizations have four means with which to influence physicians to practice in ways that serve organizational interests: selection, education, economic incentives, and utilization management. I will discuss the first three here, leaving utilization management for subsequent chapters, since it is part of a much broader change in the accountability structure of health care and is not limited to situations in which physicians are organization dependent.

One generalization can be made about all four types of approaches, however: they can be used in ways that either serve or detract from the best interests of patients. Although a legitimate role can be seen for each type, examples (either real or realistically hypothetical) can be cited in which the approach fails to serve either the interests of patients or the interests of payers.

For selection and education, the key distinction appears to be whether the aim is making care more clinically appropriate or more profitable. The implications of incentive and utilization management approaches from the standpoint of patients' interests depend on how well designed a program is, and how sensitive it is to the danger that appropriate as well as inappropriate services may be discouraged.

The particular set of physicians who provide patient care services in an organization can make a great deal of difference to both the quality of care that is provided and to the organization's economic well being. Which physicians are involved is determined by *selection:* who is included initially, and who either is dropped from or leaves the organization.

The initial selection may be based on credentials (such as board certification), reputation, ability to bring patients to the organization, and, in some cases, information about patterns of care. (A hospital that is trying to form a preferred provider network with staff physicians may know which ones' patients tend to have unusually long lengths of stay. If the hospital is to be paid fixed, per-case rates, such physicians would not be an economic asset to the network.)

Once physicians are part of an organization, the role of monitoring becomes more important. Many, perhaps most, of the organizations on which physicians are dependent have some capability for monitoring at least some aspects of their performance. HMOs and PPOs oversee such matters as use of the hospital or of diagnostic procedures, and hospitals may monitor lengths of stay. Depending on the sophistication of the records system, it may also be possible for the organization to monitor patterns that might suggest poor-quality care: unplanned returns to the operating room, readmission rates for hospitalized patients, excessive use of certain drugs, and so forth. Some organizations survey patients or monitor changes in patients' choice of physicians.

This information can be used to eliminate doctors from the organization. (As I show later in this chapter, it can also be used for the less drastic purpose of increasing physicians' awareness of their patterns of care and how they compare with those of other physicians.) The ability of an organization such as an HMO or PPO to eliminate from its network physicians whose quality of care is problematic is a potentially significant advantage over the traditional organization of practice. Many quality-of-care problems can become apparent only through the monitoring of *patterns* of care, something an organization can do that individual patients could never do. But the information can also be used to eliminate physicians whose practice patterns do not serve the economic interests of the organization—a matter that may or may not be related to quality of care.

Concern about the punitive use of such information against meritorious physicians can, of course, be exaggerated. For example, when Medicare's prospective payment system was implemented, putting hospitals at economic risk for costs incurred as a result of physicians' patient care decisions, fears were expressed that hospitals might remove the privileges of physicians who were conscientiously practicing good medicine but whose practice patterns were nevertheless costing the hospital money because of flaws in the design of the payment system. Concerns were heightened when data systems were quickly developed and marketed to hospitals to enable them to track costs in relation to DRG payments on a physician-by-physician basis.

Although some hospital administrators reportedly considered removal of physicians' privileges as an option if their practice patterns were costing the hospital money (for example, excessively long patient lengths of stay), conflicts of this sort did not become prominent. This may say less, however, about the potential for such uses of information than it does about several aspects of the implementation of the prospective payment system.[60]

When prospective payment was implemented, the need for cost containment was widely understood. It also proved possible to reduce some services without jeopardizing the welfare of patients. That is, although lengths of stay declined rapidly after the initiation of the prospective payment system, and although critics worried that patients were being discharged "quicker and sicker," early studies produced no evidence to support the claim of premature discharge.[61] This suggests that unnecessarily long hospital stays had been occurring under previous payment methods, and that when the new hospital incentives came into effect, physicians could take cost-saving steps without harming their patients. (It should be noted, however, that several more recent studies have provided inferential evidence that some underservice has resulted from the new payment system.)[62]

Several buffers were built into the system. Initially, at least, most hospitals found themselves doing very well economically both because the payment formula was relatively generous and because lengths of stay declined rapidly. Thus, hospitals initially had few reasons to take drastic action against physicians. Another safety device consisted of provisions for separate payment for "outlier" cases, which meant that hospitals were not fully at risk for the cost of caring for particular patients. Finally, the Prospective Payment Assessment Commission (ProPAC) was created as a mechanism for, among other things, evaluating the fairness of payment rates for particular diagnostic groups. The quality of ProPAC's work reduced the danger that payment rates would be set so low for particular diagnoses that hospitals would lose money when providing services ordered by physicians who were practicing good medicine.

Yet the concern cannot be dismissed that the organizational dependency of physicians may be used by some health care organizations to exert pressure on physicians to practice with the organization's economic needs rather than the patient's needs foremost in mind. The danger is illustrated by the experience of Randall Bock, a physician employed by a chain-owned walk-in clinic.[63] The organization monitored the number of services that each physician was ordering (and for which the organization was therefore billing patients or third-party payers), provided the physicians with a monthly report in which they were ranked by amount of charges per patient, and pressured or fired those at the bottom of the list.

The evaluation or selection of physicians on the basis of evidence derived from monitoring patterns of care has many potentially attractive aspects, in terms of both rewarding quality and discouraging waste. At present, however, organizations may find it much easier to monitor physician-generated services in terms of their economic consequences than their quality. Indeed, that may be the primary concern of some organizations. Under such circumstances, economic factors may assume too much importance in the evaluation of physicians' performance by organizations. As the measurement of quality of care continues to improve, it can be hoped that the problematic aspects of the use of information on patterns of care will be discouraged and the benefits will increase. This may not occur, however, in organizations that are motivated more by greed than by the desire to provide high-quality services at a fair price.

*Educational approaches* by which organizations can seek to influence physicians' behavior can be lumped into two broad categories: those that emphasize practice guidelines and those that emphasize feedback. As we shall see in the next chapter, practice guidelines have been developed in recent years for a growing number of technologies and clinical situations. Such guidelines have arisen under many auspices: researchers, third-party payers, professional associations, and medical specialty societies. The general intent is to distinguish appropriate from inappropriate (or unnecessary) care. Thus, practice guidelines may lend themselves to use by organizations within which physicians provide services. Indeed, those organizations can and often do develop their own internal guidelines for different situations.

The danger, emphasized by the old canards about "cookbook medicine," is that the guidelines could be applied too rigidly, without regard for the full range of variability among patients. Other shortcomings stem from the shallow research basis that underlies much of clinical medicine—a shortcoming that additional, focused research can address.[64] Even so, the development and use of practice guidelines is a way both to identify areas of clinical medicine in which better evidence is needed and to translate knowledge into practice.

Through an extensive literature review of attempts to change physicians' behavior via educational approaches, John Eisenberg found that success is most probable when the effort takes place in a supportive environment, when the information is provided by (or backed by) respected figures, and where there is a perceived need for the information.[65] This suggests that, among the organizations discussed in this chapter, the educational use of practice guidelines seems most likely to find success in prepaid group practices because of their structure of centralized provision of services and their comparatively large degree of physician-to-physician contact. Physicians who are part of PPOs or IPAs can be as isolated from peer contact as are doctors in traditional forms of practice.

The second type of educational approach—often used along with practice guidelines—is feedback to physicians concerning their own practice patterns. Providing physicians with compilations of information about the services they have provided and their patterns of care compared with quality standards or other physicians' patterns of care is one of several areas in which utilization management activities can contribute to quality of care as well as cost control. It is worth considering ways in which such information may be useful.

Despite physicians' membership in a profession that is knowledge based and has strong ethical traditions, their behavior is far from uniform owing to variations in training and experience, the uncertainties of medical knowledge, and the characteristics of medical work.[66] (This lack of uniformity is documented in some detail in Chapter 10.) Medical practice contains a self-validating bias that encourages physicians to continue to do what they have done before.[67] Furthermore, practicing physicians often do not have full information about the outcome of the treatment they provide and are often unable to distinguish the results of treatment from the natural course of the disease.[68] Thus, individual physicians often develop characteristic and even idiosyncratic responses to particular clinical situations which they may be unaware of until they are shown how their practice patterns compare with those of their peers. Until the relatively recent development of patient classification taxonomies and computerized data systems, such information about their own practice patterns was seldom available to physicians.

Although doctors may generally be unaware of distinctive or unusual patterns in the care they provide, they do not seem indifferent to such information when it becomes available. Several researchers who have studied patterns of medical care advocate using insurance claim data and hospital discharge abstracts to document variations in patterns of care and outcomes, and providing the results to state medical associations, specialty societies, and individual hospitals and their medical staffs. As a result of his observations of such efforts in Vermont, Maine, and elsewhere, John Wennberg believes that "when information is presented in an objective fashion, physicians will respond by accepting responsibility for the outcome implications of the practice variation phenomenon."[69]

Nevertheless, experience with providing feedback to physicians has been uneven for a variety of reasons. John Eisenberg concludes that "information about practice patterns alone is usually necessary but often not sufficient to change physicians' practice patterns."[70] Stronger tools are available to organizations on which physicians are dependent. Informational feedback is most likely to play a leading role in collegial environments such as prepaid group practices, but even there it may be only the first stage in a progression that includes economic penalties or stronger sanctions against the individual physician whose patterns of patient care consistently deviate from clinical or economic norms.[71]

The advantages and dangers of the educational use of data on physicians' practice patterns are basically the same as those identified in the discussion of the use of such information to eliminate selected physicians from an organization. That is, the use of information to improve the clinical aspects of care has very different implications from the use of information to encourage patterns of care that serve the organization's economic interests. The extent to which such information is used—and for what purposes—is not now documented.

Finally, patterns of care have always been influenced by *economic incentives* created by payers.[72] The incentives that accompanied third-party payment in a fee-for-service health care system encouraged not only the provision of needed services but also of marginal or even unnecessary services.

In recent years the use of economic incentives for cost-containment purposes has become widespread. Using incentives to influence physicians' patient care decisions—to encourage desired behavior or discourage undesired behavior—is a tool that is available to any organization that controls the flow of dollars to physicians. Organizations such as ambulatory care centers presumably structure their compensation arrangements in a way that rewards physicians for providing *more* services, since these organizations are generally paid on a fee-for-service basis. The effects of different compensation arrangements in such organizations have, unfortunately, received very little empirical study.

Much more attention has been given to the use of economic incentives by alternative delivery systems that are at risk for the cost of services generated by affiliated physicians. Many alternative delivery systems have a degree of control over payments to physicians and can, therefore, structure the compensation system to encourage parsimonious care.

In prepaid group practices physicians are generally salaried, a payment method that eliminates the fee-for-service system's incentive to provide additional services. If the organization generates surplus revenues, bonuses are commonly used as a reward. Little documentation is available about the size or impact of such bonuses. (I have heard the bonuses distributed by the very large and reputable Kaiser-Permanente HMO described by executives as "symbolic" and by critics as "Mercedes money," but these statements could refer to different years.)

In IPAs the compensation arrangements with physicians can be much more complex but are always designed with cost containment in mind.[73] Depending on how the plan is organized, patients' access to certain services may be controlled by a "gatekeeper" physician to whom they are assigned. Depending on how compensation arrangements are structured, the physician who admits a patient to the hospital or makes a referral to a specialist or specialized services (for example, substance abuse) may be unaffected economically or may suffer a considerable loss of income. Concern about the nature and effects of such arrangements has led to a series of studies to document the payment methods or financial risk arrangements used in HMOs.[74]

The lack of standardized terminology to describe the different aspects of these arrangements—and the resulting variation in definitions used in the surveys—prohibit a brief summary of results. What is clear, however, is that the arrangements in some plans create some very strong disincentives against physicians' making patient care decisions (regarding hospitalization, diagnostic services, specialist referrals) that would cost the plan money. The most worrisome arrangements (from the standpoint of patients' interests and the fiduciary ethic) create a close, direct connection between a physician's decisions about *particular* patients and a substantial financial penalty or loss of income. Full capitation (whereby each doctor receives a set payment for *all* physician and hospital services that each patient might receive over a period of time) would be the most extreme example and appears to be rare. It would ignore the basic risk-spreading idea that underlies insurance and would put the individual physician at more economic risk than many would be willing to accept, even if they bought insurance to protect themselves. But less extreme versions exist, with different surveys reporting that from 20 percent to 60 percent of plans make use of individual physician incentives.[75] The least worrisome arrangements are those in which the financial stakes are relatively small, in which they are attached to cumulative patterns of care (rather than to decisions regarding individual patients), and in which they are indexed to the performance of a group of physicians rather than to individual performance.

## Challenges to the Fiduciary Ethic

In Chapter 8 I discussed the stress that physicians' own economic investments can place on the fiduciary ethic. Similar concerns arise with economic incentives that are designed to contain costs. Again, the effect can be to magnify the financial consequences of different patient care decisions for the individual who is making those decisions and providing patients with advice.

Even if the most worrisome arrangements—those in which the physician is at full economic risk for expensive diagnostic, hospital, or specialist services provided to individual patients—are uncommon, the fact remains that large numbers of alternative delivery systems use their compensation arrangements with physicians as a way to encourage the economical use of services. This may well be a necessary element in delivery systems that have significant other advantages.

Available evidence shows that such incentives do influence patient care decisions, but the impact on quality of care is uncertain.[76] Problems can nevertheless be foreseen in some circumstances—for example, when the level of economic competition among systems in a locale is very fierce, when systems try to rely too heavily on physician incentives as a way to control costs, and when the immediate bottom line is more important to the organization than its long-term reputation.

Where is the boundary between incentive arrangements that encourage physicians to be aware of the cost implications of clinical alternatives and those that prevent needed services from being provided? What types of risk or compensation arrangements within an alternative delivery system are incompatible with realistic assumptions about the working application of the fiduciary ethic by physicians within that system? These are issues about which concern may grow in the future and which signal the need to supplement reliance on the fiduciary ethic with new concepts of organizational responsibility and new types of monitoring systems. These are themes to which I will return in Chapter 12.

Financial arrangements within alternative delivery systems are not the only challenges to the fiduciary ethic that are presented by the new organizational dependency of physicians. Two more subtle conflicts are suggestive of the variety of issues that may arise.

I have suggested that, notwithstanding their advantages in terms of cost containment and oversight of practice patterns, alternative delivery systems may affect a physician's ability to act as the agent of the patient. They may also discourage physicians' inclinations to do so. David Ottensmeyer, a physician who went from heading a large multispecialty group practice to taking a leadership position in an investor-owned health care company (Equicor), assessed the matter thus: "The marketing of medicine [by organizations of which physicians are a part] lessens the physician's proprietary feelings toward the individual patient. It also lessens bonding between patient and physician. Instead, the patient forms ties with a health care system (such as an HMO) or a team of physicians (such as a group practice). The doctor-patient team is defined no longer by personalities, but by a contract."[77]

Or, as the health services researchers Donald Madison and Thomas Konrad have written, instead of thinking about "my patients" or "our patients," the physician may begin to think in terms of providing services to "their patients."[78] This is most likely to occur when the organization, not the individual physician, controls the volume of work and the flow of patients, and when the physician's identification with the organization is relatively weak. The first could happen in a staff model HMO, where productivity norms (for example, four or five patients per hour for primary care physicians) are used to keep costs in line with revenues. The latter could occur in IPAs or PPOs, particularly when the system provides only a portion of the physician's patients and has the power to negotiate a substantial discount from his or her normal charges.

The circumstances in which physicians obtain only a small number of patients through participation in an alternative delivery system can also present other challenges to the fiduciary ethic. The details of these arrangements can conceal some difficult conflicts of interest. The internist Robert Berenson has written about this circumstance from his own experience in an IPA that had a contract to care for Medicare patients.[79]

Under a program that was implemented nationally in 1985, Medicare beneficiaries may enroll in an HMO.[80] Patients who take the option may have broader benefits, lower out-of-pocket expenses, and less paperwork. A physician who is a member of an IPA that secures a Medicare risk contract may thus care for some Medicare patients under the traditional fee-for-service arrangement and for other patients under the IPA's capitated system.

Particular patients' choices about staying with fee-for-service or joining the IPA may have significant financial consequences for the physician and the IPA.

An ethical difficulty may arise because, although the IPA, and perhaps (depending on the economic arrangement being used) the physician, will be paid a set amount of money to care for a patient, the treatment costs for each patient are not the same, and not all patients require the same amount of the physician's time. As little as 5 percent of patients may account for half of the charges for physicians' services in a program such as Medicare.[81] Obviously the IPA (or physician) that treats the sickest patients will receive much less money than would a physician who treated the same patients on a fee-for-service basis. (The rationale that the losses on the sickest patients should be recouped by profits on other patients is, of course, central to the theory of this payment method, but, as I shall discuss, this actuarial viewpoint may not come into play when a particular patient is being encouraged to enroll or discouraged from enrolling in the IPA. This reduces the likelihood that the Medicare risk-contracting program will actually save the anticipated 5 percent of costs.)

Berenson notes that the doctor is often the major source of advice for elderly people about how to negotiate the health care system.[82] The physician also has knowledge of the patient's health status. From the standpoint of fiduciary responsibilities to patients, physicians should perhaps urge their sickest patients to join the IPA because of the broader benefits that it provides. To do so, however, would mean that the payment the physician receives would be less than under fee-for-service. It could even be lower than the physician's expenses.

In ordinary fee-for-service practice the physician's decision to provide some uncompensated services would affect only his or her own income. But if the physician who is a member of an IPA were to advise a chronically ill, high-utilizing patient to enroll in the IPA, it would put the organization itself at risk for the costs of all of the patient's care, including hospitalization. Such a physician would likely show up as a poor performer in the IPA's records on days of hospitalization generated, number of specialist referrals, amount of ancillary services used, and so forth. The physician might be viewed by professional colleagues as drawing disproportionately on the pool of funds from which all are compensated and would risk being dropped from the IPA (and from access to its patients) for being a high-cost provider.

Can the physician's adherence to the fiduciary ethic in advising patients withstand such pressures? Will physicians come to view the fiduciary ethic as simply impractical in the face of such realities of medical practice? Can patients and health policy makers continue to assume that physicians represent their patients' interests first and foremost? Because of such questions, a search for alternatives to reliance on the fiduciary ethic is under way.

### Physician Groupings and the Fiduciary Ethic

Although this chapter has emphasized the growing organizational dependence of individual physicians, it is obvious that physicians often deal with these changing circumstances as members of groups. Because the matters that I have been discussing are concerned with bargaining power, the significance of physicians' acting as groups must be considered. Groups obviously have more power than individuals, and group practice brings with it the possibility of both formal and informal social control, based on mutual observation, development of group norms, and so forth. (Of course, the possibilities that reside in a particular form of organization are not necessarily realized, and groups may not necessarily be willing to exercise discipline over individual members.)[83] Conflicts with the fiduciary ethic can also arise.

The power of "organized medicine"—including state and county medical societies—to defend the status quo of individual, fee-for-service medical care has been diminished by a series of legal cases and by fragmentation (for example, the growth of specialty societies). Yet, several other types of aggregations of physicians have been factors in the developments discussed in this chapter.

### *Provider-Controlled Alternative Delivery Systems*

I noted earlier that some IPAs were created by county (or state) medical societies as a defense against other alternative delivery systems. Some PPOs were also created by providers (hospitals and affiliated physicians) for similar purposes. (Physicians were, of course, involved in the creation or administration of many of the other types of organizations that I have discussed. A distinction should be made, however, between physicians' acting as entrepreneurs or executives and physicians' acting as a group to create an organization that will serve or protect the interests of its members.)

The medical-society-based IPAs (and provider-controlled PPOs) have faced a number of difficulties and have, by and large, not become a prominent part of the industry. Several reasons can be identified. First, the establishment of such an organization generally did not keep competitors out. The U.S. Department of Justice and the Federal Trade Commission took an unfavorable view of providers' forming an organization for the purpose of restricting competition. As the American Bar Association noted, "Independent, third-party, 'brokered' HMOs and PPOs are inherently safer [from an antitrust perspective] than provider-sponsored systems."[84]

Physicians in private practice have thus been able to join several IPAs or PPOs. From their standpoint, being a member of many plans can mean that no particular plan controls a large percentage of the practice's patients. This obviously has contributed to physicians' independence from external control and limited their loyalty to any of the organizations of which they were a part. But as a practical matter it has also meant that the physician-controlled organizations were ineffective in keeping competitors out and would eventually have to face economic competition.

Also, problems arose in managing costs. As part of their philosophy, many of these plans were open to any (and as many) physicians who wanted to join, whereas alternative delivery systems have found generally that selectivity is essential to good management and cost containment.[85] Furthermore, because they were often established as a way to preserve the autonomy of individual physicians, these organizations were reluctant to put into place the kinds of information systems, incentive structures, and other tools necessary for controlling costs in a system in which per-patient income would be fixed. Too many of their physicians (who, after all, were accustomed to practicing under the incentives of fee-for-service) continued to practice as before.

Indeed, in many cases they were continuing to be paid on a fee-for-service basis by the IPA.

As a consequence of these factors, many of the medical-society-based plans were financially unsuccessful, either because they were unable to set competitive prices or because they were not able to keep expenses in line with revenues. The choice these organizations have faced is either to go out of business, sell, or start managing in a way that uses the tools described in this and the next chapter. This means that the organizations that were intended to preserve the autonomy of individual physicians would have to start monitoring their member physicians' patterns of care, establishing incentives to discourage utilization, and selectively adding physicians to, or dropping physicians from, the network of IPA members.

An interesting but at present unanswered empirical question is whether, as competition has grown, physicians find that the experience of being members of a medical-society-controlled IPA (or PPO) is substantially different from being a member of a system that is controlled by, say, an investor-owned corporation.

## Unionization of Physicians

A movement that signifies the changing conditions of medical professionalism is the creation and growth of unionization among physicians.[86] Although critics once saw unionlike elements in the activities of the American Medical Association on behalf of its members, antitrust and price-fixing laws set very real limits on the extent to which physicians in private practice can join together on behalf of their shared interests. Even among employed physicians there may be questions about the extent to which they are covered by the National Labor Relations Act, which does not apply to "supervisors."[87]

The movement toward unionization of physicians in the United States involves physicians who work in salaried positions. There have been examples of strikes among resident physicians, employees of municipal hospitals, and employees of staff-model HMOs. Such strikes illustrate an ambiguity in organizations whose purpose is to represent the interests of physicians: to what extent do they give voice to such professional concerns as the fiduciary ethic and science-based standards of care, and to what extent do they speak for physicians' economic interests and working conditions?[88]

At this point physicians' unions are found in only limited circumstances and are more of a curiosity than a matter of broad public policy concern, although they can certainly be important to the particular organizations in which they exist and the populations that they serve. How much the growing organizational dependence of physicians will result in their finding themselves in a relatively powerless, employeelike position is open to speculation. National organizations that provide (or contract for) health care clearly grew in number in the 1980s, but in most cases the services they offer are provided by physicians who contract with the organization as individuals or members of group practices. At present the growth of physician unions seems to be a much less noteworthy development than the growth of group practices.

*The Rise of Group Practice*

Group practices are increasingly significant elements of our health care system. The percentage of physicians who practiced in groups of five or more rose by one-third between 1975 and 1983 to reach almost 23 percent.[89] The number of group practices of three or more physicians grew by 143 percent between 1969 and 1984, reaching 15,485 (with 140,392 positions in 1984).[90] The size and numbers of large group practices has also been increasing. For example, between 1969 and 1984 the number of groups with more than 25 physicians grew from 147 to 660, the number with more than 50 grew from 50 to 306, and the number with more than 100 grew from 17 to 158.[91]

There are good reasons to expect this trend to continue. Not only do group practices provide advantages in terms of more regular hours and more consistent case loads, but also a group can generate enough patient volume and cash flow to attract more sophisticated management, gain better access to capital to pay for new technologies and alternative delivery sites, absorb certain costs such as liability insurance, and market more effectively. In a multispecialty group, specialists have a source of referrals, and primary care physicians do not face the specter of losing patients once they make a referral. Joining a group practice is an attractive option for young doctors emerging from training with large debts and facing the costs of setting up their own practices, and for many female physicians who wish to accommodate family circumstances. Collegiality, ready availability of consultants, ease of referrals, more adequate capitalization, and economies of scale may all enhance the quality of care in group settings, as may the group's interest in maintaining its reputation and avoiding lawsuits. A large group may also be in a strong position to negotiate with HMOs or PPOs and may even be in a position to establish one.

Although group practices have significant advantages, they do not solve—and may even complicate—some of the problems of accountability. The financial arrangements in group practice create income-related and expense-related dependencies that engender informal (but very real) feelings of mutual accountability and, perhaps, formal structures for monitoring the financial performance of group members. Group practices also create opportunities for income-enhancing decision making. For example, referrals to colleagues can generate income for the practice under certain payment arrangements.

Many of the same trends that have changed the accountability structure of individual practices are mirrored in group practices. For instance, group practices may make substantial capital investments that generate pressure for utilization.[92] Economies of scale and opportunities for revenue enhancement encourage the development of ancillary services such as pharmacies, laboratories, radiology services, and electrocardiography capabilities.[93] The need to generate a return on capital investments and opportunities for producing additional revenues may influence individual physicians, the corporate culture of a practice, and the balance of forces that affect the sense of being responsible first and foremost to the patient. These possibilities have not received much empirical study.

In a health care system increasingly dominated by large organizations, group practice increases physicians' ability to maintain areas of control and to influence other parties. Generalizations are not warranted, however, because of the diversity of types and circumstances.

A number of useful concepts for distinguishing among group practices have been developed by Donald Madison and Thomas Konrad.[94] *Reactive* groups try to operate in the "traditional 'open market' (unrestricted price setting with fee-for-service payment from an undefined client population)" and resist involvement in managed care systems. *Proactive* groups "desire greater definition of their service populations and seek involvement in 'managed-care' arrangements."[95] Which stance a group adopts will in part be a function of two other factors, both of which have consequences for the internal organization of the practice and the practice's position vis-à-vis external control.

One is the extent to which the practice's capacity is committed to the care of defined populations (for example, as a staff-model HMO is to its enrollee population). In general, the more a practice's capacity is committed, the more its individual physicians will work within a formal, hierarchical structure. The second factor is the number of *clients' agents* who purchase care directly from the organization. Traditionally, each patient was his or her own agent; in HMOs and PPOs, however, there are agents who speak for *many* clients. As Madison and Konrad observe, "Agents with little power (e.g., individual patients acting in their own behalf) negotiate only minor issues, such as setting an appointment time for a physician visit. The more powerful agents, who may represent from hundreds to many thousands of patients, negotiate progressively larger issues: questions of quality and use of service, the hours a facility will be open, even the physician staffing pattern."[96]

A group's stance toward the marketplace (a matter which, it should be apparent, it only partially controls) is just one factor that determines its effect on the autonomy of individual physicians. Another is how the group believes the work of medical practice should be administered. This factor is influenced by marketplace forces, but it also has much to do with the group's history—whether, for example, it was founded by practicing physicians or on the initiative of another organization (hospital, government agency, insurance fund, consumer cooperative, medical school, industrial firm). Madison and Konrad distinguish the *autonomous* tradition of the former situation with the *heteronomous* (subject to control of another law) tradition of the latter. As autonomous groups get larger, as they deal with fewer patients' agents, and as larger portions of their capacity are committed to defined populations, *individual* autonomy is likely to be replaced by *administered* autonomy, with a clinical hierarchy of physician officers and committees. "The tradition holds that the group's welfare is more important than the individual physician's preference, and that such hierarchy is needed to achieve the professional and economic goals of the organization. Applied in the clinical arena, this principle also gives some notion of legitimacy to monitoring—if not explicit supervision—of the work of each individual practitioner."[97]

This brief discussion suggests that the growth of group practice as a way of preserving the voice of the physician is indeed a complex matter. Some group practices are controlled by non-physicians, and the physicians in other group practices are subject to some degree of control by others. None of this is necessarily bad, but it is a significant change in the tradition of autonomy. The implications of group practices with regard to the fiduciary ethic may lie in how they are controlled and by whom, and how and to what end the performance of individual physicians is monitored and even manipulated.

Although physician autonomy has often been pictured as essential to the ability of doctors to ensure that the interests of patients are being served, past conceptions of individual autonomy and freedom are rapidly becoming obsolete. For growing numbers of physicians, their ability to practice medicine has become contingent on their establishing and maintaining a relationship with an organization.

These organizations themselves have goals, interests, and corporate cultures which may influence the end toward which the work of the physician is oriented. For example, the organization may give primacy to the highest standards of professional practice or to the generation of short-term profits. To what extent are the doctors and nurses who actually deal with patients given a voice in setting organizational policies that affect patient care? And with what tools does the organization seek to monitor and/or influence their professional practices? Around such matters will turn the answer to the question of the extent to which the changed circumstances of medical practice serve the interests of patients and of payers.

Research has shown that physicians' patient care decisions are influenced by many factors in addition to their training—by economic incentives, by the presence of monitoring, by procedural requirements. (Some of this evidence was presented in Chapter 8; more is in Chapter 10.) It is reasonable to expect that physicians' patient care decisions will be influenced by various aspects of their linkages with organizations on which they are dependent— by the economic incentives that are built into their relationship to the organization, by the methods these organizations use to contain costs or to generate business, by corporate cultures, or by other factors. It has been shown, for example, that the patterns of patient care decisions by physicians who practice in *for-profit* facilities for treatment of patients with end-stage renal disease differ from patterns in nonprofit and public facilities, with patients in for-profit facilities being less likely to receive kidney transplants or to receive dialysis treatment at home.[98]

As is the case with the entrepreneurial activities that were discussed in Chapter 8, physicians' relationship to an organization can sometimes magnify the personal consequences of making certain decisions for their patients. Depending on the circumstances, the consequences may pertain either to the physician's immediate economic interests or to his or her continued relationship with colleagues or to the organization. The consequences may be attached either to a particular patient care decision or to a pattern of decisions.

How all of this will affect the interests of patients (and of payers) will likely depend on a variety of factors. It may be influenced by the environment in which the organization operates— for example, the degree of economic pressure it faces as a result of the competitive situation and the power of large purchasers of care. Organizations that are under a great deal of economic pressure may behave in uncharacteristic ways. The effects may also depend on the tools being used to manage care, the sophistication and skill with which they are used, and, perhaps most important, the end to which they are used. These considerations suggest the importance of safeguards—at two levels.

First, because methods of containing costs, organizing care, and influencing physician behavior can all have unanticipated consequences, the organization needs internal safeguards—ways of detecting departures from desired performance. The management of professional work is difficult, however, and our ability to measure quality of care is still limited. Organizations that are able to put into place a structure of incentives that reward physicians for limiting the services provided to patients are not necessarily also able to, or interested in, establishing a sensitive monitoring system for detecting whether patients are receiving needed services. Indeed, it cannot be assumed that all organizations put the welfare of individual patients ahead of even their short-term economic interests.

This suggests the need for a second level of safeguards external to the organization. These may be regulatory (such as disclosure requirements or prohibitions on certain arrangements), or they may be carried out by (or on behalf of) the purchaser of services. These are topics to which I will return in Chapter 12.

# · 10 ·

## Payers and Physicians'
## Patient Care Decisions:
## Steps toward a New Accountability

In the 1980s the work of physicians and the institutions that provide medical services came under growing scrutiny by parties concerned with costs. This scrutiny ranged from bill audits and retrospective review of services to prospective attempts to determine the appropriateness or necessity of services. Third-party payers, whose creation had originally been bitterly opposed by the medical profession on grounds of potential interference with the doctor-patient relationship, no longer limited their role to paying for the services provided or ordered by physicians.[1] Indeed, given that the patient care decisions made by physicians trigger most health care expenditures, cost-containment efforts have begun to focus on those decisions. The traditional roles and responsibilities of payers and providers in determining what services will be offered to patients and in what settings are changing in very significant ways, and physicians are experiencing a marked decline in the individual autonomy that the profession has customarily enjoyed.

---

Because of some overlap in content, a note of explanation is warranted about the relationship of Chapters 10 and 11 to the Institute of Medicine (IOM) report on utilization management (Bradford H. Gray and Marilyn J. Field, eds. *Controlling Costs and Changing Patient Care? The Role of Utilization Management* [Washington, D.C.: National Academy Press, 1989]). Chapters 10 and 11 of this book were originally drafted before the initiation of the IOM study, which I directed. Much of the material in those drafts eventually found its way into the IOM report. Chapters 10 and 11 underwent a substantial revision subsequent to the publication of the IOM report.

Consider the following description of the health care cost management approach of a company that administers health benefit plans for self-insured employees:

> At U.S. Administrators, nationally prominent physicians serve as consultants and help to develop and continually update a series of computerized model treatment screens for specific diagnostic codes. Any discrepancy between services rendered and what is deemed appropriate by the treatment screen is flagged for analysis while the claim is being processed, often leading to denial of payment. If the provider challenges a payment decision, U.S. Administrators will defend its analysis, in court if necessary.
>
> When a patient enters the hospital, hospital staff are expected to complete and file a predetermination form that identifies the admitting diagnosis and the attending physician. Failure to do so can result in reimbursement being denied. Upon receipt of a diagnosis, an appropriate length of stay is assigned based on the model treatment screens and transmitted on the same day to the hospital, attending physician, and individual patient. Subsequently, if a hospital bill is received that deviates from the length of stay determination, the excess days will not be reimbursed until additional clinical justification is received from the provider. If the excess days still cannot be justified, payment is denied, and the patient is held harmless.[2]

Even allowing for the possibility that the company promises more than it can deliver, the strategies described convey a marked change in accountability and physician autonomy.

The doctor-patient relationship has traditionally been imbued with a moral quality that discouraged oversight or intervention by anyone else. Norms of privacy rendered medical decision making practically invisible to regulators and payers (and also, incidentally, to researchers). The invisible has now become more and more visible—at least to payers—and the work of physicians and medical institutions is coming under a degree of external oversight that has few parallels elsewhere in society.[3]

Two integral characteristics of medical care as it is provided in institutions make this oversight possible. First is the need to keep detailed records—because of the fallibility of memory, because care is provided by teams for whom the record is a means of communication, because of the specter of liability actions (it can be difficult to prove that a service that was not recorded was actually performed), and because services provided must be documented for payers.

Second, third-party payment gives somebody other than the doctor and patient a strong and legitimate interest in the services that are being provided. It also makes feasible some activities that would never be possible if the providers and recipients of the service were the only parties to the transactions. The information that is conveyed to third-party payers as a part of routine billing and review procedures provides a rich source of data about what is going on between doctors and hospitals and patients. When computerized, the information conveyed by providers to payers permits the latter to aggregate the experiences of individual patients into information about patterns of care, to compare providers with one another or against objective standards, and to seek ways to use the information for cost-constraint purposes.

The former reluctance of third-party payers to intrude into the doctor-patient relationship has clearly yielded to active efforts by payers to influence the services that patients receive either by dealing directly with patients' physicians or by putting pressure on hospitals to do so. Third-party payers have taken on new responsibilities. The term *management* abounds. Corporate benefit managers talk of "managing" their health benefit plans, and they contract with "managed care" plans and organizations that provide "utilization management" services for "managed fee-for-service" plans.[4]

The object of all of this management is, of course, health care costs. The tools used include an assortment of incentives, data systems for monitoring patterns and costs of care, and procedural requirements. The use of incentives was discussed to some extent in the last chapter. After a discussion of the cost problem and the changing orientation of purchasers of care, this chapter will concentrate on utilization review. Chapter 11 will focus on utilization management methods in which a third-party becomes involved in patient care decisions prior to the provision of services.

The active effort by payers to influence patient care raises large questions. How do these new cost-containment approaches actually work? What effects do they have? Do they selectively eliminate only unnecessary or inappropriate services? If so, that would have both cost and quality benefits. On the down side, consequences range from increased administrative expenses to the possibility of harm to patients if more than "unnecessary" services are discouraged.

And what are the responsibilities of the various parties? The parties who are demanding greater accountability are clearly not the ones—patients—whose interests physicians (and perhaps hospitals) have traditionally been expected to serve. The fiduciary obligations of employers and third-party payers are at best undefined, as are the obligations of providers in situations in which their conceptions of appropriate care differ from the utilization managers' conceptions. Are patients' interests adequately protected? In short, utilization management raises some new issues of accountability, as well as some new versions of old ones.

### Reasons for the Rise in Accountability to Payers

In view of the themes of this book, it is tempting to argue that payers were convinced of the need for new modes of accountability by the rise of investor-owned providers and multi-institutional systems, the increased commercial behavior of nonprofit institutions, and growing physician entrepreneurship. Those developments may have had an effect on the environment, and they contributed to the problem of health care costs. But it is the cost problem itself that has been the most direct and proximate cause of third-party payers' demands for new forms of accountability.

Even so, the suspicion that providers and medical decision makers are excessively influenced by economic incentives is close to the surface when purchasers, payers, and utilization management organizations describe the problems they are seeking to correct.[5] Older cost-containment policies such as the health planning program of the 1970s reflected a perception that was characterized by the health services researcher Milton Roemer in terms that became known as Roemer's law: that a hospital bed built is a hospital bed filled. Yet occupancy rates have declined (to around 65 percent), but the cost problem has not abated.

One need not talk to many corporate health benefit managers before one discovers that a new perception—related to Roemer's law but different—is widely afoot. They believe that a service that will be paid for is a service that someone will provide. Whether or not this perception should be elevated to the status of a law, payers who believe it are faced with a vastly expanded conception of their own responsibility. Whereas Roemer's law implied an agenda of assessing communities' needs for hospital beds and putting in place a regulatory mechanism (certificate of need) for controlling unnecessary expansions, this new law has much more radical and far-reaching implications because it suggests that the payer bears some of the responsibility for whatever services the patient receives.

The reason that payers have begun to take on this responsibility—one, incidentally, that few seem to welcome—boils down to one word: costs.

### The Effort to Control Costs

With medical costs rising at twice the rate of inflation and growing faster than the national economy, health care now accounts for about 12 percent of the gross national product, up from less than 6 percent in 1965. For the public programs, Medicare and Medicaid, costs have been an issue ever since the first compiled figures showed costs to be rapidly outstripping projections. The cost of these programs led to a whole series of cost-containment methods: health planning and certificate-of-need programs; rate-setting programs in some states; freezes in payment levels; changes in eligibility and coverage; support for the development of HMOs and a program to enable Medicare beneficiaries to enroll in HMOs and competitive medical plans; the adoption of Medicare's prospective payment system; and, most recently, physician payment reform under Medicare. None of these programs, however, contains the key elements of utilization management: case-by-case decision making prior to the provision of services.

Regarding utilization management, the earliest steps were Medicare's utilization review requirements and the professional standards review organization (PSRO) program, in which many of the tools of utilization management were developed and first applied. Utilization *review* was required of hospitals from the outset under Medicare regulations and had existed in some Blue Cross/Blue Shield plans and hospitals even earlier. Such activities were essentially advisory and educational forms of peer review and proved to be too weak as a means of influencing the use of services and containing costs. Hospital-based utilization review for Medicare was supplemented by the quasi-independent activities of PSROs under legislation passed in 1972.[6]

The PSROs were physician-controlled organizations whose responsibility was to review the appropriateness of services—particularly the use of the hospital. Such review was either retrospective (taking place after the services had been provided) or concurrent (as with determinations of whether the continued hospitalization of a patient was appropriate). Because such concurrent review was used to make determinations about the appropriateness of a particular patient's continued hospitalization, it was one of the first activities to fit the definition of utilization management.

For review purposes hospital records were abstracted by nurses employed by PSROs. Early on, PSROs' review activities made heavy use of statistical norms (diagnosis-specific average lengths of stay) and the professional judgment of reviewing physicians regarding the appropriateness of services. There was interest not only in the care of particular patients but also in patterns of care (such as trends, comparisons among providers, and, eventually, variations from objective standards). Indeed, it was through their work in PSROs that many physicians became aware of how commonly and how extensively doctors differed from one another in their use of services. Interest developed in documenting, understanding, and reducing this variation, particularly when it reflected inappropriate care.

For a variety of purposes, therefore, it was desirable to develop patient classification systems and objective criteria against which the medical necessity or quality of a patient's care could be evaluated. Accordingly, research activities associated with the PSRO program (as well as research elsewhere) were moving to develop patient classification systems and criteria of appropriateness. These were tasks of great complexity,[7] but they were of fundamental importance to the eventual development of utilization management. A number of patient classification systems were eventually developed (not all in the PSRO program, it should be noted) based on diagnostic and procedural taxonomies, combinations of diagnostic and resource-consumption categories (for example, diagnosis-related groups), organ system involvement, objective clinical findings, and stages of disease and indices of severity. Numerous criteria sets have been developed for use in evaluating the appropriateness or quality of care. Such work, under a variety of guises (most recently the development of so-called practice guidelines), has grown into a very active area of research.

The development of classification systems and evaluation criteria required outlays of research and development funds, which became available substantially because of the concentration of economic stakes brought about by third-party payment. Most of the utilization management systems now in use grew out of systems that were developed in the PSRO program, although systems were also developed by private insurers, third-party administrators, and utilization management organizations.

Leaders and physician-participants in the PSRO program always emphasized its potential to improve the quality of care, but it was the inability to demonstrate cost savings and the perception that PSROs were insufficiently independent of providers that led to the program's elimination in 1984 legislation. Under the same legislation, however, a new review program, to be conducted by "utilization and quality control peer review organizations" (known, mercifully, as PROs), was established to assume the Medicare utilization review function. But meanwhile many of the PSROs, as well as spin-off organizations, had begun to provide data analysis and utilization review services for private third-party purchasers of medical care.

By the late 1970s the private sector had become interested in finding ways to contain health care costs. Employers' costs were increasing rapidly and were often depicted vividly, as with Joseph Califano's characterization of health care costs for employees, retirees, and dependents as accounting for 500 dollars of the price of every car made by the Chrysler Corporation. The implication that this was hurting competition with the Japanese may have been misleading,[8] but the problem of costs was very real.

Table 10.1 shows employment-based health care costs expressed as a percentage of corporate profits and as a percentage of costs of employment compensation. Health care costs, which

*Table 10.1.*   Health spending by business as a percentage of pretax
corporate profits and of total labor compensation,
1965–1987

| Year | Health costs as share of pretax profits | Health costs as share of total compensation |
| --- | --- | --- |
| 1965 | 8.7 | 2.1 |
| 1970 | 20.2 | 3.2 |
| 1975 | 22.8 | 4.1 |
| 1980 | 28.7 | 5.2 |
| 1985 | 51.0 | 6.0 |
| 1987 | 48.6 | 6.2 |

Source: Katherine R. Levit, Mark S. Freeland, and Daniel Waldo, "Health
Spending and Ability to Pay," *Health Care Financing Review* 10 (Spring 1989): 9.

had been equivalent to less than 9 percent of profits in 1965, had
risen to the equivalent of 50 percent of profits by the mid-1980s,
and had tripled (from about 2 percent to about 6 percent) as a
portion of companies' total labor costs. It is not surprising that
expenses of this level began to attract the attention of corporate
leaders and led to a variety of cost-containment strategies including, eventually, utilization management.

The most significant early signal of a new determination by
private employers to address the problem of health benefit costs
was the publication in 1978 of a thirty-seven-page report with the
unprepossessing title "Labor-Management Group Position Paper
on Health Care Costs." The "labor-management group," however, was a most formidable and influential aggregation which
included former Secretary of Labor John Dunlop, the chairmen of
eight major corporations, and the presidents of seven influential
labor unions. The report, issued after nine months of meetings
and staff work, supported prospective reimbursement methods,
HMOs, health planning, technology assessment, medical malpractice reform, and health education, as well as such utilization
management precursors as preadmission testing, piloting
second-opinion programs, introducing utilization review into
health benefits programs, and expanding alternatives to inpatient
hospital treatment.

Many notable approaches to controlling health care costs developed among payers in the private sector during the late 1970s and early 1980s, including:

· the Blue Cross/Blue Shield Medical Necessity Project, which began with the American College of Physicians in the mid-1970s and later expanded to involve other medical specialty societies. Various tests and procedures were evaluated to guide Blue Cross administrators in determining what services they should pay for. This program was apparently the first attempt to link professional societies' educational efforts and professional opinion to the reimbursement process;[9]

· the development of local "health care coalitions" such as the Midwest Business Group on Health, created by 120 companies in eight midwestern states to "motivate and assist corporations to develop and implement health cost management tools";[10]

· the widespread development of new employee benefit packages with increased cost sharing by employees and incentives for them to use HMOs or preferred providers who offered discounts to the employer;

· the implementation of hospital bill auditing programs (errors have been reported on 30 to 80 percent of all bills), reported in 1986 to be in use by 44 percent of companies;[11]

· the development by employers, health care coalitions, and insurance carriers of methods for analyzing health care utilization data in forms that allow comparisons of providers and identification of unusual patterns in the utilization of, and charges for, health care services.

Another development that had particularly broad ramifications was for large employers to self-fund their health benefit plans—to pay beneficiaries' medical costs as an ongoing expense rather than purchasing insurance plans. The number of self-insuring companies increased from 19 percent to 59 percent, according to surveys by the Wyatt Company in 1980 and 1986. Most employers hired insurance companies or specialized organizations to administer their benefit plan. Self-funded health benefit plans enabled employers to maintain more control over their funds, tailor their benefits as they saw fit, and avoid state mandates regarding what services health insurance should cover.[12] A key secondary effect was to tighten the link between health care costs as incurred by beneficiaries and as experienced by the company. This helped to prepare the market for utilization management services when they became available.[13] Many of the organizations that provide those services also serve as the third-party administrator of employers' health benefit plans.

Seen in the context of all these developments, the rise of more direct efforts to modify medical practice patterns was not a surprising step. But several factors in addition to the need to control costs underlie the particular approaches that have been developed. These factors include (1) the emergence of research evidence that suggested to payers that the cost problem was to some degree mutable because it developed from questionable medical decision making; (2) the growing economic power of purchasers vis-à-vis providers and their realization that their own policies and practices had contributed to the problem; and (3) the rise of organizations willing to provide cost-containment services for purchasers.

### The Mutability of the Cost Problem

The direction that utilization management has taken has been strongly influenced by evidence that many services are unnecessary or inappropriate and that less costly ways of providing care can be found. Studies of variations in patterns of medical care, research on unnecessary or inappropriate services, and evidence that medical decision making can be changed through education and incentives have all led to the belief that health care costs can to some extent be managed.

*Variations in patterns of care.* One source of support for this view is studies showing wide and largely unexpected variations in patient care patterns across geographic areas. For example, several studies have linked the amount of surgery performed in a population to the supply of surgeons.[14] Other studies have found that hospital stays averaged two days longer on the East Coast than on the West Coast; that the percentage of Vermont children who have had tonsillectomies ranged from 8 percent in one hospital market to 70 percent in another; that the proportion of seventy-year-old Maine women who have undergone a hysterectomy ranged from 20 percent in one area to 70 percent in another; that the rate of cesarean section as a percentage of all deliveries in 1981 ranged from 10.5 percent in Detroit to 24 percent in Washington, D.C.; and that the chances of an eighty-five-year-old man having had a prostatectomy varied from 15 percent to 60 percent in different areas of Iowa.[15] Wide variations in the incidence of medical and surgical services are the *norm*, not the exception.[16]

Although differences among populations in the use of particular services could reflect differences in the incidence of the medical conditions for which those services are provided, many variations in the patterns of services appear to be due to differences among physicians in what John Wennberg, the leading researcher in this area, calls their "practice styles"—the characteristic and sometimes idiosyncratic ways physicians respond to medical problems for which there is little professional consensus about appropriate treatment. For conditions associated with a high degree of professional consensus about diagnosis and treatment (for example, appendicitis, cancer of the bowel, or hip fractures), geographical variations in the incidence of procedures are much smaller than for those for which consensus about treatment is lacking, such as conditions resulting in hysterectomy or prostatectomy.[17]

An important implication of the studies on variations in patterns of medical care is the suggestion that whether or not certain services are provided to particular patients depends on much more than their objective needs. At one time this implication might have had little effect. Indeed, the uncertainty involved in medical decision making has been one of the justifications for physician autonomy. But variations have come to be seen as clues for use in reducing unnecessary services, even though the data on variations in patterns of care reveal nothing in themselves about appropriate levels of utilization.[18]

*Documentation of inappropriate utilization.* Documenting variations in patterns of care requires data on services, providers, and, ideally, place of residence of patients (so that population-based rates can be calculated). Developing population-based statistics about the use of various procedures is no small task in our system of multiple payers and multiple reporting systems. Unfortunately, such statistics do not distinguish appropriate from inappropriate utilization. That requires comparing actual with "correct" use of services.

Several approaches have been developed for this task, including two that have come to be used in many utilization management programs. An assortment of studies has shown that as much as 25 percent or more of expenditures for medical care is for unnecessary or inappropriate services. This has led to the hope and belief that some aspects of the cost problem can be addressed without depriving patients of needed services.[19]

An early approach to documenting unnecessary care involved the review of pathological evidence after surgery. For example, examination of tissue removed in surgery at five Baltimore hospitals in the late 1950s showed that more than 25 percent of the appendectomies at the two university hospitals had been "unnecessary" or of "doubtful necessity," with even higher rates at the three community hospitals.[20] Although it is generally agreed that the goal should not be to reduce the rate to zero, which could be done only at the expense of too many errors of omission (complications of perforations and peritonitis), subsequent studies showed that through education, peer review, and changed conceptions of indications for surgery, the rate could safely be reduced to less than 2 percent.[21] This approach to documenting unnecessary care is highly labor intensive, applicable only after the service has been provided, and suitable for a relatively small portion of medical care. Nevertheless, the use of such approaches to pursue reductions in unnecessary surgery was an important step in the effort to contain costs through the application of objective criteria regarding what services were needed or appropriate.

Of much greater public policy impact than tissue studies by pathologists were the early results from the original surgical second-opinion studies begun in 1972 under the direction of Eugene G. McCarthy, M.D., at Cornell–New York Hospital. His finding of a 17 percent nonconformance rate for elective operations in a second-opinion program implemented by a New York City labor union was interpreted by a congressional committee and the press as a measurement of the extent of unnecessary surgery.[22] Although a nonconfirmed opinion for an *elective* surgical procedure cannot properly be construed as evidence that the original surgeon had recommended an *unnecessary* operation, the sensation caused by the national extrapolations of 2.4 million needless operations at a cost of $3.9 million and 11,900 deaths was credited (or blamed) by the American College of Surgeons with providing "strong impetus for government and insurers to develop second-opinion programs as a way to reduce 'unnecessary' operations and expenses."[23] Such programs have become an element in many cost-containment efforts.

Better documentation of unnecessary or inappropriate care has come from audits of medical records. In the earliest studies experts reviewed records for evidence that in their judgment documented the need for the services that had been provided. Much unnecessary utilization was found.[24] In later studies objective criteria that justified the provision of a given service were developed, and patient records were abstracted to determine whether the criteria had been met. Using such methods, various studies have shown that between 20 and 40 percent of laboratory testing and ancillary services in hospitals—as much as 65 percent of some laboratory services in one teaching hospital—were unnecessary or inappropriate.[25] Other research has documented unnecessary prescriptions.[26] More recent work by Rand Corporation researchers at hospitals that were *not* selected for "poor performance or questionable practices" found that one-third or more of coronary angiographies and coronary artery bypass surgeries may have been performed in patients for whom the risk was as great as the procedure's benefit.[27] Similarly, carotid endarterectomies (a procedure to remove clots in the arteries leading to the brain) were found to be clearly warranted in only 35 percent of cases.[28]

Although the provision of inappropriate services generally entails unnecessary costs and risks, hospitalization itself also involves significant risks (and costs) because of the problem of nosocomial (hospital-acquired) infections and other iatrogenic diseases (caused by medical care). Researchers using patient records and the criteria set known as the Appropriateness Evaluation Protocol (AEP) have found inappropriate hospital utilization in the range of 20 to 30 percent or more among admissions and days of hospitalization.[29] Some inappropriate use of hospitals is probably inescapable, but a number of researchers believe that it would be possible to reduce rates of inappropriate admissions to below 5 percent and to reduce unnecessary days of care for patients whose admissions were appropriate to 5 to 10 percent.[30] The matter of the definition of "appropriate" services is of obvious importance, and we will return to it later. The point that I want to stress here is that researchers have found much evidence of unneeded and inappropriate services and that this has been seen as providing clues to opportunities for reducing services without harm to patients.

*Responsiveness of physicians to feedback and incentives.* The perception that something can be done about costs has also been fed by experiences showing that physicians' utilization patterns sometimes change quickly when they receive feedback about how their practice patterns compare to some norm (usually a statistical one),[31] or when their decisions are monitored.[32] Moreover, the perception that patient care patterns can be changed is also fed by the belief (which seems ubiquitous among payers) that health care providers (individual and institutional) are responsive not only to the objective needs of patients but also to economic incentives. That belief was fueled by the cost increases that occurred while providers were being paid under cost-based and charge-based payment methods and by research showing that physicians' patterns of practice vary in accordance with how the economic incentives affect them. This is not the place for a full review of such research, but a few examples suggest its flavor.

One study of ambulatory testing of uncomplicated hypertension patients found that after controlling for patients' age and sex, duration and severity of disease, and doctor's year of medical school graduation, there were 50 percent more electrocardiograms and 40 percent more chest radiographs among the patients in fee-for-service group practices than among the patients in prepaid group practices.[33] The fee-for-service groups of course received additional income each time an additional service was provided; the prepaid groups experienced additional services as an expense that would deduct from the revenues received from their fixed per-enrollee fees. Another study found a positive association between the physician-to-population ratio in an area and the rates of *physician-initiated* patient care visits (which account for 43 percent of all patient visits to physicians).[34] Another study showed that Colorado physicians responded to a decrease in Medicare reimbursement rates in the mid-1970s by doing more surgery and more laboratory testing; such changes

were not found among physicians who had not been affected by
the rate changes.[35] Similarly, physicians in California responded
to a 1971 Medicare price freeze by increasing virtually all types
of services—patient visits in hospitals and offices as well as
various types of ancillary services—so much so that higher billings resulted; after price controls were lifted in 1975, physicians
raised their fees substantially, and the quantity of services provided decreased.[36] Similar increases in surgery followed a 30 percent reduction in Medicaid surgical fees in Massachusetts in
1976.[37]

*Low utilization levels in HMOs.* Also very influential in suggesting that health care costs might be mutable to some extent
has been the low rate of hospital use among enrollees in prepaid
group practices (averaging 30 percent lower than conventionally
insured populations) and the fact that these low rates have been
achieved without deleterious health effects.[38] The HMO experience has long been used to buttress arguments that fee-for-
service payment encourages unnecessary hospital admissions,
but not all evidence supported this interpretation. Harold Luft
has noted that hospital admission rates among HMO enrollees
appear to be lower for *all* causes of admission, not just causes for
which high rates of unnecessary utilization are known to exist.[39]
Furthermore, differences in hospitalization rates could occur
because HMOs provide greater coverage for preventive services,
although there is little evidence to support this possibility.[40]

In addition, it is possible that HMOs attract comparatively
healthy people. The Rand Health Insurance Experiment provided
solid evidence that differential incentives, not differential selection of patients, accounted for the variations between prepaid
and fee-for-service health care in the use of hospitals in the HMO
that was studied. In that experiment patients were randomly
assigned either to an HMO or to a fee-for-service physician of
their choice. After three to five years, hospital admissions were
40 percent lower among HMO patients, although ambulatory
visit rates were similar.[41] The reasons are not altogether clear.
The results could be due to peer pressure, to selection of physicians who practice a certain style of medicine, to utilization
controls, or to incentives. Two lessons have been widely drawn,
however: that much lower use of hospitals than occurs in conven-

tional fee-for-service medicine can be safely achieved, and that incentives influence medical decision making.

In summary, evidence of physician responsiveness to economic incentives—together with the evidence on variations in patterns of care and on the extent of inappropriate services—has shaped the perception that the health care cost problem is to some degree mutable. These same factors have also influenced the methods that have come to be used for utilization management purposes.

### Changing Power and Orientation of Purchasers

In the last decade large employers' views of health benefits have undergone significant shifts. On a broad scale, employers concluded that part of the problem was the way health care was being purchased. As one employee benefits manager put it: "In the past, many of us in the business community simply were not prudent purchasers of medical care benefits. We routinely paid bills for medical care with no questions asked. Unknowingly, we contributed to the continuation of many abuses in the medical care system by simply signing the check and looking the other way—and by purchasing benefits that tended to encourage more costly forms of health care."[42]

In part as a consequence of analyzing patterns in their health care expenditures, some demystification of medical care has occurred in the eyes of corporate management. An illustration is the assessment by Lee Iacocca, chief executive officer of the Chrysler Corporation, of Chrysler's health care committee, made up of himself, Joseph Califano, a lawyer and former secretary of Health, Education and Welfare, former governor of Michigan William Millikin, and Douglas Fraser, then president of the United Auto Workers. "As a foursome," Iacocca wrote in 1984, "we probably know as much about health care as any four guys in the world."[43]

Many purchasers have come to view health care costs as just another corporate expense that requires management. For most large corporations, a first stage was to make some changes in benefit plans (more cost sharing by beneficiaries) and to self-insure, moving from insurance contracts to "administrative service only" contracts. The latter step enabled companies to manage the 5 to 10 percent of costs that was due to administration, and it set the stage for the attempt to manage the rest. More and more corporate benefit managers began to talk about health benefits as a complicated instance of a familiar problem—the procurement of the supplies and services needed in the production of the company's products.

Such a shift was described vividly in a 1986 speech by Patricia Nazemetz, Xerox's benefits development manager. Characterizing the traditional health benefit programs of Xerox and other companies as involving the "purchase of poorly defined products and services at undefined prices," she described changes that were under way to correct the problem. The model followed was a program that Xerox had adopted for acquiring the "commodities" needed by the company. This program involved reducing the number of suppliers by 90 percent (from 5,000 to 450 in the previous five years) and developing detailed specifications that suppliers must meet. Adapting this approach to health benefits meant that Xerox could define its own requirements regarding "benefit levels, service requirements, quality standards, and price," request proposals from health care providers, and select those "who can conform best to our specifications."[44] All of this is easier said than done, of course, but this was the direction in which Xerox and other companies set out to move during the mid-1980s.

Indeed, the idea of *purchaser-developed* specifications against which the performance of providers can be evaluated has become commonplace in corporate managers' discussions of health care. This reflects not only a changed view of what the purchase of health care is about but also a shift in power.

The ability of large purchasers to gain increased control over the conditions of their purchase of medical care comes in part from the fact that the element in shortest supply in the health care system is no longer hospital beds or physicians but patients who have the means to pay for care—insured patients. The role of purchasers' *power* in bringing about change is suggested by the fact that the precursor of many approaches now being used by payers to effect modifications in patterns of care came from the most powerful payer—Medicare and its associated utilization review efforts. The first use of utilization review requirements by private purchasers appears to have been in situations where those purchasers were in a particularly powerful position vis-à-vis health care providers, such as manufacturers with large facilities in midsized cities.[45] Corporate efforts to persuade hospitals to accept independent, concurrent utilization review (UR) activities were marked by conflict and the use of corporate economic power.[46]

## Industry Restructuring to Manage Health Care Costs

The determination of large public and private purchasers of care to control their health care costs has created two new markets that are transforming the provision of health services. The first is for organizations that integrate utilization and cost management with the provision of medical services. The second market is for organizations that offer utilization review and management services to purchasers (and providers) who seek to contain costs.

### Cost-Containing Provider Organizations

The demand has grown in both the private and public sectors for health care organizations that have cost-containment incentives built in—particularly by contracting to provide a set of defined services for a beneficiary population for a set amount of money. Thus, the past decade or so has seen considerable growth of HMOs, PPOs, and new insurance-provider hybrids, which must either have cost-control mechanisms in place or shift the economic risk to providers. The growing prominence of HMOs and PPOs was described in Chapter 9, as were some of the associated cost-containment methods—particularly the use of practitioner selection and incentives. The utilization review and management methods that will be discussed later in this chapter and in Chapter 11 can be used *within* such organizations, as well as in benefit plans that pay on a fee-for-service basis.

Price competition for the business of large purchasers has also produced changes among the country's largest insurers and multi-institutional systems of providers. In the mid-1980s those organizations began to market plans that relied on incentives and utilization management techniques to control costs. To gain marketing advantages and create internal incentives for cost control, several insurance companies, hospital chains, and HMOs took major steps toward integration of the insurer and provider functions.[47] By 1986 nine of the largest ten group insurance carriers (plus Blue Cross/Blue Shield), all six of the largest multihospital systems (including Voluntary Hospitals of America and American Healthcare Systems), and six of the eight largest HMO systems had developed an integrated product.[48]

Many vertically integrated insurance companies, HMOs, and large hospital chains developed so-called triple-option plans, which allow employees to enroll in an HMO, a PPO, or an indemnity plan, making their own tradeoff between price and freedom of choice in provider selection. Because premiums in those plans are typically based on the group's utilization experience, there is a close relationship between utilization levels within an employee group and the insurance rates paid by the employer.

The establishment of large, vertically integrated organizations that market different types of health plans to large employers in a highly competitive environment clearly created powerful incentives for the insurer-provider to control costs, with hospitalization itself heading the list of costs requiring control. Gaining such control, however, has not been easy. Earnings in insurer-provider hybrids in the first two or three years were very disappointing to sponsors and investors, and as a result some organizations moved out of the market while those remaining sought to reduce expenses through more vigorous utilization management.[49]

*Development of a Utilization Management Industry*
In the 1980s the success of large government and private purchasers of health care in finding ways to put all other parties at some economic risk has created new incentives for cost control. Hospitals have been put at risk by Medicare's prospective payment system and by their contracts with HMOs and PPOs. Economic risk is built into the contracts that HMOs and some PPOs have with enrollees and employers. Insurance companies and third-party administrators must have effective methods of utilization control to compete for the business of large employers.

The need to control costs has created a substantial and growing market for utilization management services for insurers, corporations, business coalitions, unions, and providers. A trade source listed more than 150 private independent utilization review organizations in 1987, a figure that did not include the utilization management programs of many insurers.[50] A 1989 industry survey by *Business Insurance* listed 125 utilization review organizations whose business covered as few as 10,000 and as many as 11 million individuals. (Again, utilization review departments of many insurers were not listed.) The number of Blue Cross plans that reported using utilization management methods increased from 28 to 95 percent between 1982 and 1986.[51] For hospitals and physicians (particularly those whose practices included a significant amount of hospitalization of patients) the work of utilization review organizations became omnipresent. The Mayo Clinic, which draws its patients from all over the country, reported that it had gone from dealing with a Medicare utilization management program in 1984 to dealing with more than a thousand utilization review plans four years later.[52] The American Hospital Association says that individual hospitals deal with anywhere from 50 to 250 such programs.[53]

Some utilization management organizations are descendants of the PSROs, many of which were marketing utilization review services to private customers by the early 1980s.[54] In addition, new organizations—some of which were spin-offs from PSROs—entered the market for utilization review and management services. Insurance companies, coping with the loss of business that resulted from employers' decisions to self-insure, saw the need to offer new services. The same was true of third-party administrators hired by self-insuring companies to process claims. Many of the largest utilization management organizations are now third-party administrators or insurance companies or their subsidiaries.[55]

The strategies, lines of business, market niches, and sophistication of organizations in the utilization management field are quite varied. Some organizations specialize in a specific service,. such as second-opinion programs; others offer a broad range of services. Some organizations have developed technologies and software packages that other organizations can use to analyze claims data or assess the appropriateness of services. A few such companies have gained enormous influence by developing and publicizing the methods that are used by many other companies.[56] Other organizations are primarily or exclusively engaged in the actual conduct of utilization management services for employers, insurers, or third-party administrators.

The services offered by the various organizations include comparative analyses of claims data for assessing the performance of providers against one another or against external standards, reviews of medical records to document inappropriate or poor care, and actual intervention in the patient care decision-making process through such programs as preadmission or preservice certification, continued-stay review, surgical second opinions, and case management. The methods, criteria, standards of appropriateness, and computer programs used by each organization is its own peculiar combination of invention, borrowing, adapting, and purchasing from other organizations. Many small organizations apparently use relatively simple systems derived from information in published sources.[57] Others have developed sophisticated computerized systems of their own, using criteria and standards borrowed and adapted from numerous sources.

## Medical Decision Making and the New Approaches to Cost Containment

Efforts of recent years to contain costs by influencing physicians' patient care decisions have led to the creation of new organizations, the shifting of economic risk, the collection and analysis of data, selective contracting, and the addition of new parties into patient care decisions. In one way or another all approaches affect the incentive structure that has been seen as the culprit behind payers' health care cost problems, but the different approaches vary in how they affect the doctor-patient relationship and the accountability structure of health care.

Major approaches that are designed to influence physicians' patient care decisions in ways that help control payers' costs fall into three categories: (1) approaches that rely primarily on incentives, (2) approaches that are based on retrospective review of services, and (3) approaches that involve interventions before services are provided. Although these approaches are often used in combination, it is convenient to treat them separately. I discuss the first two in the remainder of this chapter and the third in Chapter 11.

### Incentive Approaches

The creation of private and public third-party payment programs was seen as a way of enabling patients to get care without facing financial ruin, not as a way to create a set of financial incentives that would stimulate providers of medical care to act in accord with payers' goals. Yet, an unintended effect of the effort to facilitate access by removing financial barriers in a fee-for-service system has clearly been the creation of incentives that encouraged the provision of services, including services that were only marginally useful or even unnecessary.

As awareness has grown that these incentives were contributing to the health care cost problem, payers and organizers of services began to make use of new incentives designed to encourage physicians and hospitals to provide fewer services and less expensive care. Incentives that reward providers for containing costs can be structured in a variety of ways. Many approaches involve payments for groupings of services. Paying hospitals on a per-admission basis encourages the hospital to control the expenses incurred during the admission, for example, by minimizing testing and discharging the patient as early as possible. Incentives against hospitalization can be created through the use of capitation methods in which an HMO is paid an annual per-patient rate to provide a broad package of services including whatever hospital care is needed. Within HMOs incentives are commonly used for utilization management purposes, as when physicians contract to share responsibility for the total cost of the medical-surgical care to enrollees and receive bonuses when utilization or financial targets are met.[58] As I discussed in Chapter 9, many of the organizations that have created and used incentives for such purposes have their own economic interests and have fostered a growing physician dependence on them for access to patients. The cost-containment approaches of organizations such as HMOs with which physicians have a direct relationship are designed to give the physicians on whom patients rely for advice an economic stake in the control of costs.

The use of incentives to shift the economic risk also shifts the problem of controlling costs. From the payer's or HMO's standpoint, incentives can be used instead of monitoring or interventions to encourage providers to be cost conscious. But incentives that reward providers for cost containment also give them a reason not to provide all the services that were supposedly contracted for, so a need to monitor services remains. As monitoring has become less necessary for purposes of cost control, its role in quality control has become more apparent.[59]

Taxpayers and employees have an interest in containing health care costs, but the same individuals, when illness strikes and services are needed, undoubtedly hope that the physician will act in accord with the fiduciary ethic. Incentive arrangements that reward the physician for providing fewer services potentially conflict with the interests of individual patients. The question is how to reconcile the fiduciary ethic with efforts by the payer to manipulate the physician's behavior through the use of economic incentives. Lending importance to this question is the fact that patients often may not understand either the incentives or the physician behavior that they reward and, thus, may be in a poor position to protect their own interests.

### Retrospective Review

Because of the record-keeping practices associated with providing medical care and obtaining payment, medical care lends itself well to monitoring after services have been provided. Retrospective review (or utilization review, as it can be called) designed to deter payment for unnecessary services has been in use in the Medicare and Medicaid programs since the early 1970s, and the review of claims arising from particular episodes of care has spread in the private sector, as has the analysis of patterns of care. Such utilization review can be used to verify billing information, to identify unusual patterns of care that merit additional investigation or intervention, to compare providers by costs or treatment outcomes, to verify whether criteria of medical necessity have been met, and to assess quality of care.[60] Parties whose concern is cost containment or, in some cases, quality of care now commonly review care retrospectively.

In Chapter 9 I discussed the use of information on patterns of care to provide feedback to physicians (or institutions). Providing individual physicians with compilations of information that show how their patterns of care compare with quality standards or other physicians' patterns of care is one of several ways in which utilization review can contribute to quality as well as cost control. The results of retrospective utilization review activities can be used in a variety of other ways as well.

*To determine whether payment should be made.* Claims for payment can be compared with patient records to determine whether services that were billed for are shown. This may be useful in maintaining the financial accountability of providers of health care. Of much more significance from the standpoint of medical decision making are reviews aimed at determining whether criteria of medical necessity were met. Although the former determination may be useful in maintaining the financial accountability of providers of health care, the latter is of much greater significance from the standpoint of medical decision making.

The denial of payment on the basis of such audits has been much more characteristic of public programs than private ones.[61] But because it lends itself to use wherever a contractual relationship exists between payer and provider, retrospective review and payment denial is also commonly used in IPA-type HMO settings. Results to date are based much more on oral reports than on independent research. For example, one company estimates that its retrospective review program for outpatient services in an IPA throws approximately 20 percent of billings into a "questionable" category, of which about half are ultimately denied on the basis of a record review or the physician's failure to submit records for review.[62]

Interest in denying payment for unnecessary or inappropriate services has stimulated the development of criteria against which those matters can be judged. Work to develop criteria or "criteria maps" has been taking place for at least a decade, and for a growing number of conditions and procedures clear criteria have been developed by means of various types of professional consensus processes. Even where such criteria have been developed, however, there is often a need to apply judgment either because the criteria themselves have a subjective element or because it is difficult to cover all potentially relevant circumstances (clinical, individual, social) in a set of formal criteria.

The more specific, objective, and reliable those criteria are, the more applicable they become either before or after the provision of the service.

*To focus more intensive utilization review efforts.* Retrospective data analyses can be used to identify unusual patterns of care for additional study or intervention and to identify institutions or situations where more intensive utilization controls (such as prior authorization of services) may be cost effective. Profile analysis—aggregating utilization data to profile institutions, practitioners, or types of patients—was part of the PSRO program from the mid-1970s and can be used to identify possible quality problems or unnecessary services, information which can then be investigated further.[63]

A more recent approach is the development of screens to identify questionable services. A well-known set of such screens was developed for outpatient physician Medicaid claims in California and was subsequently marketed under the name "Patterns of Treatment."[64] In using a computerized version of this set of screens, Metropolitan Life found that 75 percent of "screen failures" were accounted for by only 5 percent of physicians.[65] By focusing their utilization review program on this small group, they reported that they were able to minimize employee disruption and achieve a savings-to-expense ratio of about four to one.[66] Another set of proprietary screens is used by a managed care firm called CAPP CARE, which sends out letters to physicians whose patient care practices trigger the screen. Physicians are said to be "highly responsive."[67]

Other interesting uses of utilization data have been reported by private employers. For example, when insurance claims data for workers, retirees, and beneficiaries covered by General Motors' health benefits were aggregated and analyzed, it was learned that there were very high hospitalization rates among employees in New Jersey, very high use of podiatry services in the counties surrounding Detroit (podiatry costs are 6.5 times higher there than in other urban areas of Michigan), high rates of cesarean deliveries in Michigan, and "a disturbingly high recidivism rate among alcohol and drug abusers, with some employees going through treatment centers dozens of times."[68]

A Ford Motor Company study of 20,000 hospital admissions of

persons covered by its health plan in southeastern Michigan in 1984 found that the company had paid for over 27,000 possibly unnecessary hospital days at a cost of $15 million and had paid an additional $5 million in excess costs for services rendered. The total amounted to 21 percent of Ford's payments for inpatient care at southeastern Michigan hospitals in 1984. The hospitals were asked to submit corrected bills and corrective-action plans that addressed all identified problems. Several hospitals were earmarked for further "intensive follow-up activity."[69]

Such examples convince purchasers of the wisdom of increasing their oversight of health care providers and have resulted in a growing interest in using claims data to identify patterns of care that deserve closer attention. Once questionable patterns are identified, a variety of strategies can be used to deal with them—persuasion, benefit plan changes, implementation of prior authorization programs, or creation of preferred provider networks that exclude certain providers.

*To select providers for contracting or to determine whether a contract will be renewed.* Contracts between purchasers of care and providers are becoming more common in both public programs, such as California's Medi-Cal program, and among large employers (such as Honeywell, Inc.). Also, HMOs typically provide for the hospitalization needs of enrollees through contracts with selected hospitals, and selectivity is part of the very rationale of preferred provider arrangements.

Selective contracting is a necessary but not sufficient condition for movement toward a health care system in which large purchasers buy medical care based on providers' past performance. Accounts to date suggest that providers have not been selected on the basis of past performance but on the basis of price (as with Medi-Cal) or of submitted bids that, in the Honeywell case, were evaluated on criteria that included "design flexibility; a working case management program; cost sharing and financial flexibility; legal compliance with government regulations; willingness to be audited; and customer services such as a grievance mechanism."[70] In the first generation of PPOs, which were generally sponsored by *providers* to enhance or protect their market share, business was sought by offering purchasers discounts from charges, not by providing data on performance. Increasingly, however, PPOs are sponsored by employers and other insurers,[71] and "selective contracting with cost-effective providers" now receives mention as an element of cost containment in these arrangements.[72]

Vendors now offer the services of data systems that will allow employers and insurers to compare providers' performance and make some rough assessments of cost effectiveness. Tables 10.2 and 10.3 are examples of the kind of data that can be produced using available data systems. Table 10.2 compares the cost and complication rate for a surgical procedure at nine hospitals and also provides a means for evaluating whether the differences are due to the severity of cases on admission. The combination of cost, complications, and severity suggests which hospitals a purchaser or patient might wish to use. Table 10.3 provides information of a similar nature for childbirth.

Access to such data enables purchasers to select hospitals not only on the basis of cost but also on some tentative indicators of quality and effectiveness. Insofar as the purchaser's data are gen-

*Table 10.2.*    Costs, severity index, and complications for gallbladder surgery (total cholecystectomy) in 9 hospitals

| Hospital | Total $ | Severity index[a] | Complication rate (%)[b] |
|----------|---------|-------------------|--------------------------|
| A | 4,906 | 1.57 | 4.7 |
| B | 2,900 | 1.46 | 2.5 |
| C | 5,390 | 1.39 | 9.1 |
| D | 3,585 | 1.38 | 3.4 |
| E | 6,008 | 1.38 | 3.2 |
| F | 2,756 | 1.33 | 1.9 |
| G | 4,916 | 1.28 | 6.7 |
| H | 3,374 | 1.17 | 1.9 |
| I | 3,129 | 1.13 | 4.3 |

Source: Copyright © 1986 by MediQual Systems, Inc. All rights reserved. Used with permission.
a. Based on MediQual's MedisGroups severity score.
b. Based on the MedisGroups morbidity indicator.

Table 10.3. Hospital-specific profiles of obstetric care: deliveries (DRGs 370–374)[a] in one city

| Hospitals | Average total $ | Average length of stay (days) | Cesarean section (%) | Hypoxia/asphyxia rate per 1,000 |
|---|---|---|---|---|
| A | 1,428 | 3.5 | 18 | 12 |
| B | 1,538 | 3.6 | 20 | 11 |
| C | 1,635 | 3.6 | 25 | 28 |
| D | 1,841 | 3.7 | 19 | 38 |
| E | 2,101 | 4.4 | 34 | 53 |
| F | 2,174 | 4.3 | 33 | 11 |
| G | 2,481 | 3.9 | 15 | 8 |
| H | 2,512 | 4.2 | 19 | 8 |
| Overall average[b] | 1,809 | 4.0 | 25 | 18 |

Source: Copyright © 1986 by the Health Data Institute™. All rights reserved. Used with permission.
a. N > 750 cases in DRGs 370–374 (high length-of-stay outliers trimmed).
b. All averages are age-adjusted.

erated through the claims payment process, however, the more a purchaser contracts selectively, the more a particular purchaser's ability to make comparisons among providers will decline. In the long run, the benefits of such analyses will best be realized through data systems and reporting requirements that are available publicly.

Several factors now discourage providers from making available data that would enable purchasers to compare costs and outcomes.[73] The high costs of documenting and ensuring quality might put a provider at a disadvantage if purchasers wanted to buy on price alone.[74] Providing purchasers with information about quality might also entail the risk of creating physician dissatisfaction, and documentation of the degree of conformity to quality standards could generate fears of liability in influential quarters. Serious efforts to control quality would also require more of a top-down management structure than now exists in hospitals. For all of these reasons, few hospitals may take the steps that would be necessary to compete on the basis of documented quality and efficiency unless there were strong pressure from purchasers to do so.

Purchasers may be reluctant to make such demands. Employees would have to be convinced that they were not selecting certain providers merely to save money. Some employers might face a loss of business from providers who are important customers if they were not selected. Valuable personal and social relationships between hospital and business leaders might be jeopardized.[75] The necessary data systems often do not exist. Also, bureaucratic factors, such as the division of responsibilities between purchasing and personnel departments and the reward structures for executives, could make it difficult to address the issue.[76]

Nevertheless, through the activities of local health care coalitions and organizations such as the Washington Bureau Group on Health, the Midwest Business Group on Health, and the U.S. Chamber of Commerce, and through an accumulation of experience, corporations are becoming more sophisticated and innovative in seeking to control health care costs. In some locales, such as the Twin Cities, Des Moines, and Worcester, Massachusetts, the aggressiveness of purchasers, the competitiveness among providers, and the growing availability of data are creating environments in which selective purchasing based on quality and efficiency can develop. Legislation was passed in 1986 in Pennsylvania to create a Health Data Council to collect and analyze data on both the price and quality (readmission, mortality, morbidity, and infection rates) of health care services from facilities and physicians, and to make such data publicly available.[77] A project is under way in five Pennsylvania cities to help providers learn to use the data to improve their performance and to help purchasers develop methods whereby they can shift patients to institutions that perform best.

In sum, although utilization review data about quality and efficiency are not yet used by employers and third-party payers to select their health providers, trends toward selective purchasing and the development of increasingly sophisticated data systems increase the likelihood that such an approach to purchasing medical care will emerge.

## Utilization Review and Public Disclosure

The health care cost problem has led to a series of developments that increase the oversight of the providers of health services. Third-party payment has led to the use of data systems that have the potential for increasing the consequences for providers of high costs and poor quality. The use of these data systems creates pressure for their improvement.

The full potential for making purchasers of care more knowledgeable and rational has not yet been realized. There are obstacles to be overcome, but data systems that are useful sometimes take on a life of their own.

The use of monitoring systems in which claims or discharge data are collected and analyzed makes possible another form of accountability: to the public via the publication of comparisons of the costs and outcomes of care provided by different institutions and practitioners. Advocates argue that public disclosure of such information would help patients (and their physicians) to make more informed choices of hospitals or HMOs.

Utilization review organizations and health care providers have generally opposed the release of such data because they believe that the public will be unable to make intelligent use of it and that disclosure can be unfair to providers. The information may not mean what it seems to mean.[78] Excellent institutions or practitioners could have high mortality rates because they attract the most difficult cases.[79] The review organizations that collect and analyze utilization data tend not to reach conclusions based solely on institutional profiles but, instead, use those profiles to identify targets for closer and more valid reviews; thus, they find the idea that patients might select providers solely on the basis of profile data (for example, mortality rates) alarming.

Private organizations that collect and analyze utilization data for private clients have little reason to release data, as do their clients. Why give away proprietary information that was costly to develop, particularly if there is the possibility of being sued by a provider whose reputation may be harmed? Nonetheless, much utilization information is collected and analyzed with the support of tax dollars, by federal or state government payers, regulators, or data collection agencies, or by government contractors, most notably PROs. Here the questions of liability and proprietary interests in the data are much less germane. Furthermore, arguments for disclosure can be made on the basis of government sunshine laws and/or on the government's responsibility for the health and welfare of the people.[80]

Until 1986 those who objected to the release of utilization review data about identified institutions generally prevailed, although there were public disclosures of data on institutional performance in a few cities.[81] In early 1986 it became known that the Health Care Financing Administration (HCFA) had compiled lists of institutions with unusually high and low mortality rates. The lists had been compiled for use by PROs, but in response to public pressure, on March 10, 1986, they were published and received widespread publicity. In general, consumer groups applauded the action ("a major victory for health-care consumers" according to the People's Medical Society),[82] while providers pointed out that a high mortality rate at an institution could have many causes, including the presence of a hospice.[83] In August 1986 California Medical Review, Inc., a PRO, released hospital-specific data, including mortality rates, based on the analysis of 826,000 Medicare discharges over a one-year period,[84] and in 1987 HCFA released its second analysis of mortality data on identified hospitals. This detailed and more methodologically sophisticated analysis filled seven thick volumes.[85] By 1989 the release filled thirteen large volumes.[86] (In May 1990 HCFA released a ninety-three-volume report on nursing homes, based on thirty-two quality indicators assessed during one-day surveys of the 15,000 skilled nursing facilities in the United States.)[87] With the issuance of the hospital mortality data and the report on nursing homes, the debate shifted from the desirability of the public release of data by the Health Care Financing Administration and/or PROs on facilities and outcomes of medical care to the question of how to improve the quality of the data that *are* released.

Third-party purchasers of medical care have responded to the problem of costs in ways that have great significance for the accountability structure of health care. Developments include implementing new payment methods that create different kinds of incentives, contracting with selected providers, and undertaking monitoring activities that are unprecedented in their scope and detail. A whole industry has been created that markets cost-containment services to purchasers. The most significant development, however, has been the widespread adoption of cost-containment methods that operate on a case-by-case basis prior to the provision of services. Those methods are the subject of Chapter 11.

# · 11 ·

# Utilization Management
# by Third Parties

Many medical services are unnecessary or are provided in unnecessarily expensive ways or settings. That is the lesson that payers and other parties who are concerned with health care costs have drawn from the studies and corporate experiences that were described in Chapter 10. Until recent years, however, third-party payers—particularly those in the private sector—had few practical ways of avoiding paying for unnecessary or inappropriate services or even of identifying them. Bills from health care providers do not announce which, if any, services were not really needed. And attempts by an insurer to deny payment may leave the patient on the hook for the bill, with consequences that could range from employee dissatisfaction to a bad faith lawsuit against the erstwhile payer.[1] Questions of fairness are endemic. Many private payers have not found retrospective denials a feasible approach to cost containment. Yet the work of researchers, PSROs, and insurers showed that it was possible to develop some relatively objective tools for distinguishing necessary or appropriate care from unnecessary or inappropriate care.[2]

These circumstances provide the background for the emergence of a group of cost-containment methods that share an element that would have been unthinkable a decade or two ago: a party other than the physician and patient is introduced into the decision about whether (and where) particular services should be provided to particular patients. Such *utilization management*[3] (UM) is designed to preclude payment for unnecessary or inappropriate services and to see that services are provided in a manner that minimizes costs (for example, on an outpatient rather than an inpatient basis). UM is carried out by many organizations that have an interest in cost containment—government programs such as Medicare and Medicaid, insurers, third-party administrators, specialized UM companies, HMOs, and PPOs. I will use the term *utilization management organization* (UMO) to refer to any organization that carries out UM.

The discussion in this chapter is based both on the published literature (much of which is in trade sources rather than in peer-reviewed journals) and on information I obtained as director of the Institute of Medicine's two-year study of utilization management.[4] The IOM report was based on discussions at eight meetings of a study committee that included several leaders in the field, a public hearing, a group of commissioned papers, and site visits to twelve UMOs, including independent UM firms, insurance company subsidiaries, PROs, and HMOs.[5]

## The Methods of Utilization Management

Three utilization management approaches—second-opinion programs, discharge planning, and high-cost case management—rest primarily on the involvement of specialized personnel. In two other approaches—preadmission (or preservice) certification and concurrent review during hospitalization—patients' needs for services are evaluated against objective criteria in a process that is designed to be implemented by nurses, with physician backup. The criteria-based approaches have great potential for shaping the medical decision making of the future because of their relatively low cost as well as flexibility and widespread applicability. Criteria of appropriateness or necessity are being developed for a growing number of procedures and patients' circumstances.

The UM programs for particular patients may be triggered in different ways. Depending on the program, the involvement of a UMO may be triggered by hospitalization, the decision for an elective hospitalization (or hospitalization for an elective procedure), or, in a growing number of programs, the decision that the patient will undergo certain diagnostic or surgical procedures even if hospitalization is not contemplated. Beneficiaries of third-party payment plans are put on notice that full coverage by their health benefits is contingent on their getting prior authorization for elective hospitalization or for certain procedures. Because hospitals and physicians have an important stake in the health benefit plan's coverage of a patient's expenses, they have learned to inquire about these matters and frequently initiate the UM process themselves. For patients with unplanned admissions to the hospital, the review process is initiated after admission, with the hospital often taking the initiative. Once the UMO has been notified, the applicable UM methods can be brought into play.

## Approaches that Rely on Expert Personnel

### Second-Opinion Programs

Second-opinion programs are the oldest form of utilization management, having been in use since the early 1970s. In these programs patients are required or encouraged to obtain an opinion from a second physician before undergoing procedures that are believed to be subject to unnecessary use. Strictly speaking, such programs do not involve third-party *management* of utilization; rather, they usually increase the amount of information available to patients in making decisions regarding elective procedures. For many payers second-opinion programs were their first foray into UM, but they have at most a relatively small place in most current UM programs.

As with all methods of UM, much variation exists among programs. The process is generally activated in a preadmission (or preservice) review program in which patients or providers must obtain authorization prior to the provision of services. UMOs have lists of procedures for which second opinions may be required. Patients for whom a second opinion is required are generally given the names of specialists who can provide the consultation. This is not a standardized matter, however, and it can raise significant issues. One is whether patients will be referred to a physician with the same specialty as the original physician. (The referral physician might be either more or less "qualified" than the original, but in either case controversy can result.) Another is whether the referral physician will be one who is known by the UMO to be conservative regarding the use of the procedure in question. One of the UMOs visited during the Institute of Medicine study was marketing (with apparent success) a program in which the "second opinion" was provided by a staff physician at the UMO who did not even examine the patient.

Programs may be voluntary or mandatory. Voluntary programs encourage second opinions by covering their cost; mandatory programs require second opinions as a condition of payment. The voluntary programs generally have low rates of participation— only 1 to 2 percent of those eligible[6]—but the percentage of nonconfirming opinions (30 percent is typical) is about twice as high as in mandatory programs, presumably because of patient self-selection.[7] In most instances, after the second opinion has been obtained, the patient (and the original physician) can decide whether to go ahead with the procedure. In a few programs, however, differences may have to be resolved by a third opinion.

Second-opinion programs lend themselves to simple though potentially misleading calculations of results—percentages of opinions that are confirmed and percentages of patients who undergo surgery within some time period (usually six months or a year). Most studies of second-opinion programs have reported a savings of two to four dollars for each dollar they cost, though one study showed a loss.[8] In the first eight years of the pioneer Cornell–New York Hospital program, two-thirds of patients whose first opinion was not confirmed had not had surgery six months later, compared to 16 percent in the group who received a confirming second opinion.[9] In the first three years of this program, surgical claims decreased by 9 percent; annual decreases of 10 percent were reported by another mandatory program.[10] Calculations of savings are generally based on the costs of surgery not performed. This is most readily calculated for surgeries not confirmed and not performed, but advocates believe that savings also result from a sentinel effect, which causes less surgery to be proposed when a second-opinion program is in place.[11]

There is, nevertheless, room for doubt about the effects of second-opinion programs. The number of people who do not have recommended surgery outside of second-opinion programs is not known, and nothing is known about the number of people who would have declined surgery after one opinion but were persuaded to proceed by a confirming opinion.[12] Only data from a randomized trial would measure both these factors and the full effect (including the sentinel effect) or lack of effect of a second-opinion program.

The impact of second-opinion programs also depends heavily on how the program is focused (that is, to what procedures or circumstances the requirement is attached). For many procedures the percentage of confirming second opinions is so high that the cost of the program would exceed any savings. And even for conditions where there is a payoff (for example, tonsillectomies), some percentage of patients will have symptoms that leave little doubt that a second opinion would confirm the first. For this reason many UMOs use screens and waive second-opinion requirements for patients whose history or symptoms suggest that a second opinion is likely to confirm the first. It is clear that focusing can be used to increase the payoff per dollar invested. But the more tightly focused a second-opinion program is, the fewer the patients to whom it will apply and the smaller the role that second opinions will play in the overall cost-containment program.

Discussions with industry leaders and the site visits conducted during the IOM study suggest that second-opinion programs are coming to play only a limited, though perhaps still important, role in utilization management programs. Second opinions may prove to be most useful in situations in which the evidence suggests to the UMO that a procedure is unnecessary but the UMO is reluctant to deny coverage without independent confirmation by an examining physician because of the risk of liability if the decision is wrong. Used in this manner, a second-opinion program is an element in prior-authorization programs (discussed later in this chapter).

### Discharge Planning Programs

Another approach involves discharge planning programs, which are designed to minimize hospital lengths of stay by helping patients and their families, physicians, and hospitals arrange for services at home or in skilled nursing facilities. The discharge planner may be an employee of the hospital. Hospitals may use discharge planning to ensure that patients' needs are being met; in fact, Medicare requires hospitals to use discharge planning as a safeguard against the danger that the prospective payment system's incentives (payment on a per-case basis) will result in neglect of the needs of patients who can be discharged from the hospital but still need some services. The discharge planning efforts of UMOs are generally part of broader concurrent review or case management programs and as such have not been evaluated separately.

### Case Management Approaches

At least two distinct cost-containment approaches are referred to as case management. Both can be distinguished from the social work version of case management, which is aimed more at the coordination of services than at cost containment. Some HMOs and state Medicaid programs use case management to control the use of specialists or specialized services by making payment contingent on their having been recommended by a "gatekeeper," or primary care physician to whom each patient is assigned.[13] This physician may be given economic incentives not to make such referrals. For example, the physician may receive a set amount from which all physician services must be paid. Although the obvious intent is to discourage the excessive use of specialists, the danger is that the gatekeeper will become too reluctant to make referrals. In any event, this approach involves the organization of services rather than the introduction of a third party into patient care decisions and thus does not fit my definition of utilization management.

Many UMOs use a very different type of case management that does involve third parties. It is commonly called *high-cost* or *large* case management. The focus is on selected types of high-cost patients. These may be patients who have suffered a sudden catastrophic event (a stroke or an automobile accident) that may require a long hospitalization, or they may be patients who have serious, often fatal, chronic conditions (certain cancers, AIDS) that require repeated hospitalization. In any insured group a relatively small percentage of cases accounts for a disproportionately large share of expenses.[14] The idea of high-cost case management is to seek savings in the care of such patients. A 1987 trade survey of large employers found that about half were using what was termed "case management for catastrophic illness," up from almost none only a few years earlier.[15]

Although large expenditures for individual patients are sometimes difficult to avoid, costs can often be reduced in complex cases. A fragmented health care system is at its worst in providing care to patients with chronic conditions who need various types of services. Overlapping and redundant services are common, as are gaps in services. Moreover, the prevailing fee-for-service mode of payment does not create attention among providers to the cumulative patterns and costs of the services that the patient receives. Worse, it encourages the overuse of services. And patients with chronic diseases or conditions that require extensive rehabilitation may initially be in the hands of physicians whose relevant training and experience is limited.

For all of these reasons, some UMOs (including HMOs) find that specialized attention to the management of services provided to certain types of patients can significantly affect costs. Patients diagnosed with conditions that have the potential for incurring extraordinarily high costs can be identified early and assigned to a case manager, who can arrange for such patients to receive the most suitable combination of services, including care in less expensive settings than hospitals. UMOs that use high-cost case management programs contend that because they have much greater experience in managing potentially catastrophic cases than the average practitioner, they can contribute to "better quality care through appropriate planning and intervention" and can "establish the payer as a patient advocate who ensures high quality care."[16]

As a practical matter, however, it appears that the case management efforts of most UMOs have a relatively narrow goal: to find ways of getting high-cost patients out of hospitals and into less expensive settings. This may require locating sources of skilled nursing or home care, educating patients and physicians about emerging alternatives (for example, in 1988 some case managers were conveying information about the feasibility of doing continuing infusions of antibiotics at home), and getting employers to waive benefit plan restrictions (for instance, on home care) that can have the effect of making it costly for the patient to leave the hospital.[17]

The basic elements of high-cost case management are relatively straightforward. Cases can be identified by the case management program on admission (through reporting requirements attached to hospitalization) or when bills begin to arrive. (Obviously, the former method contains a much larger potential for savings, since the payer may not start receiving bills for several months.) In most UMOs the case managers are usually experienced nurses who operate via telephone. In the dozen organizations visited in the IOM study, however, several variations were found. One organization used physicians as case managers, and another's nurses actually visited the patients, families, and doctors. UMOs that operate by telephone may deal only with the patient's physician (obtaining information and offering advice about alternatives) or with the patient, family, *and* physician.

Despite these differences, most high-cost case management programs share an element that departs philosophically from the prior-authorization methods described later in this chapter. At least as reported in 1988, their logic was to generate alternatives that could be offered to—not required of—patients, families, and physicians. Aversion to a lengthy hospitalization appears to open the way to consideration of other options.

Despite the claim that high-cost case management *both* improves quality and contains costs, most supporting information comes from case management vendors who have a stake in reporting positive results.[18] Virtually all of their evaluations are based on comparisons of the care (and its costs) that patients actually received with the vendor's estimation of the care and costs that would have occurred in the absence of case management. These accounts can be very convincing, but as evidence they are far removed from a controlled study.

Such a study would be very difficult to conduct, however, so most evidence will likely continue to be of the sort that the Institute of Medicine was able to identify: the 13 dollars saved in averted costs for each dollar spent in a case management program conducted for the Service Employees International Union in Oregon (the savings ratio subsequently dropped to 4 to 1); the $1.2 million saved (for $155,000 costs) in the first year of the Bank of America's case management program for people with AIDS; the nearly $2 million that Blue Cross of Philadelphia saved on thirty cases in 1987.[19] The only independent study that the IOM committee found (by Mary Henderson and colleagues at Brandeis University) had independent consultants do case-by-case evaluations of the impact of one UMO's case management program. As the IOM report characterized the result, "In general, the consultants were considerably more conservative in their projections of savings than the case managers."[20]

Reasonable skepticism notwithstanding, many of the claims of case management programs have considerable plausibility. Furthermore, nothing that came to light during the IOM study contradicted the claims of the UM firms that case management programs are accepted well by patients and their families. The situations in which case management is introduced, the voluntary nature of most programs, and the specialized knowledge that case managers can apply all lend plausibility to the generally positive assessment that is reported in most high-cost case management programs. Although more evidence is needed before any self-respecting health services researcher would draw conclusions about the value of case management approaches, the anecdotal accounts of success have stimulated widespread acceptance among UMOs and their clients.[21]

## Criteria-Based Approaches

Chapter 10 described the development of criteria or decision rules for determining whether the services received by a particular patient were necessary or appropriate. In utilization *review* programs, in the terminology that I am using, criteria are applied *after* services are provided either to determine whether payment should be made or to measure the extent to which services are inappropriate or unnecessary. In utilization *management* programs, the criteria are applied *prior* to the provision of services.

The utilization management approach that has the most far-reaching implications and has generated the most controversy involves prior-authorization programs—programs that make payment (in whole or in part) contingent on the patient's or provider's (whether doctor or hospital) obtaining authorization (or precertification) from a party concerned with cost management before covered services are provided to the patient. (Services provided in an urgent or emergency situation are handled differently.)

Prior-authorization programs are designed to eliminate payment for services that are unnecessary and to encourage the use of less expensive alternatives to hospitals.[22] The scope of a prior-authorization program may be broad (covering all planned hospital admissions) or it may focus on particular diagnoses or providers where there has been evidence of inappropriate services. Though most commonly applied to admissions to or continued stays in the hospitals, prior-authorization requirements can be applied to any service that is costly enough to justify the expense.

Prior authorization often also serves as a tool for implementing other cost-containment approaches. For example, a widely used step for reducing hospital use in the 1980s was to change the established practice of admitting patients to the hospital a day or two in advance of surgery for testing and other preparations. To encourage that such testing be done before admission, many prior-authorization programs refused to certify the necessity of days of hospitalization preceding surgery, except under special circumstances. In a similar fashion, pressure was brought to bear that encouraged the shift from inpatient to outpatient surgery for many procedures. Prior-authorization requirements are also often used in conjunction with other UM or cost-containment approaches—for example, as a way of identifying potential cases for high-cost case management or a highly focused second-opinion program, or for conveying to the patient that the amount of payment may depend on whether or not services are obtained from hospitals that are part of a preferred provider network.

Although prior authorization is used in some government programs, the most widespread, advanced, and controversial uses of this approach to cost containment have been among private insurers and self-insured employers that purchase services on a fee-for-service basis (hence the term *managed fee-for-service*). The impact reported by the companies that experimented early with UM was so dramatic that the use of these approaches (and the size of the industry that provided them) grew at an extraordinary rate. A 1987 survey of large employers showed that more than 60 percent were using preadmission review and about half were using concurrent review.[23] Such programs had been in use among only a handful of companies three or four years previously. Moreover, another survey showed that preadmission certification or continued-stay review was used in 80 to 90 percent of preferred provider organizations,[24] and a study of "determinants of HMO success" found that successful HMOs generally "have strong administrative controls on utilization and/or strong incentive programs."[25] Changed incentives (particularly Medicare's prospective payment system) have also caused many hospitals to establish or strengthen their internal systems, particularly continued-stay reviews for hospitalized patients. The various forms of prior authorization have clearly become a normal part of the purchase of medical care by third parties in the United States.

Physicians experience these requirements as an interference in the doctor-patient relationship. They have complained that this interference is coming from someone who does not even see the patient and may not even be an appropriate specialist—or even a physician. The industries that provide or purchase UM services describe the process in more innocuous terms. They note that health benefit plans generally cover only medically necessary and appropriate services, and that prior-authorization requirements let the doctor, hospital, and patient know whether services that have not yet been provided will be deemed eligible ("certified") for payment under those provisions. However preauthorization processes are viewed, they have obvious potential for shaping medical decision making and influencing the services that patients receive.

*How the process works.* In the traditional fee-for-service context involving employee health benefits, prior-authorization requirements are implemented in the following way.[26] Provisions are built into employees' health benefit or health insurance plans that tie payment for services to the employees' compliance with preauthorization requirements.[27] Thus, not surprisingly, the leverage that makes the system work is financial, with both patients and providers having an interest in ensuring that required steps are followed. The employer or insurer contracts with a UMO to provide the service. This organization may be a subsidiary of an insurance company, a third-party administrator hired by self-insuring companies, or an independent UMO.

For the self-insuring employer, the financial benefits of reduced utilization levels are obvious. But employers who contract with the insurance carriers that underwrite their health care expenditures and bear the financial risk also benefit financially either through discounts or lower experience-rated premiums. In both cases the UMO is directly accountable to a payer whose interest is in controlling health care costs.

Although many accounts in the trade press and elsewhere describe how a "typical" review program works, my major impression from visiting twelve UMOs during the IOM study of utilization management was of significant variations among programs.[28] These variations would appear to have implications for the efficiency and rigor of programs, the burdens that they place on providers, and the safeguards that exist for patients, but no studies are available to document in any systematic way the consequences of the differences. In describing the prior-authorization process, I will try to convey something about the variations among organizations that are engaged in UM.

Typically, before a nonemergency hospitalization (or the use of certain procedures), the patient, a physician, or an employee of the physician or hospital must contact the UMO (usually by telephone), learn whether prior authorization is required as a condition of payment, and if so, provide the information—diagnosis, plan of treatment, estimated length of stay, and complicating medical factors—that the UMO requires for making its decision whether to certify the service.[29] For unplanned admissions, the process begins after the patient is already in the hospital and focuses on the appropriateness of a continued stay, as does the concurrent review process used with all hospitalizations. In concurrent reviews, contacts are usually initiated by the UMO, which may check with the physician's office or the hospital either daily or less often to request status reports for assessing the need for continued hospitalization.

Certification for admission is often accompanied by authorization of a specified number of days of stay; separate approval may have to be obtained if the patient is to be kept in the hospital longer.[30] Nonetheless, continued-stay review programs are not necessarily based on lengths of stay assigned before admission. For example, U.S. Administrators, which administers health benefit plans for self-insured employers, bases continued-stay decisions on daily calls to attending physicians.[31] Continued-stay review programs often use standard norms—most commonly diagnosis-specific average length-of-stay figures from the Professional Activity Study (PAS) of the Commission on Professional and Hospital Activities—to trigger the review of a patient's need for continued hospitalization. The decision whether additional days of hospitalization are warranted may be based on objective criteria, the reviewer's clinical judgment, and justifications provided by the attending physician.

At the UMO the information on a planned admission or service (or the initial review of an unplanned admission) is received by a reviewer—a nurse in most cases. UMOs all value experience on the part of their review nurses, and the majority seem to have been successful in recruiting a cadre of knowledgeable nurses. There is, however, a great deal of variation among UMOs in how much training they receive, how much authority they have (some UMOs encourage their nurses to negotiate with physicians; others forbid it), how much work they are expected to handle, and how they are supervised and monitored.[32]

Generally, while still on the telephone with the physician's office or hospital, nurse-reviewers assess the information about proposed services against the policies the UMO has adopted regarding how such cases should be handled. Do the symptoms justify hospitalization? Should the procedure be done on an outpatient basis? (For some procedures certain UMOs have begun asking whether the procedure itself is necessary.) Is a second opinion warranted? How long should the patient be in the hospital? Some UMOs even consider questions such as the number of surgeons that should be involved in a case. The UMO's answers to those questions are built into a set of screens, decision rules, criteria of appropriateness, and length-of-stay norms.

In the early days these policies, screens, rules, and criteria were contained in manuals, and the information about the patient was recorded by hand. Now industry leaders use computerized systems. The information obtained from the physician is entered into the computer along with basic information about the employee, the insured group, the physician, and the scheduled date of the service or hospital admission. The computer compares the information with the screens and criteria that are built into the software.

If proposed services pass the screens and meet the criteria, approval is conveyed immediately. If not, the nurse-reviewer makes this known and indicates that the case will be referred to a physician-adviser (or consultant physician), who may then discuss the case with the attending physician. UMOs vary enormously in the percentage of cases that are referred to physician-advisers. Two UMOs in the IOM study said that only 1 or 2 percent of cases go to advisers, while five organizations said that this happens with 10 or 15 percent of their cases.[33] By contrast, an industry leader that was visited reported that 40 percent of its cases are referred to a physician-adviser, and one firm advertises 100 percent physician review, although this seems to be something of a matter of terminology (screening by computers is still used) and of marketing strategy. Obviously the more cases that pass through the first set of screens, the smaller the burden a UMO's program places on providers, and the smaller the likelihood that the UM program will change the care that patients would otherwise receive.

The organizations visited during the IOM study all indicated that they would never deny authorization without review by a physician-adviser. In most of the organizations—PROs seem to be the exceptions, having a history of physician review based on the documentation supplied by review nurses—the physician-adviser contacts the patient's physician to discuss the case, seeks information that might justify an exception to the criteria, and tries to get the physician to accept the UMO's determination. From the point of view of the UMOs, these exchanges are "collegial." At least, that is the tone that most say they strive for.

As the physician-adviser's role is generally described, their determinations are based on their knowledge and experience, not just on application of the UMO's criteria. It is probably true that physician-advisers do not find it necessary to refer to the organization's criteria or to formal lists of allowable exceptions. Yet this does not mean that the criteria are irrelevant to the physician-adviser's evaluations. In some UMOs the advisers themselves have developed or approved the criteria and are responsible for updating them. Also, some UMOs have monitoring processes and regular discussion sessions among physician-advisers for purposes of ensuring quality control and consistency of decisions. At the other extreme, the advisers in some UMOs are office-based physicians who work by telephone from their own offices, are subject to minimal oversight, and have little if any contact with one another. In such programs the scope of the application of the physician-adviser's clinical judgment is maximized, and the amount of consistency is doubtful. Such advisers may also tend to identify more with the point of view of the patient's physician (and to be comparatively unwilling to deny certification) than advisers who are regular employees of a UMO and who work on site and regularly meet both formally and informally.

In circumstances in which a physician-adviser does not authorize the course a patient's physician proposes, an appeals process is generally available. This usually involves review by another physician—often but not necessarily in the same specialty as the attending physician—who is employed by or is a consultant to the UMO. (Some UMOs have panels of physicians for this purpose.) A few UMOs, perhaps reluctant to accept responsibility for actually denying authorization, apparently use the appeals process and its attendant delays as a substitute for denials, counting on the fact that a certain number of physicians will not follow through on appeals.

Most UMOs visited during the IOM study reported that denials occur in no more than 1 or 2 percent of cases, although they indicated that modifications of proposed care are negotiated with patients' physicians in a much larger proportion of cases. If certification is actually denied, the doctor and patient can choose to proceed anyway, but the patient faces financial penalties, and the provider faces the risk of not receiving full payment. No one seems to know how often this occurs.

How willing are UMOs to make exceptions to their criteria (for example, allowing preoperative stays or a hospital admission for a surgical procedure that is usually authorized only on an outpatient basis)? In the early days of UM it was commonly said that determined physicians could generally prevail and obtain the decision they sought through the appeals process,[34] although little documentation is available to verify this. Discussions with UMOs in 1988 during the IOM study suggested that UMOs differ in how firm they are willing to be with physicians. (Physicians also undoubtedly vary in their willingness to invest the time and effort involved in gaining authorization from a UMO.) Some UMOs take pride in their willingness to adopt a hard line against making exceptions to their criteria, unless clear justification (such as some unusual aspect of the patient's condition) is present. Other UMOs make a virtue of not injecting themselves between the doctor and patient, which they see as the effect of denying coverage. (Significantly, National Medical Audit, a firm that evaluates UMOs for corporate clients, lists "reviewer courage" as one of six elements that characterize effective UMOs.)[35]

How readily UMOs will yield to a physician's wishes may also depend on the expectations of the organizations for which they work. One UMO that was visited in the IOM study indicated that it always ultimately acceded to a determined attending physician's wishes because the mostly unionized companies for which it provided services did not want to risk the labor discontent that might arise from denials of coverage. But that is not typical. Nevertheless, some employers make it clear that they do not want to subject employees to conflict when they have medical problems. Other employers may make it clear that they will not renew their contract with the UMO unless certain economic goals are met. The decisions made by a single UMO about similar cases may thus vary depending on who the patient's employer is. (The telephone systems at some UMOs are set up so that calls from different benefit plans come in on different lines. The UMO may even answer the telephone differently depending on what line a call comes in on. In some UMOs calls from particular plans are routed to a specific group of review nurses who are familiar with whatever special circumstances may be involved and who may even start forming telephone relationships with some employees.)

UMOs that work in a relatively circumscribed geographic area or that deal with a relatively small number of physicians—as in a PPO or IPA—may develop profiles that show which physicians appear to have patterns of providing inappropriate services. Such UMOs might deal differently with those physicians whose patterns of care are questionable or who consistently report that their patients have complications that justify exceptions to the UMO's criteria.

Finally, a UMO's toughness is undoubtedly affected by concerns about liability, particularly in decisions that could have life-or-death consequences. (One insurance company visited during the IOM study was undertaking a prior-authorization program that focused on the necessity of surgical procedures. The initial group of procedures was selected for attention because of perceived overuse, because it was feasible to develop a set of criteria, *and* because they did not present circumstances in which a denial could lead to death or disability.) UMOs are all aware of court decisions that suggest that they bear some responsibility for what happens to patients.[36]

*Criteria and decision rules.* The decisions made by UMOs are based on several different screens and criteria of appropriateness, including:

· lists of procedures that will not be approved either because they are not useful or because they are excluded under the applicable benefit plan (for example, cosmetic surgery);

· lists of procedures that are ordinarily authorized only on an outpatient basis;

· factors that may justify exceptions (for instance, a history of bleeding disorders may justify an exception to a rule requiring that a surgical procedure be done on an outpatient basis);

· procedures or services for which second opinions are required and the bases (which may be procedure specific) for allowing the requirement to be waived when the probability is high that the second opinion would confirm the first one;

· criteria that justify admission to or continued stay in the hospital;

· length-of-stay norms, which the UMO has either developed itself or has borrowed from the averages published by the Commission on Professional and Hospital Activities;

· criteria of necessity for specific procedures.

The existence of such criteria, decision rules, and norms prompts a number of questions. Where do they come from? How are they used? How are they revised? How consistent are they from UMO to UMO? The answers to such questions have obvious implications for the effect that UM has on the cost and quality of patient care, and the burden UM places on providers.

The screens and criteria used by UMOs have generally been adapted from many sources—from the work of researchers, professional associations, third-party payers, various types of consensus panels, and review organizations. Most UMOs use a combination of screens, lists, and criteria that they developed themselves, that they borrowed from elsewhere, or that they purchased or leased from firms whose business it is to develop systems for use by UMOs.

Different systems start from different places and have their own logic. Some criteria sets begin with a diagnosis (or symptom) and work from there to determine if the proposed service is appropriate. Some begin with the body system that is involved. Some rules are purpose oriented—focusing on the justification for a particular level of care (such as admission to the hospital or to an intensive care unit) or for a particular service.[37] An example is the widely used Appropriateness Evaluation Protocol (AEP) for medical admissions to the hospital, a version of which is shown in Table 11.1. This is a list of eighteen types of symptoms or services, any one of which would justify a patient's being admitted to the hospital. Purpose-oriented criteria can be much more specific, however, as with the criteria for defining the combination of indications that would justify a particular procedure.[38]

The field is clearly moving toward computerization. This facilitates keeping track of the information reported about the patient and noting when further monitoring is needed, is useful in integrating the UM information with eventual payment decisions (for example, regarding which services were authorized), and generating letters to patients and providers. More important from the standpoint of medical decision making, it permits the use of computerized criteria sets that incorporate logical processes that have been determined (usually by expert panels) to be appropriate for physicians to use in deciding whether to hospitalize or perform surgery on a patient with a given set of signs and symptoms. In theory at least, computerized systems based on diagnoses (or on symptoms, which are reported more reliably than diagnoses) could be used to apply state-of-the-art knowledge to the care of patients. Thousands of protocols are reputedly built into the preadmission certification software that some companies have developed.[39]

The best-known and probably most widely used sets of criteria for utilization management are the Appropriateness Evaluation Protocol (AEP),[40] the Intensity of Service, Severity of Illness, Discharge, and Appropriateness Screening Criteria (ISD-A),[41] and the Standardized Medreview Instrument (SMI).[42] The original versions of these were all developed with public funds in the 1970s

*Table 11.1.* The Appropriateness Evaluation Protocol criteria for hospital admission

---

*Patient's condition*

1. Sudden onset of unconsciousness or disorientation

2. Pulse rate < 50 or > 140 per minute

3. Blood pressure: systolic < 90 or > 200 mm Hg or diastolic < 60 or > 120 mm Hg

4. Acute loss of sight or hearing

5. Acute loss of ability to move a body part

6. Persistent fever with oral temperature >100°F for more than 5 days

7. Active bleeding

8. Severe electrolyte or blood gas abnormality (8 different objective abnormalities are defined in the criteria)

9. Acute or progressive sensory, motor, circulatory, or respiratory embarrassment sufficient to incapacitate the patient (Back pain is excluded.) (An intensity of service criterion must also be met.)

10. Electrocardiographic evidence of acute ischemia; suspicion of a new myocardial infarction

11. Wound dehiscence or evisceration

*Intensity of service*

12. Intravenous medications and/or fluid replacement (not including tube feeding)

13. Surgery or procedure scheduled within 24 hours requiring general or regional anesthesia or equipment, facilities, or procedures available only in a hospital

14. Vital-sign monitoring at least every 2 hours

15. Chemotherapy requiring continuous observation for life-threatening toxic reaction

16. Treatment in an intensive care unit

17. Intramuscular antibiotics at least every 8 hours

18. Intermittent or continuous use of respirator at least every 8 hours

---

Source: Health Data Institute, Appropriateness Evaluation Protocol (a six-page instrument designed to be used by a utilization reviewer). See note 40 in this chapter.

Note: As the system is designed, any single criterion justifies an admission. The Appropriateness Evaluation Protocol also includes 27 criteria for evaluating the appropriateness of days of hospitalization.

and early 1980s to meet the needs of PSROs in assessing the appropriateness of services that had already been provided. Now all are being used prospectively and have been built into software that is marketed by three industry leaders—the Health Data Institute (owned by the publicly traded Caremark, Inc., which was acquired by Baxter-Travenol Laboratories in 1987), MediQual Systems, Inc. (a for-profit affiliate of InterQual), and SysteMetrics (a subsidary of McGraw-Hill). The evolution of the utilization review methodologies developed by health service researchers working in nonprofit settings into large-scale utilization management services marketed by investor-owned corporations itself says a great deal about the changes in this field.

How consistent with one another are the criteria used by different UMOs? The information that a UMO seeks and the sequence in which it wants that information may depend to some extent on the criteria sets that it uses and the logic that inheres there. This may well contribute to the lack of consistency perceived by some physicians and hospitals that deal with many UMOs. But more than a perception is involved. There are in fact differences among UMOs in what they are willing to authorize, what factors they consider, and what they take to be appropriate services under different circumstances. This should not be surprising, of course, in view of the wide variations among physicians in how they handle different clinical situations and in view of the fact that UMOs have different markets and histories and have done a great deal of independent invention.

No comprehensive examination of the criteria used by UMOs is available, but some inquiries about this topic were made during the IOM site visits to twelve UMOs. To get a sense of the consistency across organizations, they were asked how they handled two types of decisions. These two were chosen, it is important to understand, because they were known to be difficult ones about which there was no consensus. The answers are summarized in Table 11.2.

Regarding whether their organization would authorize a planned admission to the hospital of a child who was going to undergo a tonsillectomy and adenoidectomy operation, the variation was very wide. One organization treated this routinely as an inpatient procedure, while others said they would authorize admission if the physician requested or "insisted" on it. Some

*Table 11.2.* Circumstances under which 12 utilization management organizations reported that they would approve hospitalization for 2 conditions, 1988[a]

| Organization | Condition |
|---|---|
| | *Tonsillectomy and adenoidectomy for a child* |
| 1 | Distance from home to facility, complications |
| 2 | Physician insistence on admission |
| 3 | Complications |
| 4 | Age; co-morbidities |
| 5 | Physician insistence; high risk; 2+ hours travel time |
| 6 | Bleeding disorders; distance |
| 7 | Physician request for admission |
| 8 | Patient's history |
| 9 | None specified |
| 10 | One-night stay routinely permitted |
| 11 | Physician request for admission |
| 12 | No special conditions required |

a. Responses of heads or medical directors of 12 utilization management organizations visited by the author and colleagues during the Institute of Medicine study of utilization management.

could not specify what they would consider in making this decision, while others said that they would consider the patient's distance from the hospital and potential complications. A question about the circumstances under which they would authorize hospital admission for a patient with lower back pain also produced a wide variety of responses.

Differences in the standards applied by UMOs are so substantial that they have been classified. Arnold Milstein, Linda Bergthold, and Leslie Selbovitz of National Medical Audit, Inc., a company that reviews the work of UMOs for corporate clients, describe the criteria used by different UMOs in terms of three levels of rigor, which they say are "explicit in the written screen-

*Table 11.2.* (continued)

| Organization | Condition |
|---|---|
| | *Lower back pain* |
| 1 | Need for intramuscular injections for pain control; inability to move |
| 2 | Need for intramuscular injections for pain control; motor defects |
| 3 | Pain; complications |
| 4 | Severe pain; need for traction |
| 5 | 3 days of traction allowed for pain |
| 6 | ISD-A Criteria (nature not specified) |
| 7 | Failure of outpatient treatment |
| 8 | Neurological deficit |
| 9 | Physician request, after outpatient treatment |
| 10 | Physician insistence |
| 11 | Physician request |
| 12 | Rarely approved, and only for hospital-level intensity of service |

Source: Bradford H. Gray and Marilyn J. Field, eds., *Controlling Costs and Changing Patient Care? The Role of Utilization Management* (Washington, D.C.: National Academy Press, 1989).

ing criteria and implicit in the physician-adviser decisions of every UR program," and which they describe as follows:

· Level 1 is the loosest, most inefficient level, representing the most extravagant forms of fee-for-service practice and obliviousness to the considerations of cost effectiveness. This level is typically associated with over 700 annual hospital days per 1,000 covered lives in a group health plan for active employees with average enrollee demographics.

· Level 2 is consistent with adherence to "average" or "prevailing" utilization practices and reflects elimination of the most deviant types of overutilization. Level 2 standards are found in many UR programs, and their use is consistent with 450 to 550 annual hospital days per 1,000.

Level 3 represents the most efficient practices compatible with patient safety and is embodied by the most successful HMOs. The result is 200 to 350 annual hospital days per 1,000. This approach makes wider use of practices such as morning admission for surgeries that require subsequent overnight hospitalization, outpatient settings for complex surgeries, and early discharges, often with home care, than do programs with Level 1 or Level 2 standards. The standards of American UR programs generally fall at widely disparate points along the spectrum between Level 2 and Level 3.[43]

The authors provide examples of differences between Level 2 and Level 3 standards. Overnight hospitalization would be routinely approved following cardiac catheterization under a Level 2 but not a Level 3 standard. Preoperative hospitalization would be routinely approved for abdominal hysterectomy under Level 2 but not under Level 3. Target lengths of stay for single-level lumbar laminectomy or for elective cholecystectomy would be five days under Level 2 but two to three days under Level 3.[44]

It is clear, then, that substantial variations exist in the care that different UM organizations find to be appropriate. Is this a serious drawback? Variations in decisions rendered by UMOs are undoubtedly sometimes disturbing to physicians and hospitals and are a reasonable-sounding basis for criticism of UM. Yet, it is unlikely that the variations across UMOs even begin to approach the variation that exists among the physicians whose work has become subject to review. Stated differently, even with the variations among UMOs, their involvement in patient care decisions has most likely narrowed the physician-to-physician, hospital-to-hospital, specialty-to-specialty, and region-to-region differences in how similar patients are treated in the United States.

Although some of the criteria that UMOs apply will no doubt prove to be poorly founded and unwise, that is true of medical decision making generally. But, unlike the judgments made by individual physicians on the basis of their clinical experience, the decision rules and criteria applied by UMOs generally reflect some type of expert consensus and, in many cases, an up-to-date examination of the clinical research literature. Indeed, the creation of UMOs has helped to identify areas where the foundations for medical decision making are weak and has resulted in a demand for better criteria of appropriateness. This demand has helped stimulate efforts by professional associations, specialty societies, government agencies, and research firms to develop better data, to reach consensus about the use of technologies and the handling of different clinical situations, and to identify areas where a better research base is needed.

Also, UMOs do not make decisions in a vacuum. Their routine work generates constant feedback on the criteria, decision rules, and screens that they use. A UMO that tries to apply a criterion that is broadly unacceptable to physicians will encounter a great deal of resistance. Also, many UMOs are part of firms that also pay medical claims, so they have an ongoing source of data on actual patient care patterns. One UMO that was visited in the IOM study mentioned that it changed its criteria on a particular procedure—categorizing it as outpatient rather than inpatient treatment—when claims data showed that a majority of physicians were already doing the procedure on an outpatient basis.

A largely unrealized potential also exists for UMOs to monitor the relationship of their decisions to some types of patient care outcomes (readmission to the hospital; return to work) and to modify criteria on that basis.

## Issues Raised by Prior-Authorization Programs

### Lack of Standardization

UM programs have been implemented by a wide variety of organizations that have done a great deal of independent inventing. Furthermore, there is no regulatory framework to shape the operation of organizations. It is thus not surprising that the most striking lesson from the IOM site visits to twelve UMOs concerns the variations among them.

Certain elements are common, if not universal. These include reliance on telephones, the application of criteria of various types, and the use of a two-stage approach, with nurses doing initial screening for authorization and with physicians reviewing cases that do not pass the initial screen. But many key elements are far from standardized. UMOs vary enormously among themselves on such matters as the qualifications and training of nurse-reviewers and physician-advisers; the numbers of physician-advisers and nurse-reviewers per number of cases; the number of cases per unit of time dealt with by physicians and nurses; the percentage of cases referred to physician-advisers; the relationship of advising physicians to the organization; the oversight and monitoring of both nurse-reviewers and physician-advisers; the degree of computerization of the system; the strength of the commitment to cost containment and attitude toward providers and beneficiaries; the degree of integration with claims payment systems; and the nature and operation of appeals processes. Not surprisingly, the outcomes—generally measured in terms of number of days of hospitalization per one thousand employees or covered lives— also vary enormously.

*Effects on Costs*

The rapid adoption of different UM methods occurred because of accounts of a handful of companies' positive experiences with these methods in the early to mid-1980s. These experiences were conveyed not in the health services research literature but in the trade press and at conferences of employee benefit managers and others (HMOs, PPOs) concerned with cost containment. Most were before-and-after accounts of the introduction of a UM method, usually as part of a broader change in a health benefit plan (for example, the introduction of cost sharing). The actual methods used were often not described at all, and little or no awareness existed that programs with similar names might be very different from one another. Table 11.3 summarizes some of these reports and conveys well the gist and flavor of this evidence about the impact of programs on the cost and use of services. Other similar reports can be found.

Notwithstanding the limitations of the research design, the results were very dramatic and more than sufficed to stimulate widespread adoption of the approach by benefit managers desperate to control their health care costs. Furthermore, when more rigorous studies began to be done, they also produced evidence that utilization management has had a significant impact on hospital use and costs.[45] (No studies have used *both* control groups and before-and-after comparisons.)

Notwithstanding this evidence, there are troublesome ques-

*Table 11.3.* Summary of reported effects of utilization management programs

| Organization | Year | Program type | Reported effects |
|---|---|---|---|
| Health Maintenance Life Insurance Co.[a] | 1980–1981 | Preadmission review | Reduced hospital days by 204 days/1,000 covered individuals in first year. Actual days/1,000 were 450 after 2 years. |
| Blue Cross/Blue Shield, Iowa[b] | 1981–1984 | "Mandatory utilization review program" | Hospital use declined by one-third. Premiums were reduced 3 times. |
| Deere & Company[c] | late 1970s | Utilization review, including preadmission certification | Hospital days/1,000 employees were reduced by 30% (by 400 days/1,000 employees) over "several" years. |
| Caterpillar Tractor[d] | 1980s | Utilization review by Peoria PSRO | 17% decline in hospital days/1,000 employees. One-day decline in average length of stay in first year. |
| Employer coalition, San Diego[e] | 1982–1984 | Utilization review | Reduced incidence of evening admissions prior to elective surgery from 80% to 20% of cases. |
| Blue Cross of Northeast Ohio[f] | 1983–1984 | Preadmission review | 23% decline in inpatient hospital days in first 5 months. |
| Blue Cross of Central Ohio | 1982 | Preadmission review | 30% decline in elective admissions. |
| Blue Cross/Blue Shield of Kansas City, Missouri | 1982–1984 | "Cost-control program" | 6.8% decline in admissions; 16.5% shift to outpatient surgery; 9.3% decline in hospital days/1,000. |

*(continued)*

*Table 11.3.* (continued)

| Organization | Year | Program type | Reported effects |
|---|---|---|---|
| Blue Cross/Blue Shield, North Carolina | 1983 | Preadmission certification | Decrease of 37% in days/1,000 in pilot group. |
| Blue Cross/Blue Shield, South Carolina[g] | 1982–1983 | Preadmission review | Reduced inpatient use of 10 surgical procedures from 62.5% to 33.9% of time. |
| All Blue Cross/Blue Shield Programs[h] | 1984–1985 | All managed care programs | Saved $6 billion in 1984 and $9.7 billion in 1985. |
| CIGNA[i] | 1985 | "Cost management and utilization review programs" | Saved customers $400 million (17% of paid claims). Saved $9 for every dollar spent in preadmission/concurrent stay review program. |
| CostCare[j] | | Utilization management program | Reduced one large corporate client's hospital use from 579 to 389 days/1,000 covered individuals in 2 years; reduced another's from 627 to 416; reduced a third's from 1,065 to 703. |
| General Motors[k] | 1985 | HMO, PPO, or indemnity plan with preadmission and continued-stay review and review of necessity of emergency admissions | Total health care costs declined from $2.3 to $2.1 billion after increasing an average of $200,000/year for previous 3 years. |
| Chrysler Corporation[l] | | Chart audit; data compilation; education program; monitoring | Reduced hospital admissions for lower back pain by 64% in one year at 8 target hospitals. |

| | | Utilization management program | Larger inpatient decline among group covered by program; 3.8% net decline in benefit costs in covered groups, compared to 6% increase in other groups. 4:1 return on investment in UM programs. |
|---|---|---|---|
| RCA Corporation[m] | 1985 | | |
| Blue Cross/Blue Shield, Massachusetts[n] | 1984 | Offered utilization management option in fee-for-service plans | Between 1983 and 1985, hospital days dropped from 680 to 520 in managed plan and 600 in traditional plan. |
| One insurer's contracts with a utilization review firm[o] | | Utilization management program | Attributed reductions owing to utilization management to be 12.3% of admissions, 8% of days of hospitalization, 11.9% of hospital expenditures, and 8.3% of total expenditures. |

Sources: a. *Hospital Peer Review* 5 (February 1980): 1; b. Nancy S. Bagby and Sean Sullivan, *Buying Smart: Business Strategies for Managing Health Care Costs* (Washington, D.C.: American Enterprise Institute, 1986), pp. 29–30; c. Glenn Richards, "Business Spurs U.R. Growth," *Hospitals* 58 (March 1, 1984): 96; d. Richards, "Business Spurs U.R. Growth," p. 96; Sean Sullivan, *Managing Health Care Costs: Private Sector Initiatives* (Washington, D.C.: American Enterprise Institute, 1984), p. 11; e. Richards, "Business Spurs U.R. Growth," p. 96; f. Teri Shahoda, "Preadmission Review Cuts Hospital Use," *Hospitals* 58 (August 1, 1984): 54; g. "SC Plan Sees Hospitalization Drop for Review Program Participants," *Hospitals* (November 16, 1983): 54; h. "Blue Cross and Blue Shield Plans Save $9.7 Billion for Subscribers," press release, Blue Cross & Blue Shield Association, Washington, D.C., June 5, 1986; i. G. Robert O'Brien, president of the CIGNA Employee Benefits and Health Care Group, remarks at Government Research Corporation's Tenth National Health Leadership Conference, Washington, D.C., March 17, 1986; j. CostCare, "Performance Results" (mimeograph, n.d.); k. Suzanne Powills, "GM's Managed Care Program, One Year Later," *Hospitals* 60 (May 20, 1986): 44–46; l. Walter B. Maher, "Controlling Low Back Pain at Chrysler," *Business and Health* 2 (May 1985): 20–23; m. Peter S. O'Donnell, "Controlling Costs under a Fee-for-Service Plan," *Business and Health* 4 (March 1987): 38–41; n. Jacob Getson, "Reforming Health Care Delivery: the Massachusetts Blues' Role," *Business and Health* 4 (February 1987): 30–34; o. Paul J. Feldstein, Thomas J. Wickizer, and John R. C. Wheeler, "The Effects of Utilization Review Programs on Health Care Use and Expenditures," *New England Journal of Medicine* 318 (May 19, 1988): 1310–14.

tions about the results of prior-authorization programs. Controlled studies that isolate the effects of such programs have not been carried out. The lack of standardization of programs makes it difficult to generalize. There are also major problems involving measurement of effects. The inadequacies of measuring impact in terms of "days saved" (which UMOs calculate on the basis of days or hospitalizations requested minus days or hospitalizations approved) are obvious, although that has been the basis of some organizations' claims about impact. More sophisticated measures of cost savings sometimes suffer from the problem that shifts from inpatient to outpatient settings may produce misleading results if one's measurement is focused on hospital use and costs.[46] Savings from reduced use of the hospital can be outstripped by increases in prices or in the use of outpatient facilities.

These are among the reasons for the relatively mild claims by the IOM Committee on Utilization Management by Third Parties about the impact of UM on costs. The committee noted that UM has "helped to reduce inpatient hospital use and to limit inpatient costs for some purchasers beyond what could have been expected," but that UM's "impact on net benefit costs is less clear," and that UM has not "altered the long-term rate of increase in health care costs."[47] Regarding this last point, an additional comment seems warranted. The methods that have been described in this chapter are designed to focus on unnecessary and inappropriate services and cannot be expected to affect cost trends that are due to other factors (new technologies, the aging of beneficiary groups). To expect otherwise is unreasonably demanding of a set of methods that have limited purposes, no matter how much those methods alter the traditional accountability structure of health care. So long as these methods provide a means that is otherwise lacking for questioning the necessity of services that physicians, hospitals, and ambulatory care centers wish to provide and be paid for, it is likely that these methods will continue to play a role.

### Effects on Quality of Care

Few if any organizations in the field of private UM have done formal evaluations of the effects of their programs on quality of care. (Two studies of the limited preadmission review program in Medicare have found no evidence of harm.)[48] During the two years of the IOM study—which involved work by more than twenty people who are active in the field, a public hearing, site visits to a dozen organizations, and a commissioned paper on the legal status of UM—no documented cases of quality problems linked to prior review came to light.[49] Nonetheless, almost one-third of the physicians who responded to a 1988 AMA survey said that they had patients who had suffered an aggravation of an illness or injury as a result of delays or denials in a prior-authorization process.[50]

Yet a search for harm is a most inadequate way to assess the impact of UM on quality. Even if an occasional patient is harmed—as seems inevitable in a program designed to change patient care patterns—other patients may avoid harm because of UM. The methods, after all, are designed to minimize exposure to the risks of hospitalization and, in the case of some programs, to discourage the provision of unnecessary surgery. Discussions with doctors and nurses who work in UMOs produce many examples of situations in which, by their account, they were able to identify and prevent a tragedy in the making. Given all that is known about physician-to-physician variations in patterns of care (and in quality of care), it seems very likely that a review process that demands that proposed services be justified and that applies sophisticated algorithms and criteria maps will prevent harm to some number of patients.

The potential impact of computerized criteria sets on the quality of patient care can be illustrated by a recent study of the cost effectiveness of the care provided to patients with pharyngitis (sore throat).[51] In this study the actual care given to a series of patients by ten experienced physicians in a student health service was compared with the treatment prescribed under four different sets of decision rules. These rules covered whether it was appropriate to obtain a throat culture and whether the patient should be treated for a streptococcal infection based on objective patient characteristics, such as temperature, recent exposure to streptococcal infection, a recent cough, pharyngeal exudate, and enlarged or tender cervical lymph nodes, to which empirically derived probabilities and weights had been assigned. The study found that the patient care decisions indicated by one of the statistically based sets of rules were better than the decisions actually made by the physicians. If this set had been used, the result would have been fewer tests, less overtreatment, and no undertreatment. Each of the other three sets was better in some regard than were physicians' decisions. All sets made more cost-effective decisions, but two would have resulted in the under-treatment of a small number of patients.

This study shows that the types of decision rules that can be built into UR and UM programs can improve medical decision making, but it also shows that they will not *necessarily* do so. That depends on what rules are adopted. It also illustrates that the choices made when decision rules are developed may incorporate explicit trade-offs of cost containment and the risk of negative patient outcomes. Although such trade-offs are not new, the application of decision rules in UM programs formalizes them, potentially affecting large numbers of patients. UM also entails an important change in who makes the trade-offs. In balancing costs, benefits, and potential harm of services, patients and physicians may not reach the same conclusions as the payer. Indeed, they may not even agree on what a particular patient's "needs" might be.

Definitions of necessity are always influenced by societal and cultural factors and personal values. Is cardiopulmonary resuscitation an appropriate and medically necessary intervention for a patient whose heart has stopped beating? The answer to this question is not inherent in the technology and the patient's condition; it depends on a variety of factors, including the scarcity of resources and the personal values or wishes of the patient. Cost also influences definitions of necessity. The distinction between the recipients of service (who have the "needs" in question) and the purchasers of care (who make key decisions about what they will pay for) may gain significance if economic factors come to influence definitions of what services are or are not deemed necessary.

The development and application of utilization criteria by purchasers of care seem sure to reduce the wide variations in patterns of use for certain services, which were discussed earlier. This may well be desirable. Yet there is a difficult dilemma involved. In general, those services whose use exhibits a high degree of variation that seems not to reflect differences among patients are services for which there is relatively little professional consensus about appropriate use. But these inappropriately used services are the best target for UM programs. In the absence of scientifically validated knowledge that reflects a high degree of professional consensus, it is difficult for UM programs to push toward the positive goal of improving the appropriateness or cost effectiveness of the use of services. Instead, UM efforts generally exert pressure for providing fewer services. This approach rests on the reasonable assumption that such high levels of unnecessary or marginal services have been provided under prevailing methods of payment that significant reductions can be made without affecting quality. At some point, however, this will cease to be true. There is clearly no guarantee that UM efforts devoted to reducing the use of services will be consistent with all parties' conceptions of quality, particularly if the maintenance or enhancement of quality is not an explicit goal.

How much harm or benefit UM produces may be a function of several factors. These include the quality of the criteria and the procedural soundness of UM programs, the willingness of physicians and hospitals to take issue with UM determinations that could jeopardize a patient's health, and the overall effects of UM, UR, and other forms of managed care on the structure of accountability in health care.

### Morale and the Responsibilities of Physicians

Statements by doctors that they would not again choose medicine as a career or would not recommend it to their children have become commonplace. Utilization management is cited among the leading causes for complaint. "Physicians are often left watching while clinical decisions about their patients are being taken out of their hands by insurance companies, employers and consultants. The irony is that, in talking with this new class of arbitrators, I've yet to meet one who wishes to or feels competent to practice medicine."[52] Cost-containment methods that come into play after the physician has examined the patient and made recommendations about what should be done can disrupt the doctor-patient relationship. The fact that someone else has to concur before the physician's recommendations can be implemented clearly signifies a loss of physician autonomy and may also cause a loss of status in the patient's and the physician's own eyes. As the president of the Kentucky Medical Association put it a few years ago, "Most of us think that we can walk on water. Now we're being told that we have to ask permission to go to the little boys' room."[53]

One source of complaint and disquiet among physicians is the annoyance of dealing with bureaucracy which has accompanied the proliferation of UM programs. Stories of busy telephone lines at UMOs and of seemingly poorly trained and unreasoning reviewers are common.[54] Here are two such complaints (about *retrospective* review programs, it should be noted) from the experience of one practicing internist:

> [I] treated a young woman for a bleeding ulcer. Unlike most ulcer patients, she required two examinations to treat the problem successfully. When she presented her bills to her insurance company, the claims representative informed her that the insurer would pay for only "one look into the stomach." When she protested, the clerk stood firm. When she said, "I have bills for two examinations. What should I do?" the claims representative replied, "Why don't you just give your doctor a bleeding ulcer."
>
> I recently diagnosed a patient suffering from cancer of the bowel. On the day after he underwent emergency surgery, I received a computer-coded note from yet another part of the new medical bureaucracy—an oversight agency contracted by the patient's employer. The document said he was suffering from a kidney disease and required no surgery. I took it upon myself to investigate where this misdiagnosis originated, but nobody seemed to know. When I finally received a call from the medical director of the agency, he told me: "Doc, we're not trying to tell you how to practice medicine. Just fill out the papers."[55]

Such are the inevitable problems of dealing with bureaucracies and computerized systems. The rise of utilization management systems provides an additional setting in which misunderstandings and errors can occur.

Irritation with the utilization management process can also arise because the logic of the systems being used does not necessarily match the physician's thought processes. Definitions and categories that work well for utilization management purposes (or even for payment purposes) can be inconsistent with the way that physicians think.[56] For example, a UM system that is keyed to diagnoses (as some are) may create difficulties in situations in which the physician has not yet settled on the diagnosis. Similar problems may be created when secondary diagnoses or complicating factors are present. Although increasingly elaborate computerized systems that incorporate clinical logic are in use, physicians' dealings with UMOs can still take on the flavor of working with an alien and unreasoning intelligence.

Also affecting physicians' morale are the increasingly voiced concerns that some methods for controlling costs create conflicts with the physician's most fundamental ethical obligation: the responsibility and duty of loyalty to the patient.[57] The use of economic incentives that reward the provision of fewer services has led to such concerns, as has the use of threats to hospital privileges, membership in a group practice, or employment status in an alternative delivery system. Although the expression of such concerns can conceal motives of defending a status quo that has served physicians' economic interests very well, physicians increasingly complain of pressures on them to divide their loyalty to the patient. In some parts of the country doctors have organized to voice these concerns and to oppose HMOs and other organizations that attempt to manage health care.[58]

All approaches used for utilization management and cost containment have drawbacks from the standpoint of physicians. Denials of payment for services that have retrospectively been determined to have been unnecessary create questions of fairness. Prospective utilization control methods are seen as disruptive of the doctor-patient relationship. Incentive approaches are seen as introducing new and more powerful conflicts of interest than have existed in the past (although this argument usually glosses over the incentives present in fee-for-service compensation).

As yet, little is known about how different approaches and combinations of incentives, retrospective review, and prospective utilization controls compare in terms of their impact on physician decision making, on their sense of ethics and personal responsibility, and on their morale and sense of pride. With the growth of increasingly powerful organizations using increasingly powerful tools to monitor and shape patterns of care provided to patients, these are possible consequences that should not be overlooked.

The rise of utilization management could affect physicians' sense of personal responsibility for patient care decisions. This can be illustrated by the leading legal case to date regarding utilization management—the *Wickline* decision by the California Court of Appeals.[59] The court held that the state's Medi-Cal program was not liable for the harm of complications suffered by the patient (resulting in the amputation of her leg) after her allegedly premature discharge from the hospital at the end of the length of stay that had been authorized for payment by Medi-Cal's utilization review program.[60]

A key question in *Wickline* was who was responsible for the decision to discharge the patient from the hospital. Medi-Cal contended that its UM program did not shift control of decision making away from the physician. The California Medical Association (CMA), in an amicus brief, argued that requirements that the doctor obtain prior authorization as a condition of being paid blurs responsibility for patient care decisions: "Traditionally, decisions concerning medical care have been based on the treating physician's personal knowledge of the patient's condition and the patient's informed consent. This personal involvement and responsibility disappears when third parties assume a decision-making role . . . The potential conflict between profit motives and concern for the patient is real and ominous."[61]

In reversing a lower court's decision in favor of the patient and against Medi-Cal, the appeals court gave important hints about the extent to which the rise of utilization management complicates the legal question of responsibility for patient care decisions. Although explicitly acknowledging the legitimacy of payers' efforts to contain costs, the court stated that physicians who believe utilization managers' decisions to be wrong are obliged to argue the patient's case. This had not happened when the stay authorized by Medi-Cal expired and the patient was discharged from the hospital. The reason for this, according to testimony at the trial, was that experience had taught physicians that appeals to Medi-Cal were pointless. As the argument was put in the CMA brief: "Physicians' best efforts to protect their patients' interest may well be futile where the individual or committee which makes a prospective utilization review decision has inadequate resources, whether in time, information or expertise . . . [Physicians] cannot spend unlimited amounts of time

doing battle with insurance carriers, utilization review coordinators, Medi-Cal consultants, or hospital administrators."[62]

Such sentiments on the part of physicians may help explain
the reportedly high level of physician compliance with the determinations of utilization managers. As one medical journalist put
it: "Companies often do not need to enforce their nonpayment
policies when concurrent review determines that further hospital care is not medically necessary. In almost all cases, the
attending physician will discharge the patient, say review agencies and companies alike."[63]

### The Fiduciary Ethic and Physicians' Obligations

In the last several chapters I have placed considerable emphasis
on the fiduciary ethic which obliges physicians to put the interests of their patients ahead of their own interests. The introduction of UMOs into patient care decisions creates some new challenges to the fiduciary ethic. Several interrelated issues arise in
circumstances in which a serious conflict develops between the
determinations of a UMO and the physician's view of the welfare
of the patient.

What is the extent of the physician's obligation to persevere in
trying to obtain authorization? To do so carries costs in terms of
time and nuisance. (Many physicians, preferring to spend their
time seeing patients, delegate the task of obtaining authorizations to office personnel.) Discrepancies between what physicians wish to do and what UMOs will authorize may pertain to
relatively trivial matters—perhaps affecting only the patient's
(or the physician's) convenience—or they may have significant
implications for the patient's health. The physician's certainty
about the likelihood for harm may also vary from case to case.

The physician's obligation to invest effort in seeking to over-
turn an adverse determination would appear to increase with the
seriousness and certainty of harm to the patient's well-being.
UMOs implicitly operate on the assumption that physicians will
behave in this way; their procedures are designed to *respond* to
physicians' judgments about what services are necessary and
appropriate. If the physician does not bring mitigating circumstances to the attention of the UMO, it has no way of making

exceptions where they are needed. Moreover, the physician has a legal duty to care for the patient, and legal analysts see it as unlikely that a physician could avoid a malpractice claim on grounds that he or she was following a decision made by a UMO.[64] The tension between the interests of UMOs and physicians may be uncomfortable for physicians, but it may also help protect the interests of patients.

The easiest way to escape the tension while maintaining allegiance to the fiduciary ethic and minimizing the time that has to be invested in dealing with UMOs is for the physician to shade the truth to gain approval for a service that he or she deems advisable for the patient. This seems to be almost an automatic response. (Many express scorn for UMOs because it is so easy to manipulate them by telling them something that is clinically significant but difficult to verify from afar.)

No doubt many situations can be successfully manipulated by distorting patients' symptoms or conditions. But this has consequences. Because some UMOs give authorization subject to retrospective reviews of the medical records, erroneous information may be entered into the patients' records and could have consequences later. Believing that they are being lied to, UMOs have begun to request verification of some matters, such as copies of lab reports or of X rays. All of this adds to the expense and the cops-and-robbers pattern in the health care system. It also means that UMOs do not get a true sense of how practicing physicians are responding to their criteria or of the extent to which their reviewers are making bad decisions. The self-correcting aspects of UM may thus not be working very well.

If a UMO refuses to authorize payment for services that a physician believes are necessary to the patient's health, the question arises as to the extent of the physician's and the hospital's responsibility to provide the service anyway. William Helvestine argues that this situation is similar to cases where a physician has been found to have a continuing obligation to treat a patient who can no longer pay.[65] Moreover, the decision of a third-party payer concerning what to pay for is distinct from the physician's judgments about what services a patient needs. By virtue of training, ethical traditions, firsthand contact with the patient, and legal responsibilities, physicians cannot just turn over patient care decisions to payers and their agents. Furthermore, the decisions in prior-authorization programs are often made under time constraints; compliance ignores the possibility that a bad decision can be corrected later.

The stakes may be higher, however, in situations in which the physician's determinations affect other parties as well. A hospital, for example, may be unwilling to provide services that a UMO has not certified for payment. Medical staff bylaws in many hospitals include provisions that require physicians to perform in a way that permits the hospital to receive payment for its services, and at least one case (*Edelman v. John F. Kennedy Hospital* in New Jersey) upheld a hospital's decision to remove a physician's staff privileges for economic reasons.[66]

Another set of issues in situations of conflict between the physician's and UMO's views of necessary or appropriate care is whether the physician should discuss the matter with the patient (and family). Physicians may fear that this will increase patients' anxiety and perhaps undermine their confidence in the physician's judgment. Nonetheless, several factors can be identified in favor of such discussions. The refusal by a UMO to authorize a service is information that may influence the patient's judgment of the need for the service and may present patients with unexpected financial burdens. Information about trade-offs of costs, risks, and benefits is germane to patients' decisions about what services they want, and, under informed consent doctrines, they may very well have a right to it. Understanding the financial and medical implications of the situation, the patient or family may prefer either to assent to the UMO's decision or to accept the financial implications and follow the physician's advice, perhaps seeking legal redress from the UMO or payer later. (The problem is exacerbated when the costs exceed the patient's ability to pay.) Furthermore, only if patients and their families understand such situations will it be possible for them to make the employer or payer aware of the difficulties caused by the UM program. This is information that may help the employer or payer assess the effects of the UM program and make sure that the interests of patients are being given proper weight. And the involvement of patients when providers and UMOs disagree will reduce the extent to which UM shifts decision-making responsibility away from patients.

A final question that arises when the physician has to invest time and effort in seeking reversal of a UM decision is who pays for that time. Scattered reports suggest that some physicians are billing patients for the time that they invest in dealing with UMOs and payers, and the American Medical Association has held that it is ethically acceptable for physicians to bill for services that go beyond normal record keeping. (A potential for abuse can be identified; physicians could recommend unnecessary services and bill for time spent in appeals. Such thoughts arise from the logic of distrust that now often characterizes relationships of physicians and third-party payers.) Alternatively, the costs of complying with UM requirements might be built into practice overhead, although this would tend to shift the costs caused by inefficient UM programs to all payers.

### Responsibilities of Utilization Management Organizations

Patients and providers may be affected by UMOs' procedures and by the decisions they make. Their logistics, qualifications and number of personnel, and internal incentives all determine how burdensome it will be to deal with a UMO, to gain authorizations, and to exercise appeals. The UMO's philosophy, procedures, and assignment of decision-making responsibilities, the screening criteria and rules that it uses, the type of appeals process that it operates, and instructions from the purchasers for whom it provides services may all affect authorization decisions.

What are UMOs' responsibilities regarding the interests of patients and providers? How much danger is there that UMOs, in trying to save money, will take insufficient account of the legitimate interests of the patient and the provider? What safeguards exist?

*Obligations to patients.* Two factors militate against excessive callousness regarding the needs of patients. Patients may complain to employers, who may then become dissatisfied customers. Also, fear of legal liability encourages UMOs to give due weight to the interests of the patients. The language of the *Wickline* case has been widely circulated: "Third party payers of health care services can be held legally accountable when medically inappropriate decisions result from defects in the design or implementation of cost containment mechanisms as, for example, when appeals made on a patient's behalf for medical or hospital care are arbitrarily ignored or unreasonably disregarded or overridden."[67] Organizations that engage in UM may thus find themselves legally obligated to employ screening criteria and decision rules that are clinically valid and reflect a generally accepted medical consensus, provide reasonably timely and efficient means for enabling attending physicians to discuss decisions with which they disagree, and offer a genuine (not rubber stamp) appeals process about which affected parties are informed. Further case law will help spell out the substance of these requirements.

Some UMOs seek to evade their duties vis-à-vis patients by claiming that they are only certifying the necessity of care for payment purposes, not making patient care decisions. Still, their determinations will as a practical matter often decide whether services are provided, and a negative verdict may be interpreted by patients as equivalent to a judgment that the service is not needed.

A murkier area of UMO responsibility toward patients is in circumstances in which the organizations become aware of potential malpractice. Prior-authorization programs will inevitably encounter situations in which a patient's health and wellbeing are threatened by proposed interventions that seem to have no sound basis. The UMO may find itself faced with a conflict between an ethical and legal obligation to warn the patient and a potential defamation action from the provider. Notwithstanding the maxim that the truth is an absolute defense in defamation cases, the facts that confront a UMO may not be absolutely clear. Less urgent but no less consequential circumstances may arise when a pattern of questionable care is uncovered, as may occur in UM programs connected with claims payment systems. These are areas in which UM could potentially improve the quality of care but where legal ramifications are as yet undefined.

*Obligations to providers.* Other than the legal liability that a UMO may incur if it conveys information to patients in a way that defames providers, it is not clear that UMOs have any obligation to consider the interests of providers in their day-to-day operations. In contrast to patients, providers are not in a position to complain to the employer who hired the UMO, nor do providers represent the same type of liability threat as do patients. Although some UMOs have designed their systems to facilitate efficient handling of requests and appeals, providers' complaints about busy telephone lines and callbacks that never come raise suspicions that some UMOs may use inefficiency itself as a cost-containment tool, discouraging provider appeals and thus achieving savings without taking the responsibility for making negative decisions.

For their part, providers can make it easier or more difficult for UMOs to do their job by being more or less cooperative or honest. Providers have some power to engender discontent among patients, for example, by inducing them to complain to their employers about the UMO.

Whether the power of the respective parties is reasonably in balance is difficult to assess. Many providers believe that the demands of UMOs are excessive and are making it harder to provide good care to patients. Correspondingly, some UMOs have considerable cynicism about the motives and integrity of providers and believe that some physicians (and, to a lesser extent, some hospitals) make UM unnecessarily difficult. Whether tension and distrust arise more in some models of UM than in others has not been studied empirically. Nor have the consequences.

## Accountability Problems in UM Programs

Utilization management is still a relatively new field and is in rapid evolution. For example, during the course of the IOM study from 1987 to 1989, some UMOs were beginning to move beyond their initial focus on reducing the inappropriate use of hospitals to an effort to identify and discourage unnecessary procedures. The variability in the field constitutes a sort of gene pool out of which some approaches will survive and some will fail. This was an important reason why the IOM committee decided against recommending that UMOs be regulated.[68]

The procedural variability, differences in internal monitoring and external toughness, and variations in criteria that are the current status of UM have already been commented on. In addition, I see six areas of procedural weakness in the conduct of UM.

First, the criteria used by most UMOs are subject to little outside scrutiny, not even by public or private organizations that have an interest in quality of care.[69] Yet these UMOs' decisions may affect millions of patients. (Intracorp, the largest UMO in the

1989 *Business Insurance* survey, covered 11.5 million lives, and eight other organizations each covered more than 2 million lives.) In their dealings with providers, UMOs purport to speak with some authority—often referring to policies and guidelines and to the medical advisory committees that were involved in developing them. The UMOs are generally reluctant, however, to disclose their decision-making criteria to physicians, citing fears that this might facilitate gaming (whereby physicians' reports about a patient's condition are influenced by their knowledge of what is needed to gain approval of treatment. This fear quite possibly reflects a serious underestimation of the amount of gaming that already occurs). A patient's physician will often have to decide whether to accept a UMO's determination without being able to review the evidence or logic on which it is based. External parties cannot review and compare the criteria used by different organizations.

What is known about the reliability and validity of criteria sets used by UMOs? Most of the UMOs visited in the IOM study reported that they had started with either the AEP or the ISD-A for use in hospital review. (Most also said that they had made their own modifications. Some firms have developed their own computerized systems.) Of all the systems used by all the UMOs, the only reliability study I have found is for the AEP, which is, as described earlier, a generic criteria set for the appropriateness of hospitalization.[70] The large measure of agreement among independent raters that evaluate medical records using the AEP has been one of its strengths, along with its relative simplicity. Although InterQual's ISD criteria have been in use for ten years, no reliability studies have been conducted.[71]

The validity of the criteria used by UMOs is generally implicitly entrusted to the process by which they are developed—which is a combination of borrowing, consensus development by experts, and trial and error regarding what patients' physicians will accept. A study of the AEP raises questions, however.[72] Registered nurses (who typically serve as reviewers in UM programs) were asked to apply the AEP retrospectively to patient records for 1,266 random medical and surgical admissions at twenty-one acute care hospitals in southeastern Michigan. There were reasonably high levels of agreement among raters on nonacute care (care that does not require use of an acute care hospital). Levels of agreement were 75 percent for medical admissions, 60 percent for elective surgery, and 80 percent for days of stay. As a validity check, three physicians from a large teaching hospital were asked to review each case. If two of them agreed with a decision made by a nurse using the AEP, the judgment was considered to have been corroborated or validated. More often than not, the initial AEP conclusions were not validated by the reviewing physician.[73]

This suggests that it would be unfair to providers if the AEP were used retrospectively to deny payment for "unnecessary services" in the absence of physician review. If the AEP is to be used *prospectively* to authorize admission or continued stays, it clearly needs to be accompanied by physician review because of its tendency toward false positives in identifying days of unnecessary hospitalization. In addition, the study makes clear that the stringency of decisions regarding approval of hospital use can be tightened or relaxed by adding requirements for physician validation of decisions made by nurse-reviewers who use the AEP. If AEP-based decisions not to authorize use of the hospital had to be validated by a physician, more days of care would be authorized; if validation by two physicians were required, even more days would be authorized.[74]

The ways in which utilization management criteria are used can plainly influence what services are authorized and can thus affect the quality of care. Although UMOs generally claim that physician-reviewers are consulted whenever a proposed admission or continued stay does not meet review criteria, no systematic data are available about the procedural safeguards that are used in UM programs.

Other than the limited evidence on AEP that I have described, little public information exists about the performance of criteria sets that are used in UM programs. But the more such criteria are used to determine payment or authorize services to patients, the more important it will be to learn about their properties in action, and to look beyond the assurances of UM firms that their criteria were developed through a procedure involving the consensus of experts.

The IOM Committee on Utilization Management by Third Parties stopped short of clear recommendations that the criteria used by UMOs should be opened to outside review and that the reasons for review decisions should be provided to the patient's physician. It did observe, however, that such steps would improve physician acceptance of UM, and it argued that UMOs' fears of gaming by providers and of losing competitive advantages by disclosing the fruits of development efforts to competitors are "outweighed by the need to move toward open criteria and standards."[75]

A second limitation of most UMOs' prior authorization programs is that the criteria and procedures make no reference to patients' views about the type of setting in which they would prefer to receive services or about their readiness for discharge from the hospital. This is in striking contrast to the way most UMOs describe their high-cost case management programs, in which patients and families are usually parties to the process of working out alternatives to hospitalization. Prior-authorization programs are generally carried out in discussions between UMOs and physicians (or personnel in physicians' offices) and hospitals. In contrast to other trends in which patient autonomy is given increased importance (informed consent, decisions about life-sustaining technologies), prior-authorization programs may reduce patients' control over the care they receive. No published information is available about the extent to which decisions resulting from UM programs are satisfactory to patients.

Third, despite the serious consequences of their determinations, UMOs face no external requirements to offer fair appeals processes. In some cases such requirements are part of the contract between a UMO and the organizations for which they provide service. The appeals processes used if a patient's physician disagrees with the determination made by a physician-consultant at the UMO are neither uniform nor independent. Most UMOs refer appeals either to another medical consultant within the organization or to the medical director. A few UMOs refer such cases to committees, and some refer them to the employer that hired the UMO. (This is not illogical, since the question of payment may end up there anyway.)

Fourth, UMOs do not have much reason to consider the burden that their activities place on providers. Dissatisfied patients can complain to whoever provides their health benefit plans—and presumably also selected the UMO. Providers, however, generally have no recourse except, perhaps, through patients. But nothing about the structure of UM gives UMOs any reason to weigh the costs that their organizations, both individually and cumulatively, put on providers of health care, particularly those who are willing to appeal decisions and policies with which they disagree. (Many physicians say that they have had to hire extra staff to cope with this process, and the Mayo Clinic told the IOM committee that it had a department of fourteen people performing a function—dealing with UMOs—that had not existed four years before.)

Fifth, physicians may bear an unfair burden of responsibility under the current conduct of UM. Some UMOs seek to modify physicians' patient care decisions without taking the responsibility for doing so. They do this by conveying the impression that their determinations are authoritative, by making it logistically difficult to gain approvals, or by creating ambiguity about whether a proposed service will be paid for ("We *may* not be able to certify this"). Physicians who comply with a determination of a UMO may nevertheless be legally liable if harm subsequently befalls the patient. As William Helvestine notes, "in the *Wickline* decision, the judicial system blamed the treating physician for failing to protest strongly enough against the reviewer's decision."[76]

Sixth, organized systems for monitoring the occurrence of adverse outcomes appear to be quite uncommon among UM programs, in part, I am told, because few of the employers who hire UMOs are willing to pay additional fees for such monitoring. UMOs also vary as to whether and how they monitor the performance of nurse-reviewers and physician-advisers.[77] Only a few UM organizations attempt to assess the views of patients about their experiences with UM.

*Responsibilities of Purchasers of UM Services*

The account provided in this chapter suggests that oversight is needed to ensure that the interests of patients are adequately protected in UM programs. Regulatory requirements that UM organizations disclose the criteria that underlie their decisions and that they make a reasonable review process available would be one step. Calls for regulatory relief may disguise other motives, however, including providers' desire to escape detailed oversight.

Purchasers of UM services are in a position to play a leading role in the conduct and improvement of UM, particularly if provisions are made to ensure that the interests of employees are represented. If employers purchased UM services only after a careful review of procedures, and if employers took care to inform beneficiaries about the purposes and processes of UM, the availability of appeals procedures, and avenues for complaining about problems, and if employers were willing to pay for monitoring efforts to detect underservice or other problems in the health benefits provided to beneficiaries, the overall structure of accountability in the field of utilization management would be improved.

Such exhortations notwithstanding, it is apparent that there are limits to what employers can do to evaluate the quality of UM organizations before involving them in their benefit plans. There is a need for mechanisms that will assist employers in evaluating UMOs, whether done within the industry, by organizations whose business it is to evaluate UMOs for employers, or by government. The demand will no doubt grow for assistance in making sure that the organizations that provide utilization management services—services whose role seems likely to become even more important in the future—behave responsibly toward patients and employers.

Building on more than a decade of research on the necessity and appropriateness of various types of medical services, utilization management seeks the selective elimination of wasteful use of resources. It does so by bringing independent judgments and objective criteria of necessity or appropriateness to bear on patient care decisions. Differences of opinion about the necessity or appropriateness of contemplated services can be addressed in discussions between the patient's physician and a physician-consultant at the organization that does utilization management.

The operation of these programs involves the legitimate but potentially conflicting interests of several parties: payers, who wish to pay only for necessary services; patients, who want to receive services; and providers, who wish to carry out their responsibilities without unnecessary interference. Even so, the widespread and rapid implementation of UM has been relatively free of serious conflict. Perhaps because UM organizations have sought to avoid the risks of liability and of creating dissatisfaction among patients, the conduct of UM has resulted in virtually no well-documented allegations of serious harm to patients. UMOs report high levels of cooperation among patients, physicians, and institutional providers of care. The results of the process appear to have been generally acceptable, if not always completely satisfactory to patients and their physicians. Providers have tolerated the process although they complain about some aspects of the conduct of UM, and covert resistance may be more widespread than has been recognized.

In implementing methods that require authorization before the provision of services, third-party purchasers of medical care have made it clear that trust will no longer substitute for accountability, wherever it is possible to create mechanisms of accountability. We are in the beginnings of an unplanned national experiment to see how much medical care can be managed through the use of incentives and review mechanisms. It will not be surprising if the limitations of these methods become increasingly clear as our experience with them grows. Yet at the same time, once payers believe that someone is willing to provide what they are willing to pay for, what other choice will they have?

# · 12 ·

# The Profit Motive and Accountability in the Future

Economic self-interest has never been the primary basis on which the U.S. health system has been expected to operate. Although health care providers' economic interests often coincided with their ethical and social responsibilities, their behavior was supposed to be oriented toward the provision of humane care in which biomedical knowledge would be applied to benefit patients and communities, even if this required departures from economically rational behavior.

The extent to which providers actually operated by such principles was never well documented, and some observers were skeptical of the idealistic image that providers have long cultivated. Nevertheless, the public's high expectations of health care providers had enough plausibility to support a largely private health care system that relied heavily on trust and self-regulatory mechanisms. This reflected widely held presumptions about the values of competence and ethicality that professionalism was seen to connote, the service orientation of nonprofit organizations, and the social responsibility that resulted from local control of hospitals by voluntary trustees.[1]

The plausibility of those presumptions has been undermined by the changes documented in this book. Economic motivations have come to the fore among the institutions and physicians who provide medical care, and conditions that might moderate the influence of these motivations have been weakened. Third-party purchasers of medical care have concluded that reliance on altruism, professionalism, the service orientation, and self-regulatory processes leads to unacceptable levels of expenditures and the inappropriate use of many services and procedures. Manifestations of this conclusion abound.

Fraud and abuse statutes and mechanisms of detection have steadily become more elaborate, comprehensive, and tough, as we saw in Chapter 6, and private payers have also increased their attention to fraud and abuse.[2] (The growing willingness of patients to bring suit against health care providers may also have some of the same roots.) Payment systems that are premised on health care providers' responsiveness to economic incentives have been widely implemented. Private and public third-party payers continually increase their demands for documentation about the services for which providers request payment. Moreover, as I discussed in Chapters 10 and 11, many payers have adopted utilization management methods through which they actually participate in the decisions about what services will be provided to patients. All of these developments speak volumes about the extent to which distrust has replaced trust in the relationship between payers and providers.

More formal accountability has also been developing regarding the social responsibilities of hospitals. Legislation was passed in 1986 against hospitals' "dumping" uninsured patients—at least those in need of emergency services. Local governments in many parts of the country have begun to insist that nonprofit hospitals demonstrate that their tax exemptions are justified by their behavior.

As formal mechanisms of accountability are developed in areas where trust previously played a prominent role, and as payers and regulators develop means with which to monitor and control the behavior of providers of health care in ever-greater detail, it is worth reflecting about implications.

I will begin by arguing that a continuing need exists for the fiduciary ethic (or the ethic of beneficence, as Pellegrino and Thomasma call it)[3] on the part of professionals and that a valid and central role remains for *nonprofit* institutions.

## Continuing Importance of Ideals about Professionalism and Service

The movement toward a health care system that is oriented toward profitability, economic rationality, and cost containment does not eliminate the characteristics that have heretofore made accountability an especially difficult problem in health care: the vulnerabilities of both patients and third-party payers. Nor do the changes alter the fact that the market will not necessarily reward the provision of all important services. Indeed, in some ways the behavior connoted by the values that have traditionally been associated with professionalism and nonprofit organizations has become more necessary even as the plausibility of those values as substitutes for formal accountability has declined.

## Vulnerabilities of Patients

Individuals who are seriously ill come to the point where they must trust in and rely on the competence of the people who provide care, and on their willingness to put the patient's interests first. The importance of a provider's commitment to the patient has not been diminished by the increased oversight by payers. Indeed, the proliferation of incentives that reward giving fewer services to patients and the development of programs in which third parties evaluate the appropriateness of particular services present some danger that the needs of individual patients could suffer if providers do not have a high degree of allegiance to patients.

From the standpoint of meeting the needs and preferences of individual patients, several limitations of new payment and utilization management systems by third parties must be recognized. Experience with these methods is still limited, and safeguards and accountability structures are underdeveloped. The standards of care that are built into many utilization management programs—regarding what services a patient with a specific medical problem should receive and the conditions under which certain procedures are appropriate—are generally not open to external scrutiny. These standards are applied from a distance, generally over the telephone, with varying degrees of aggressiveness and, presumably, of competence. Furthermore, the interests of the party who is seeking to shape medical decision making (the purchaser) do not necessarily coincide with the needs of the patient.

For these reasons the decisions of utilization management organizations are not an adequate substitute for the physician's assessment as the basis on which care proceeds. Indeed, such programs rely on the physician's being oriented toward the well-being of the patient. Unless physicians are willing to object when a utilization management program makes a determination that conflicts with the interests of the patient (and unless utilization management takes these objections seriously),[4] this new form of accountability could result in patients' not receiving needed treatments. It appears that the courts will accept the distrustful view of physicians that legitimizes utilization management— that in the absence of such oversight physicians will provide unnecessary or inappropriate services—but will also expect them to defend patients' interests and hold them responsible if they fail to challenge a utilization management decision that results in harm to a patient.[5]

Paradoxical expectations about physician behavior are also built into those cost-containment programs that reward physicians for saving money in the care of their patients. Such approaches are based on the premise that physicians will respond to economic incentives in their patient care decisions but also on trust that they will not be so responsive as to jeopardize the interests of patients. Creating economic incentives that encourage providers to perform fewer services or to discharge patients from the hospital more quickly makes sense only if providers can be trusted not to be excessively influenced.

More and more the services received by patients are not the result of a decision of a single person who is accountable to the patient but are instead the product of negotiations between providers and payers. The interests of patients will not be served if patient care decisions are excessively influenced by payer-created economic incentives or determinations of appropriateness. It thus remains essential that the medical profession adhere to the fiduciary ethic which dictates that the patient's interest comes first, and that medical institutions maintain their commitment to quality and to values that are distinct from, even if not wholly independent of, the pursuit of economic goals.

### The Need to Balance the Objectification of Medical Care

A premise of utilization management programs is that patients' needs are so objective that information about the patient's condition and symptoms can enable a person who has never seen or talked to the patient to determine what services are appropriate or, more commonly, inappropriate. This approach is consistent with the rise of scientific medicine and has validity in many practical situations (for example, when inadequate indications exist for a proposed elective surgical procedure such as a hysterectomy or tonsillectomy). Yet this "objectification" of medical care through the development and application of criteria of appropriateness could lead to inattention to the needs of some patients. Heightening this danger is the fact that negotiations between providers and utilization managers commonly take place with no participation by the patient.

In the twentieth century, to use a nineteenth-century formulation by Henry Sumner Maine, we have steadily moved from medical care relationships based on status (with open, unbounded obligations, as among family or neighbors) to relationships based on contract (with mutual obligations legally specified). The rise of scientific medicine and of third-party payment created both the need and the ability to define with ever-greater specificity just what services would be paid for under what circumstances for patients with just what kinds of conditions. Scientific medicine gave us treatments that could seemingly be applied with little or no knowledge of the patient as an individual, and the advent of third-party payment created the question, "What should we pay for?" This has eventually led to the development and application of criteria or rules by which third parties determine whether a patient needs a particular service.

Discretion remains an essential element of medical practice, as are human interaction and the provision of reassurance. In 1975, before utilization management appeared on the horizon, Eliot Freidson wrote about why medical practice should not be "mechanized," even though some possibilities in that direction could be perceived.

> Computers could record and analyze the technical substance of patients' complaints and symptoms, could question patients systematically in the course of taking a general health history and a history of the particular complaint, could order and interpret necessary diagnostic tests, and could prescribe necessary drugs even if not, perhaps, actually perform necessary surgery. Programmed on the basis of established standards, a computer would perform exactly as intended, and the records it would keep would be absolutely reliable.

But such a technically feasible solution is obviously not acceptable on social grounds. Its virtue is only that it carries our thought to a logical extreme by representing the end result of thinking about health care in terms involving the enforcement and control of purely technical standards. Rightly or wrongly, necessarily or unnecessarily, human health care serves diffuse human needs for being comforted and cared for as much as if not more than it serves organic, technically defined needs. If the comfort of human interaction were removed from health care by mechanization and patients were treated as mere bodies in the course of such mechanization, medical care would no longer serve most of the needs of today's patients.[6]

The rise of utilization management has moved health care in the direction that Freidson wrote about, with powerful justifications in the need to reduce unnecessary services (and their attendant risks), to focus scarce resources, and to narrow some of the wide variations in how physicians practice medicine.

However necessary it may be for *payers* to adopt formal policies that state in impersonal terms who is entitled to services and to what services patients are entitled, this objectification of medical care is not the approach that most of us want our *providers* of medical services to take. Ideally, perhaps at an unconscious level, patients often want the care they receive to be open-ended, based less on contractual obligations than on unbounded responses to their needs—as if the provider of health services were acting out of love rather than from an expectation of gain.[7]

But HMOs and hospitals are adopting more criteria for the use of certain procedures, more tightly controlling staffing levels in each unit and on each shift (a method that can reduce nurses' ability to respond to individual needs), and pressing for early discharge of hospitalized patients as soon as criteria of "need" are no longer met. Ever-larger areas of medical care may come to be determined by factors that are independent of the judgments of individual physicians, nurses, and patients about what services are needed. This may reduce the provision of inappropriate and unnecessary services, but it could nevertheless be inconsistent with some ordinary notions of what constitutes good medical care: responsiveness to the needs of individual patients, the "somewhat nebulous and elusive quality usually desired and sometimes present in medical practice, variously called caring, compassion, humanitarianism, altruism, beneficence, or philanthropy."[8] One of the characteristic problems of modern health care is how to retain a caring and compassionate orientation in responding to problems that have technical solutions in settings that attach compensation not to "caring for" but "doing to."

Traditional conceptions of professionalism and a patient-service orientation, in which professionals and organizations that provide health care services define their role in terms of the patient's needs and interests, not in terms of doing what third parties are willing to pay for, continue to be essential.

No sector of the health care system appears to be uniquely compassionate and caring. Organizations such as nonprofit teaching hospitals, which are devoted to scientific and educational goals, are notoriously insensitive to patients' needs as individual human beings, while conversely, some investor-owned institutions and HMOs have been leaders in developing methods for obtaining feedback from patients about the care they received and, in turn, transmitting that feedback to the institutions and individuals that provided the care. But the heart of the problem created by the objectification of medical care is not the risk to such amenities as common courtesy, but the danger that the impersonal criteria that are set for categories of patients will be inappropriately applied to individual patients and that care will be strictly limited to that which has been contracted for. Good patient care requires that providers recognize individual differences in patients' needs and not allow patient care decisions to be excessively influenced by contractual obligations or the standards and criteria that payers use for cost-control purposes.

Some residue of the more open obligations remains in the ideals and assumptions that surround nonprofit hospitals (acting to serve, not to make money), locally controlled institutions (neighbors helping neighbors), and values of professionalism (emphasizing service and meeting patient needs). Such values provide some counterweight to the broad and probably inevitable trend toward objectification of medical care.

### Service to Patients Unable to Pay

There continues to be much that health professionals and institutions can do to benefit the society or community or individual patients that will not occur without some commitment to traditional conceptions of professional obligations and community service. One of the primary traditional expressions of the service ethic of health care providers has been in the treatment of patients who lack the means to pay.

Although the medical needs of more than 37 million uninsured Americans (plus millions more with inadequate insurance) cannot be adequately met through reliance on the willingness and ability of health care providers to raise funds for that purpose, such willingness helps to deal with the problem. The American Hospital Association estimates that hospitals provide more than $7 billion in indigent care annually, and the amount of unsponsored care provided by hospitals doubled (in constant dollars) between 1980 and 1986, a period in which the uninsured population grew substantially.[9] (According to the Census Bureau's current population survey, the number of uninsured Americans grew from 29.2 million in 1979 to 37.1 million in 1984, an increase of from 13.4 to 15.8 percent of the population.)[10]

Although Chapter 5 showed that provision of such services is not the exclusive province of either for-profit or nonprofit institutions, the latter serve more uninsured patients than do their for-profit counterparts, and they are more responsive to state-by-state variations in the need for uncompensated care.

At the same time, the limitations of relying on the willingness of private organizations to provide free care are apparent. Internal cross-subsidies from paying patients have always been a fragile basis for a system of caring for the uninsured. With the rise in profit-oriented health care, the growing number of uninsured, the very high costs of care, and the reluctance of payers to pay at levels that subsidize care of the uninsured, it is clear that providers cannot be relied on to solve the financing problem. There must be new sources of funding if the issue of caring for the uninsured is to be dealt with.

### Provision of Economically Unrewarding Services

Another expression of the service ethic is in making some services available in locales or under circumstances in which it is difficult or impossible to generate an economic return that is sufficient to attract or hold equity capital. Services that may be important or useful in a community cannot necessarily be offered profitably if they are a public good, if they are heavily used by uninsured patients, if volume is low, or if payment systems are inadequate.[11] Although there are real limits on an institution's ability to provide unprofitable services, the inevitable shortcomings of both the marketplace and tax revenues as a way to meet communities' needs make it desirable that there be institutions that are willing to generate revenues with which to subsidize these services. Such behavior, which Chapter 5 showed to be more common among nonprofit hospitals than among for-profits, may come from religious values (as with Catholic hospitals' mission to provide care to the poor and their efforts to offer alternatives to abortion), from institutions' educational or research missions (which may be enhanced if certain services are offered), or from persuasion by medical or community leaders that a given service is needed.

## Vulnerabilities of Payment Systems

Just as the changes that have occurred in health care do not eliminate the need for attention to the vulnerabilities of patients, neither have they eliminated the vulnerabilities of payment systems in which purchasers cannot make their own assessment of the need for a service or the adequacy with which it is provided. Although payers have greatly increased their oversight of the services for which they are asked to pay, many services that are provided to patients and billed to payers are beyond the reach of monitoring systems. Opportunities to exploit the vulnerabilities of payment systems will continue to exist, even as payers reduce their reliance on trust through the continued development of data systems and review mechanisms.

Dealing with providers who are determined to maximize their economic returns increases payers' costs. Nonprofit hospitals seem less likely than for-profits to price up to what the market will bear. As Chapter 5 showed, payers' costs have been much higher when hospital services are purchased from for-profit institutions than from nonprofit institutions.[12] Providers' pursuit of profits may increase payers' costs in other ways. Some providers apply much ingenuity to probing the weaknesses of payment, monitoring, and utilization control systems so as to extract maximum revenues for services. Some may skimp on quality when it is not likely to be detected by the patient or payer. Some may cross the line into fraudulent and abusive activities. It is axiomatic that the more health care providers seek to exploit the vulnerabilities of third-party payment systems, the more resources payers will have to put into monitoring providers' behavior and detecting and prosecuting fraud and abuse. Third-party payment has become much more than a mechanism to ensure that people will receive needed medical care. It has also become a cops-and-robbers game in which the individuals and organizations that provide health services probe for weaknesses and gaps in payment and monitoring systems, and payers strive to catch up.

As I argued in Chapter 6, the explosive growth of different types of for-profit organizations has contributed to this problem. Small proprietary firms that provide various types of ambulatory and home care services pose difficulties because (1) there is a direct link between revenues and the owner's pocketbook; (2) the common practice of involving referring physicians as investors can corrupt the objectivity of the doctor who prescribes a particular treatment; (3) payment rules and monitoring mechanisms are hard-pressed to keep up with the new organizational forms; and (4) the entrepreneurs who are attracted by the profit opportunities that these characteristics create will inevitably include some buccaneers. The willingness of even a relative few to take advantage of whatever opportunities exist to beat the system has implications for the level of resources that payers must invest in monitoring, investigating, and litigating.

Some of the opportunities for defrauding third-party payers have been reduced in certain fields by the replacement of small proprietary firms with larger, investor-owned organizations in which there is a much more remote link between the actions of any individual who provides services and the movement of money into that individual's pocketbook. Such organizations establish procedures and monitoring mechanisms to protect against particular types of fraudulent behavior. Nonetheless, the examples given in Chapter 6 of Westworld, International Medical Centers, and Paracelsus (and the history of the nursing home industry) illustrate that the large corporation can also spawn a kind of deviance that differs in nature and scale from the individual deviance that can occur in proprietary organizations. Such corporate deviance can be particularly difficult and expensive to investigate and adjudicate. The move away from cost-based reimbursement has removed a large area in which providers could apply ingenuity to extract illegitimate profits from a payment system, but many other areas of opportunity remain. Furthermore, as Chapter 7 showed, the larger for-profit organizations have been particularly active in using legal avenues and due process mechanisms to try to advance their interests.

All of this suggests that the more the health care system is populated by providers that are strongly profit oriented, the greater will be both the leakage of monies from their intended purpose and the expenditures by payers to try to prevent this abuse.

Beyond this, something is lost as the relationship between health care providers and the organizations that pay and regulate them becomes more adversarial—as providers look for every advantage, every loophole, every weakness in systems of accountability, and payers and regulators seek to establish mechanisms to reduce their costs and to detect the increasingly creative types of malfeasance on the part of those providers. The atmosphere of distrust between payer and purchaser can become poisonous. I recall testimony from a representative of National Medical Care, the leading corporate provider of kidney dialysis services, at a hearing held by the Institute of Medicine's Committee on For-Profit Enterprise in Health Care. He said that the company understood well who its "main enemy" was: the U.S. government's Health Care Financing Administration (HCFA). Robert Derzon, a member of the IOM committee and the first administrator of HCFA, noted the irony that this "enemy," HCFA's end-stage renal disease program, was the source of all of the revenues from the company's main line of business. How many companies would refer to their main customer as their enemy? How can this be? The combination of third-party payment and profit-oriented providers must be a key factor, although it should be recognized that payers' efforts to control their expenditures can also slip across the line from the prudent to the dubious.[13]

A cycle of response and reaction sets in when purchasers of care begin to suspect that the individuals and organizations that provide care are more interested in maximizing revenue than in receiving fair compensation for the services they offer, and when providers perceive the payers as trying unfairly to limit their expenditures by paying less than is adequate. Steps that purchasers take to control their costs can produce anger among providers, and this anger can become the justification for finding new ways to evade control mechanisms. And the cycle continues.

## Advantages of Nonprofit Institutions

Although investor ownership has provided an avenue for making capital for certain health services available more quickly or in locales where the services would not otherwise have been offered, several public policy advantages remain with a predominantly nonprofit hospital sector. First, as I have just suggested, nonprofit institutions conform more closely than for-profit institutions to a service ethic that remains central. They tend to price less aggressively, take a less adventurous stance toward payment systems, offer more unprofitable services, and be more responsive to the needs of uninsured patients.

Moreover, nonprofit institutions can be held accountable for engaging in such behavior by being required to justify the tax benefits they receive. Until recent years nonprofit institutions rarely had to document their performance. Indeed, past changes have relaxed the conditions that nonprofit hospitals have had to meet to gain exemption from federal income taxes.[14] Nevertheless, individual nonprofit institutions could be required periodically to document what they have done to justify their tax advantages. Such accountability would help meet needs that would otherwise go unmet by stimulating institutions to find more revenues in addition to payments received for services rendered.

Nonprofit institutions also provide stability in the health care system. The struggles to maintain profitability that have led most of the large hospital companies to sell many of their hospitals and that have even led some smaller companies into bankruptcy may be endemic to health care. The health care system relies heavily on government support, which means that providers must deal with a payer that has enormous power and will seek to control expenditures as much as possible, even if that means paying less than it costs to provide services to beneficiaries. For example, for hospital services Medicare's prospective payment system for hospitals provides a mechanism by which government payments can be adjusted, based on hospitals' past profitability.

There are advantages, therefore, in having health care institutions whose accountability structure does not require generation of profit levels that are satisfactory to investors, who always have the option of putting their capital elsewhere. Dependence on investor ownership makes the availability of capital-intensive health services (such as hospital care) less certain than does dependence on nonprofit organizations, particularly those that have a long-standing role in their communities. This is not an argument against the presence of investor-owned institutions, but it *is* an argument against too heavy reliance on them.

As I noted in Chapters 3 and 5, equity capital is much more mobile than is capital invested in nonprofit institutions because of the legal restrictions that apply to nonprofit organizations and because of the accountability structure that comes from investor ownership. Nonprofit organizations, particularly those with strong community ties, have the ability to call in times of crisis on the charitable and voluntary spirit of the community or church, or on government (national or local). This, along with the legal restrictions that apply to the use of the assets and revenues of nonprofit organizations, provides greater assurance of the availability of hospital services when resources are scarce than does investor ownership. As for investor ownership, experience to date suggests that there are many locales where generation of adequate return for investor capital is not possible. And the instability of public ownership can be seen in the chronic capital and budgetary problems of many hospitals owned by local government authorities. Thus, from the standpoint of the availability of capital-intensive medical services at the community level, a system of predominantly nonprofit hospitals continues to have some substantial advantages.

## Accountability and the Future of American Health Care

The changes that have been examined in this book create new problems of accountability and raise the salience of some old

ones. In the former category are questions surrounding the proliferation of new types of health care organizations and the rise of
utilization management by parties concerned with cost containment. In the latter are issues such as the obligations of nonprofit
institutions and the conditions that undercut the plausibility of
the medical profession's fiduciary ethic.

### Accountability of Nonprofit Organizations

Perhaps the greatest threat to the predominantly private, nonprofit nature of our hospitals comes not from the rise of an
investor-owned sector but from changes among the nonprofits
themselves. The changes that took place in the 1980s in the
methods by which hospitals are paid and the declining generosity
of major payers (such as Medicare) make significant, continued
increases in investor ownership of hospitals unlikely. The behavior of nonprofit hospitals, however, could jeopardize the primary
advantage of their nonprofit status: their tax exemptions.

Questions about this issue have arisen at various levels of government. At the federal level the issue is driven by large deficits,
the perception that nonprofit hospitals are behaving like for-
profits, and behind-the-scenes pressure from the investor-owned
sector, which sees itself at a competitive disadvantage because of
the nonprofits' tax exemptions. Similar factors have been
involved in property tax exemption issues in several states and
cities. In Utah the issue became prominent through a major
court case and statewide referendum; nonprofit hospitals there
must now periodically justify their local property tax exemptions.

Although the behavior of nonprofit hospitals has become a
policy issue, the question of whether the hospital sector of the
U.S. health care system would remain predominantly nonprofit
in the absence of tax exemptions has received little consideration. I have argued that a predominantly nonprofit structure is
desirable. But the possibility has grown that nonprofit hospitals
will find themselves held accountable for some degree of charitable or altruistic behavior. This would be a significant change in
the accountability structure of health care and would provide a
counterweight to the growing pressures, discussed in Chapter 4,

for nonprofit hospitals to perform well economically. Documentation requirements may increase our knowledge of the charitable activities of nonprofit institutions and may even stimulate such activities.

The problem that many nonprofit hospitals face is that, to finance the behavior that would differentiate them from their for-profit counterparts and help to justify the tax benefits they receive from federal, state, and local governments, they may have to rely on methods that do not comport with their nonprofit image and that may undermine the perceived legitimacy of those tax benefits. The money with which to serve patients who are unable to pay, to offer services that lose money, and to engage in research and/or educational activities that are not fully compensated must come from somewhere. The two traditional sources of funds—charity and surpluses from paying patients—have become more problematic.

Charitable contributions, which provided more than 13 percent of hospital resources half a century ago, have shrunk to less than 0.5 percent of the average hospital's revenues and are even less than that for most hospitals.[15] In light of past trends in philanthropic giving to hospitals, the increasing cost of care, and government tax policies that make charitable donations less attractive to taxpayers, many hospitals will find it difficult to stimulate charitable contributions sufficiently for them to become a substantial source of revenues. Success in doing so, however, may be essential to both the mission and legitimacy of institutions that wish to remain tax exempt.

Trying to generate surplus patient revenues to finance money-losing activities (so-called Robin Hood financing) has been made more difficult because of price competition and increasingly stringent rate-setting policies, particularly by Medicare. Hospitals thus have to finance economically unrewarding activities by other means. Government grants for this purpose are unlikely, and unreliable over time. Only one other option exists—the now common practice of generating income from activities other than patient care (such as business ventures). Some such activities bear a direct relationship to hospital operations (the hospital gift shop or parking lot); some pertain to health care but not specifically to hospitalized patients (the sale of hearing aids, beeper services, or office space to physicians); some involve the marketing of the institution's non–patient care services (laundry or data processing); some bear little if any relationship to the hospital (motels or other commercial property). Although the generation of such revenues now provides a very small proportion of hospital revenue (perhaps 1 percent for nonprofit hospitals), it may be a more viable future source of revenue than surpluses from patient care.

The law requires that taxes be paid on the "unrelated business income" of tax-exempt organizations. Nonprofit hospitals that have sources of such income typically have a corporate structure in which the taxable activities are located in subsidiary organizations. Even so, questions about the activities whereby hospitals generate revenues from sources other than patient care have been raised as a public policy issue by various business trade associations, whose members make charges about unfair competition with taxpaying businesses. Congressional hearings and numerous proposals for revising the rules for unrelated business income tax for nonprofit organizations raised this matter in the late 1980s.[16]

The more that hospitals generate revenues by engaging in unrelated businesses, the more questions can be expected to arise about the hospitals' true mission. Public policy may be tolerant of the businesslike activities of nonprofit organizations only as long as those organizations can demonstrate that the revenues are being used for appropriate purposes.

The recognition that nonprofit institutions have not really been held accountable for engaging in the types of activities that justify tax exemptions—providing uncompensated care, offering unprofitable services, pricing at less than the market would permit, and so forth—has stimulated attention to the problem at federal, state, and local levels of government. Although, as I have indicated, this seems quite appropriate, there are also dangers. Some expectations may be unrealistic in view of hospitals' resources, and the process may be subject to extraneous political and bureaucratic factors (for example, short-term government needs for new revenue sources). Also, requirements to justify tax benefits could focus too narrowly on uncompensated care because it is the most widely understood expectation of nonprofit institutions and is deceptively easy to measure. If uncompensated care were adopted as the sole justification for nonprofit institutions' tax exemptions, that would imply that there would no longer be a need for nonprofit institutions if government were to deal directly with the problem of uninsured patients. I do not hold that view, as I discussed earlier in this chapter, and I believe that justification can be sought on several grounds.

Because the predominantly nonprofit character of hospitals is a valuable aspect of American health care, government action to hold them accountable for engaging in certain activities seems vastly preferable to policies that would eliminate the benefits attached to nonprofit status, such as tax exemptions. Elimination of such benefits could lead to further erosion of the character of the institutions that remain the core of the American health care system.

Although nonprofit hospitals have prevailed in some of the recent disputes over the legitimacy of their tax benefits, the emergence of the issue has stimulated renewed concern among nonprofit hospitals about their proper mission.[17] The fact that questions about tax benefits have arisen coterminously with the concerted efforts by third-party payers to reduce their payments to hospitals (and thus hospitals' abilities to cross-subsidize money-losing activities) not only points to the need for realistic expectations. It also suggests the extent to which the performance of nonprofit hospitals over the past two decades has undercut the social legitimacy on which their tax advantages rested.

## Preservation of the Fiduciary Obligation

While improvements are sought in the accountability structure of health care, it should be recognized that the values of professionalism and of behavior not driven by the profit motive are valuable assets in our health care system that should be built upon, not ignored or destroyed. As I have argued, some of our highest expectations of health care providers can be met only if providers are willing to operate at times by principles other than the pursuit of economic gain. Furthermore, the accountability mechanisms needed in a system in which the economic imperative is moderated by values of professionalism and altruism are more modest than they would otherwise have to be.

Several steps in the organization of services merit consideration for preserving or reinforcing the fiduciary ethic.[18] One is to discourage physicians' investments in (or kickback arrangements with) organizations to which they refer their patients. Relatively narrow legislation—the Ethics in Patient Referrals Act of 1989— addressed some of the issues of physician ownership of referral laboratories. Opponents of such approaches to the conflict of interest problem argue that there is no real difference between physicians' charging for procedures that they have done in their own offices and their making referrals from which they will generate secondary income. Yet this argument overlooks the negative effects on quality and efficiency that tend to occur when a supplier has a captive market. It also denies that additional conflicts of interest can affect the physician's judgment, the patient's respect for the objectivity of the advice that he or she is receiving, and the payer's willingness to use the physician as the certifier of the patient's need for particular services. The more such conflicts of interest exist, the more payers will try to protect themselves with procedural requirements (such as preservice authorization) and monitoring systems; the more our health care system's extraordinary administrative costs will grow; and the more patients will seek second and third opinions or other devices to try to assure themselves that the advice they have received is objective rather than self-interested.

A second area where serious threats to the fiduciary ethic can be addressed is in incentive arrangements used within alternative delivery systems, particularly HMOs and independent practice associations (IPAs), to control utilization of services. The incentives vary enormously from those that are so mild and indirect as to be largely ineffective in influencing physician behavior to those that attach such powerful negative consequences to certain decisions that the physician may suffer a significant financial loss in trying to meet the patient's needs. At present there are no restrictions on the kinds of financial incentives that HMOs, IPAs, and PPOs may create for their physicians; no reporting requirements about what financial incentives a plan uses; little or no awareness among the employers who offer plans or the individuals who sign up with them about the incentives that are in use; and no requirements that anyone monitor patterns of service to make sure that the cost-containment incentives are not harming patients. (Of course, no such requirements exist *outside* of HMOs either.) This is an area in which better disclosure policies and increased patient awareness is needed.[19]

A third area where the fiduciary ethic is threatened is in circumstances in which physicians are employees. Physicians who work for ambulatory care facilities (or alternative delivery systems) may be pressured to act in ways that serve the interests of the employing organization but are contradictory to the patient's interest and to the fiduciary ethic.[20] Whether or not such problems are particularly characteristic of for-profit organizations, as some critics believe, it is unclear how this problem should be dealt with.[21] Possible answers range from letting the market work the problem out, to reviving laws against corporate practice of medicine (perhaps applying them only to for-profit organizations), to establishing physicians' unions. Perhaps the best balance of economic forces and fiduciary aspects will be found in HMOs that are organized in a way that gives significant voice to the physicians and nurses practicing therein and that provide a collegial setting for professional practice. Indeed, the growth of multispecialty group practices may be an important element in responding to many problems—providing accountability to patients, allowing the possibility of collegial forms of control, and creating opportunities for contracting arrangements that reward quality and efficiency.

## Accountability in the New For-Profits

Among the new proprietary health care organizations—the ambulatory care centers and home care providers—comparatively little systematic information is available about their structure and performance. The strategies that many of these organizations have adopted to obtain referrals (such as ownership by referring physicians), their internal incentive structures, their attraction to types of services for which patients' needs are difficult for external parties to review objectively, and, in some cases, their comparatively high charges for services rendered all suggest that some of those organizations are willing to exploit the vulnerabilities of patients and payment systems. The pace of change and the development of new types of organizations have been so rapid, however, that it has been difficult for regulatory and licensure processes to keep abreast in developing standards and reviewing compliance with those standards. Moreover, there have been some disputes about whether any new structures of external accountability—such as licensure and certification—are needed.[22]

Some mechanisms of accountability have nevertheless been developed. Many organizations that engage in utilization management are changing the focus of preadmission review programs to preservice review programs and applying them to certain expensive services whether or not hospital admission is involved. As of 1988, ambulatory surgery centers (and hospital outpatient departments) became subject to review by PROs for services rendered to Medicare beneficiaries. Voluntary accreditation mechanisms are being developed by organizations such as the Joint Commission on Accreditation of Healthcare Organizations and the Accreditation Association for Ambulatory Health Care. The process of developing accreditation standards and processes has proved to be complicated and contentious. The pace may also have been slowed by the fact that reimbursement systems have generally not provided advantages to ambulatory care facilities that have gone through the accreditation process.[23]

Various types of ambulatory and home care organizations are subject to various state licensure requirements and certification by Medicare or other third-party payers. There is considerable doubt, however, about the adequacy of these mechanisms in the absence of more elaborate and effective monitoring procedures that now exist, as recent reports on nursing homes and home health agencies emphasize.[24] Moreover, a 1990 General Accounting Office report on state regulation of sixteen types of freestanding ambulatory care providers concluded that "states do not license or otherwise regulate most of the 16 types," that "for those freestanding providers that are licensed, states have imposed few sanctions for deficiencies identified during inspections," and that "consumers do not have adequate assurance that unlicensed freestanding providers are offering quality care."[25]

*Accountability of Organizations Engaging*
*in Utilization Management*

Utilization management methods aimed at influencing physicians' patient care decisions raise significant questions of accountability. Surveys of physicians have shown that there is considerable frustration with the procedures of, and burdens of dealing with, the numerous utilization management organizations with which they must contend.[26] Self-corrective mechanisms that would penalize poor performance are imperfect, as I discussed in Chapter 11.

Utilization management programs have developed in a regulatory vacuum, subject neither to insurance regulations nor to regulations that apply to providers of health services. This undoubtedly contributed to their rapid widespread adoption by private payers, but it has made them vulnerable to virtuous-sounding attacks from physician groups that resent the intrusion on their autonomy. These opponents of utilization management led calls in many states for legislation to regulate the processes that utilization management organizations use and the credentials of the nurses and physicians who seek to influence patient care decisions. In response, in late 1989 the industry began work on an accreditation process.[27]

One legislative approach is to declare utilization management to be the practice of medicine, thereby prohibiting the involvement of nonphysicians. Most utilization programs achieve economy by using nurses to screen cases, referring to physicians only those cases that do not pass the screen. A requirement that fielding telephone calls and screening cases would have to be done by physicians would make most utilization management programs too expensive to be practical. Firms that operate national utilization management programs are also vulnerable to regulatory requirements that vary widely from state to state.

In the face of demands from physician groups for intervention to halt interference in the doctor-patient relationship, several important considerations may be overlooked. Utilization management is the only cost-containment approach that attempts to deter selectively the provision of unnecessary or inappropriate services. It is a method that permits the application of the practice guidelines and criteria of appropriateness that are being developed by many medical specialty societies and that are growing out of research on the effectiveness or outcomes of medical services. Furthermore, the ability of health benefit plans to provide coverage for certain services may well be reduced if methods that screen out inappropriate services are disabled. The failure of utilization management programs may lead to cuts in benefit plans or, where inhospitable state regulation is the culprit, the movement of some businesses to other states. Also, an evidentiary basis for regulating utilization management methods or personnel is lacking, as is solid evidence of harm that should be prevented. Finally, it appears that the courts will hold utilization management organizations liable for negligence in the performance of their function and that these organizations are keenly aware of such liability.

Although regulation aimed at inhibiting utilization management seems unwise, regulatory attention to certain other aspects of the conduct of utilization management seems more warranted. Organizations that preauthorize services are not required to disclose to any public agency or to providers of health care the basis on which they consider proposed services inappropriate or unnecessary, although hundreds of thousands or even millions of individuals may be subject to the organization's prior-authorization program. Also, no requirements exist for appeals processes or procedures to ensure that patients understand their rights. If regulation is warranted, it should start in these areas, not in attempts to specify how utilization management programs themselves should be organized or staffed.

The organizations that perform utilization management services are accountable to the employers and other large purchasers of medical care. The purchasers hire them, convey expectations regarding goals and aggressiveness, and evaluate their performance. The work of utilization management organizations lends itself well to auditing; and specialized organizations now exist that perform that service for purchasers. Finally, individuals who are covered by health benefit plans can make bad experiences known to the sponsors of those plans.

In short, purchasers of utilization management have a great deal to say about how well it is done.[28] Moreover, there is a growing awareness that employers whose benefit plans include (as most do) either utilization management or networks of providers may bear some legal responsibility for the soundness of those programs and managed care systems.[29] Because past levels of inappropriate services have been so high and levels of accountability for patterns of care have been so low, there is reason for cautious optimism about the possibility of maintaining or enhancing quality, even while some cost savings are being achieved. But that depends on whether purchasers of health benefit plans have a degree of commitment to the interests of beneficiaries, not just an interest in reducing costs.[30]

## Public Accountability: The Next Step?

In response to cost pressures and the declining plausibility of trust and self-restraint as shapers of the behavior of health care providers, third-party payers (and their agents) have developed data systems with which to monitor the behavior of the health care providers from whom they purchase services. Such monitoring not only focuses on particular episodes of care, but it also accumulates episodes and patient encounters to reveal patterns of care. Profiling has made possible the comparison of providers on such matters as the intensity of services provided to patients with particular diagnoses (number of tests ordered, drugs prescribed, visits made) and expenses generated or costs incurred. Such information is also useful in focusing more intensified utilization review activities. Some states, such as California and Maryland, collect utilization and charge information on hospital admissions, making it possible not only for researchers to do useful studies but also for information to be published about patterns of care and charges in different hospitals. Such programs potentially give patients information that they have not previously had.

The annual publication of hospital-specific and diagnosis-specific mortality statistics by the Health Care Financing Administration (and also by the State of California) beginning in the mid-1980s may prove to be the beginning of a kind of public accountability that will revolutionize all forms of accountability in health care.[31] In theory, the availability of both price and outcome information could enable patients and payers to make purchasing decisions on a much sounder basis than by word of mouth, or by using a list of specialists provided by the county medical society, or the Yellow Pages. The initial experience, however, has also shown how many obstacles must be overcome.

First, mortality is a very limited measure of performance and needs to be supplemented by other measures ranging from untoward events to patient satisfaction. A broad effort to improve the measurement of the outcomes of medical care is now under way among health service researchers. Both purchasers and providers of care have developed a strong interest in the measurement of quality of care. Rapid progress has been made over the past decade in the development of new quality assessment tools, including case-mix adjusted mortality rates, computerized algorithms against which the appropriateness of care can be evaluated, and patient satisfaction measures.[32] Such tools can be used by provider organizations or by payers or organizers of managed care systems. Second, for many diagnoses, institutions, and individual physicians, the number of cases in a particular year is too small to allow calculation of statistically valid mortality rates. Third, the relationship between mortality and other measures of quality of care is uncertain. A study done in New York of hospitals that had notably high mortality rates in the HCFA data found that these institutions had significantly *lower* rates of problems involving quality of care, based on an independent review of patients' records.[33] Fourth, mortality rates are affected by factors other than the quality of care that is provided to the patient— factors such as whether the hospital receives large numbers of patients through the emergency room and from nursing homes, whether it has a hospice unit, and whether it is a referral center for complicated cases (as are many teaching hospitals). Nonetheless, several groups of researchers have developed severity measures that can be built into data systems. Although there is as yet no consensus about the adequacy of those measures and their advantages and disadvantages vis-à-vis one another, this should be less of a problem as further research is done. Finally, since there have previously been few consequences attached to a hospital's mortality experience, we do not yet know how much hospitals might be able to manipulate their statistics through admissions, discharge, or coding practices.

With all of these problems and questions, it is clear that the day of public accountability by means of market mechanisms is not yet at hand. Some steps have been taken, but there are many problems to be overcome. There is much to be gained, however, if it becomes truly possible for payers and patients to evaluate and select providers based on their past performance.

A new accountability is rapidly developing in health care. Its elements are the development and use of practice guidelines, the monitoring of patterns of care, and utilization review and management. Although this new accountability is clearly a development of major importance, in my view enthusiasm needs to be qualified and tempered.

In several regards, the new accountability is a very significant development from the standpoint of the public interest, which I take to lie in the efficient provision of services combined with adherence to the fiduciary ethic. First, it is a rational and even potentially sensitive response to the loss of confidence in the traditional assumptions about medical professionalism and the motivations of institutional providers—a loss which I believe this book has shown is justified. Second, although the obvious impetus behind the new accountability is cost containment, the methods lend themselves to a focus on distinguishing appropriate from inappropriate or unnecessary services. Third, some methods make very practical use of knowledge about clinical medicine and, in so doing, are stimulating the development of additional reliable knowledge about the appropriate responses to patients' needs. Fourth, the methods lend themselves to providing oversight with a relatively light hand.

Some important qualifications are hidden within these statements. The ways in which these methods are used and the auspices under which they are applied may make a great deal of difference in the degree of intrusiveness of the new accountability and in the risk of harm to patients. Cost-containment programs vary in the safeguards that are built in, in their incorporation of new knowledge as it is developed, in the burden they place on physicians, in the priority accorded to simply saving money, and in appeals processes.[34]

It is desirable that the new accountability be overseen in a fashion that does not just attend to the impact on cost but that also takes into account the medical soundness of the activity and ensures that the interests of patients are protected. This implies, it seems to me, oversight by purchaser-based boards that include representatives of beneficiaries and medical advisers. The purchaser's legitimate interests need to be balanced by parties who are concerned that patients' interests be protected. Because neither the purchaser nor the beneficiaries' advocates will necessarily be able to judge the medical soundness of the criteria being used by the review organizations or of the determinations that it makes, medical advice is needed.

Such boards should pay attention at the outset to the types of information that are needed—not only data on utilization trends, payment denials, and so forth, but also on sentinel events (for example, rates of hospital readmissions) that might signal that a utilization management system is pushing too heavily in certain directions, on the criteria of appropriateness that are being used, on systematic patient satisfaction data, and on complaints from patients and providers.

It might be argued that this would put a burden on the entities that carry out the new accountability that never applied in, say, employers' relationships with traditional insurers. That is true. But the potential for benefit is very great in the new accountability if it is carried out to reflect a concern about cost, quality, and the fiduciary aspects of care—too much potential benefit to be wasted by a narrow focus on cost containment. And the potential for danger is also great because the activities of the organizations that carry out the new accountability affect thousands, tens of thousands, even millions of patients.

The changes that have transformed health care have raised many important issues: (1) the need for better accountability of nonprofit institutions; (2) the emergence of public accountability regarding the performance of institutions; (3) the proliferation of new organizational forms for which external accountability mechanisms are underdeveloped; (4) the need for more accountability of organizations that are engaged in utilization management; and (5) the need to reduce the conflicts of interest that undercut the plausibility of the medical profession's fiduciary ethic.

Because the incentives and controls that apply to the individual and institutional providers of health care will continue to be imperfect for the foreseeable future, it remains essential that the health care system be populated primarily by institutions and professionals who are committed to doing right by the patient, who are willing to consider factors other than ability to pay in deciding whether to serve patients, and whose commitment to ends other than economic return make them willing to offer certain services and to engage in certain activities that do not necessarily pay their own way.

Many of the conditions that have led to reliance on trust continue to exist, and alternatives to trust, though developing rapidly, are costly. Even in—perhaps particularly in—an increasingly commercial, competitive health care system, there are important reasons for public policy to support nonprofit health care organizations and to reinforce the fiduciary ethic as a fundamental principle orienting the behavior of the physician. At the same time, it seems essential that mechanisms of accountability be improved to ensure that physicians and institutions are worthy of the patient's trust, that tax-exempt institutions deserve the benefits that they enjoy, and that greater public accountability is required of physicians, institutions, and now the organizations that are purporting to manage the health care system.

# Notes

## 1 · The Changing Accountability of American Health Care

1. The hospital and physician figures are calculated from data reported in *Physician Characteristics and Distribution in the United States, 1987* (Chicago: American Medical Association, 1987), and from *Hospital Statistics, 1988* ed. (Chicago: American Hospital Association, 1988). The physician figure is an approximation. The AMA publication (p. 30) reports that of the 569,160 physicians in the United States, 21,938 are "federal"; no count is provided of physicians who work in state or local government hospitals. The AHA publication (Table 5A) includes federal, state, and local hospitals, but its figure of 28,033 government employees includes both physicians *and* dentists.

2. *Health Care Financing Review* 11 (Fall 1989): 167. The figures are for 1987. Privately financed services include 47.5 percent of hospital care, 69.1 percent of physicians' services, 50.9 percent of nursing home care, and 80.4 percent of other personal health services. The primary sources of publicly funded services were Medicare and Medicaid, which paid for 18.2 and 11.0 percent, respectively, of all personal health services.

3. The use of private sector "delivery systems" as the vehicle for government programs is a widespread pattern in the United States. See Lester M. Salamon, "Partners in Public Service: The Scope and Theory of Government-Nonprofit Relations," pp. 99–117 in Walter W. Powell, ed., *The Nonprofit Sector: A Research Handbook* (New Haven: Yale University Press, 1987).

4. Rosemary Stevens, *In Sickness and in Wealth: The American Hospital in the Twentieth Century* (New York: Basic Books, 1989), presents extensive discussions of the role that hospitals have played as *community* organizations.

5. This statement should be partially qualified in that some of the highly regulatory, "all-payer" hospital financing mechanisms that have been adopted in a few states (for example, New Jersey) have the practical

effect of spreading the cost of uncompensated services across all payers.

6. "The traditional expectation that doctors would provide their services free to all hospital patients, irrespective of income, had gone by the board by 1910, even in the oldest, most conservative hospitals, although doctors were still generally expected to provide free care to low-income patients whom the hospital treated without charge in the wards." Stevens, *In Sickness and in Wealth*, p. 21. By that time a characteristic pattern of financing charity care had already been set. Stevens notes (p. 25) that "by 1900 payment was the 'true scientific plan' for hospital charity . . . Patients who could afford to pay more were often charged at rates above cost to help subsidize the poor, while additional funds were sought through private donations and government subsidy." See also David Rosner, *A Once Charitable Enterprise: Hospitals and Health Care in Brooklyn and New York, 1885–1915* (Cambridge: Cambridge University Press, 1982); Morris J. Vogel, *The Invention of the Modern Hospitals: Boston, 1879–1930* (Chicago: University of Chicago Press, 1980). Such examples are not limited to the distant past; see, for example, Kathy Fackelmann, "Low-Cost Prenatal Maternity Program Loses Money but Fulfills Hospital Mission," *Modern Healthcare*, January 31, 1986, p. 38.

7. Chapter 6 of Stevens, *In Sickness and in Wealth*, describes how the "voluntary ideal" was created and used in the 1930s to defeat proposals for government control of the health care system. For discussions of the functions of ideals in fostering medical dominance of the health care system, see Eliot Freidson, *The Profession of Medicine* (New York: Dodd, Mead, 1970), particularly the insights conveyed in chapter 4; and Jeffrey L. Berlant, *Profession and Monopoly: A Study of Medicine in the United States and Great Britain* (Berkeley: University of California Press, 1975).

8. See Sunny G. Yoder, "Economic Theories of For-Profit and Not-For-Profit Organizations," pp. 19–25 in Bradford H. Gray, ed., *For-Profit Enterprise in Health Care* (Washington, D.C.: National Academy Press, 1986).

9. Arnold S. Relman, "The New Medical-Industrial Complex," *New England Journal of Medicine*, October 23, 1980, pp. 963–969. See also Stanley Wohl, *The Medical Industrial Complex* (New York: Harmony, 1984).

10. Leon Eisenberg, "Health Care: For Patients or for Profits?" *American Journal of Psychiatry* 143 (August 1985): 1015.

11. A key theoretical work on the tendency toward similarity of organizations in the same field is Paul DiMaggio and Walter W. Powell, "The Iron Cage Revisited: Institutional Isomorphism and Collective Rationality in Organizational Fields," *American Sociological Review* 21 (1983): 327–336.

12. Relman, "The New Medical-Industrial Complex," and Paul Starr, *The*

*Social Transformation of American Medicine* (New York: Basic Books, 1982). See particularly chapter 5, "The Coming of the Corporation."

13. This discussion owes a debt to Amitai Etzioni's analysis in his "Epilogue: Alternative Conceptions of Accountability," pp. 121–142 in Harry I. Greenfield, *Accountability in Health Facilities* (New York: Praeger, 1975).

14. Hospital Association of New York, *Report of the Task Force on Regulation* (Albany, 1986).

15. *Information on Hospital Inspection Reporting Requirements and Life Safety Code Enforcement* HRD 80 (Washington, D.C.: U.S. General Accounting Office, July 2, 1980). For a systematic attempt to document the regulatory requirements of accountability that apply to health facilities, see Greenfield, *Accountability in Health Facilities.*

16. James A. Morone, "Models of Representation: Consumers and the HSAs," pp. 207–235 in Institute of Medicine, *Health Planning in the United States: Selected Policy Issues,* vol. 2 (Washington, D.C.: National Academy Press, 1981).

17. Greenfield, *Accountability in Health Facilities.*

18. The seminal work in this regard is Kenneth Arrow, "Uncertainty and the Welfare Economics of Medical Care," *American Economic Review* 53 (December 1963): 941–969. More recent critics of the health care system have noted that the informational asymmetries that make patients vulnerable are not simply inherent features of health care but are accentuated by a private fee-for-service health care system in which the choice of a physician is left solely to the patient. Starr, *Social Transformation of American Medicine,* pp. 225–226; Alain Enthoven, *Theory and Practice of Managed Competition in Health Care Financing* (Amsterdam: North Holland, 1988), particularly pp. 31–42.

19. Malpractice suits are an idiosyncratic mechanism of accountability in that there does not appear to be a close and predictable relationship between the occurrence of serious departures from competent care and a provider's being called to account in a lawsuit. Factors such as rural as opposed to urban residence and the quality of the relationship between doctor and patient seem to be more influential in the likelihood of a lawsuit's being brought than is the occurrence of unfortunate outcomes. Also, untoward events and quality problems that arise in certain areas of medicine (for example, orthopedic surgery and obstetrics) are much more likely to trigger lawsuits than are occurrences in fields such as pediatrics, internal medicine, and psychiatry.

20. In 1987 the Joint Commission for the Accreditation of Hospitals changed its name to the Joint Commission for the Accreditation of Healthcare Organizations because an increasingly large share of its activities pertained to health care organizations other than hospitals. The JCAHO is revising its accreditation approach to focus on "clinical

and organizational outcome indicators," and the new system is being implemented.

21. Jeffrey Pfeffer and Gerald Salancik, *The External Control of Organizations* (New York: Harper & Row, 1978).

22. In my view, equity is concerned with access to basic, necessary health services—what the President's Commission for the Study of Ethical Problems in Medicine called an "adequate level"—and not with equality. In this regard my views and reasoning are similar to those set forth in some detail by Alain Enthoven in his *Theory and Practice of Managed Competition in Health Care Finance*, particularly pages 1–10. Enthoven holds (p. 2) that "a just and humane society can define a minimum standard of medical care that ought to be available to all its members: essentially all the 'cost-worthy' medical care that can effectively prevent or cure disease, relieve suffering and correct dysfunction."

## 2 · Accountability for Profitability

1. American Hospital Association, *Hospital Statistics* (Chicago, 1985), p. 7.

2. Ibid., pp. 8–11.

3. U.S. National Center for Health Statistics, *Trends in Nursing and Related Care Homes and Hospitals*, Vital and Health Statistics, ser. 14, no. 29 (Washington, D.C.: Government Printing Office, 1984).

4. *The InterStudy Edge* (Fall 1987): 10.

5. *Directory of Preferred Provider Organizations and the Industry Report on PPO Development* (Bethesda, Md.: Institute for International Health Initiatives, 1985), p. xi.

6. Robert Hoyer, National Association for Home Care, Washington, D.C., personal communication, April 8, 1986.

7. Bradford H. Gray, ed., *For-Profit Enterprise in Health Care* (Washington, D.C.: National Academy Press, 1986), p. 36.

8. National Association for Ambulatory Care, personal communication, April 7, 1986.

9. Health Care Financing Administration data published in Gray, *For-Profit Enterprise in Health Care*, p. 38.

10. Ibid.

11. Arnold S. Relman, "The New Medical-Industrial Complex," *New England Journal of Medicine*, October 23, 1980, pp. 963–969.

12. Diana Barrett, *Multihospital Systems: The Process of Development* (Cambridge, Mass.: Oelgeschlager, Gunn & Hain, 1980), p. 1.

13. Such arrangements are commonly referred to in the management literature as horizontal integration (in contrast to vertical integration, in which an organization acquires sources of supply or customers). Such systems can be distinguished from multi-institutional arrangements, which do not entail a yielding of institutional autonomy regarding

operations, strategic planning, capital expenditures, and so forth. Thus, definitions of systems generally exclude consortia and shared-service or group-purchase organizations and include only institutions (whether owned, leased, or managed) that are under the control of a board that determines the central direction of two or more institutions. Data on numbers of multi-institutional systems are published annually in the trade magazine *Modern Healthcare.*

14. *Modern Healthcare,* June 7, 1985, p. 76.

15. In 1960 there were only about 330 hospitals in such systems. Gray, *For-Profit Enterprise in Health Care,* p. 29.

16. Robert R. Alford, *Health Care Politics: Ideological and Interest Group Barriers to Reform* (Chicago: University of Chicago Press, 1975), p. 15.

17. American Bar Association, *The "Black Box" of Home Care* (Chicago: American Bar Association, 1986). See also testimony in U.S. Congress, Senate Special Committee on Aging, *Home Care: The Agony of Indifference,* 100th Cong., 1st sess., April 27, 1987.

18. Telephone conversation with Elizabeth Flanagan, director of ambulatory care, Joint Commission on Accreditation of Hospitals, Chicago, August 22, 1985.

19. See Richard B. Siegrist, Jr., "Wall Street and the For-Profit Hospital Management Companies," pp. 35–50 in Bradford H. Gray, ed., *The New Health Care for Profit* (Washington, D.C.: National Academy Press, 1983).

20. This sometimes leads to corporate behavior that does not appear to serve the interests of the average stockholder. For example, top executives customarily receive a substantial financial settlement—the so-called golden parachute—when they are replaced.

21. See, for example, "Hospital Corp. America Will Not Reply to $3.85 Bil., or $47/Share Bid by a Group of 3 Investors," *Wall Street Journal,* April 20, 1987, p. 9; Cynthia Wallace, "Industry Experts Skeptical of Investors' Bid for HCA," *Modern Healthcare,* April 24, 1987, pp. 8–9; "American Medical International Projects $1.7 Billion Hostile Takeover Bid by Pesche & Co.," *Business Week,* February 23, 1987, p. 54.

22. Paul M. Hirsch, "From Ambushes to Golden Parachutes: Corporate Takeovers as an Instance of Cultural Framing and Institutional Integration," *American Journal of Sociology* 91 (January 1986): 801.

23. Of particular importance is that group of stockholders known as money managers or institutional investors—pension funds, mutual funds, insurance companies, college endowments, and various types of financial institutions—whose decisions regarding buying and selling stock are made by individuals who are investing other people's money and who are expected to outperform the market. Because the results of money managers' decisions are readily quantifiable and highly visible to those whose money is being invested, they are under tremendous pressure to perform well, and to do so in the short run. The vast

number of shares that large institutional investors can control, combined with the money managers' high profile, means that the buy-sell decisions of relatively few money managers (or, less directly, the buy-sell recommendations of the "sell-side" analysts who work for brokerage firms) can have a significant impact on the value of a company's stock.

24. For example, in an August 31, 1983, stock research report, a leading analyst, Douglas Sherlock of Salomon Brothers, evaluated HCA as follows:

"Because of its size and decentralized organizational structure, HCA is at the vanguard of the evolving U.S. health care industry. By applying sound management principles and tools to this historically poorly run industry—aided by a strong image-building effort—HCA has established itself as a leader in the industry's development. Its dominant position has enabled the company to grow through acquisitions and to effectively use those acquisitions to foster future growth.

"As a result of its strong management and positive image, HCA has shown consistently healthy growth . . . Since we expect that HCA will continue this pattern of strong earnings growth, we regard its stock as an attractive investment for long-term appreciation."

For a useful discussion of the role of stock market analysts and their relationship to the companies that they follow and evaluate, see Siegrist, "Wall Street."

25. Even so, HCA's profit-to-earnings ratio had earlier been even higher—between two and three times the Standard & Poor's 500 average for much of the previous three years.

26. *Wall Street Journal*, November 2, 1983, p. 12.

27. Trading returned to normal after HCA issued a statement that it had reviewed and disagreed with the GAO draft and, more important, that the ultimate resolution of the matter would not have any "material effect" on HCA's financial position or operating results.

28. *New York Times*, October 8, 1985, sec. 4, p. 1. Wall Street analysts' negative reactions helped to kill the proposed merger between HCA and American Hospital Supply Corporation in March 1985. These negative reactions, which were couched in assessments of the impact of the merger on *earnings*, led some Wall Street analysts to remove HCA from their lists of recommended stocks. As an example, here is the assessment of a leading analyst of health care companies: "We do not believe HCA will be able to maintain its pre-merger third-year growth rate expectation of 15–20 percent without subsequent acquisitions. From what we assess to be acquirable in the health care arena, further mergers would either be dilutive or a further drag on earnings growth. Then why is HCA taking such risks? We are still unsure, but unless, or until, the new proposed combined entity can justify higher growth expectations, we think its long-term expansion rate (assuming that the merger is consummated) will hover over 12 percent. Thus, *we are removing Hospital Corporation from the Recommended List.*"

Seth H. Shaw, "Hospital Corporation of America," Equity Research Company comment, Shearson Lehman Brothers, New York, May 2, 1985 (emphasis in original).

29. Richard B. Siegrist, Jr., "Humana, Inc.," Harvard Business School case study, Cambridge, Mass., 1981.

30. "HCA," Harvard Business School case study, Cambridge, Mass., 1984.

31. James F. Freundt and Marion E. Krotzer, "A Comparison of Executive Incentive Compensation in Health Care and General Industry," *Topics in Health Care Financing* 16 (1989): 7–18. In addition, the incentive compensation in for-profits is much more likely to be based on *profitability* than in nonprofits. Indeed, profit sharing by nonprofits could jeopardize their tax-exempt status. See Fred F. Harris, Jr., Stephen Robbins, and J. Larry Tyler, "Incentive Compensation Creates Questions of Inurement," *Healthcare Financial Management* 41 (May 1987): 38–41.

32. Jessica Townsend, "Hospitals and Their Communities: A Report on Three Case Studies," pp. 458–473 in Bradford H. Gray, ed., *For-Profit Enterprise in Health Care* (Washington, D.C.: National Academy Press, 1986).

33. Ibid.

## 3 · The Evolution of Investor-Owned Hospital Companies

1. Bruce Steinwald and Duncan Neuhauser, "The Role of the Proprietary Hospital," *Law and Contemporary Problems* 35 (Autumn 1970): 817–838.

2. Ibid.; Warren P. Morrill, "Proprietary to Nonprofit," *Trustee* 1 (October 1947): 30.

3. Steinwald and Neuhauser, "Role of the Proprietary Hospital"; Federation of American Health Systems, *1990 Directory of Investor-Owned Hospitals, Hospital Management Companies, and Health Systems* (Little Rock: FAHS Review, 1989), p. 22.

4. Morrill, "Proprietary to Nonprofit," p. 30.

5. Data from the 1977 National Medical Care Expenditure Survey, National Center for Health Services Research, cited in Gail R. Wilensky, "Underwriting the Uninsured: Targeting Providers or Individuals," in Frank A. Sloan, James F. Blumstein, and James M. Perrin, eds., *Uncompensated Hospital Care: Rights and Responsibilities* (Baltimore: Johns Hopkins University Press, 1986), p. 149.

6. Return-on-equity payments, designed to compensate investors for the use of their capital, were based on a company's investment in plant, property, and equipment related to patient care plus net working capital maintained for necessary and proper patient care activities.

7. The same dynamic stimulated sales of nursing homes. See Bruce Vladeck, *Unloving Care: The Nursing Home Tragedy* (New York: Basic Books, 1980), pp. 111–112.

8. J. Michael Watt et al., "The Effects of Ownership and Multihospital

System Membership on Hospital Functional Strategies and Economic Performance," pp. 260–289 in Bradford H. Gray, ed., *For-Profit Enterprise in Health Care* (Washington, D.C.: National Academy Press, 1986); Ross Mullner and Jack Hadley, "Interstate Variations in the Growth of Chain-Owned Proprietary Hospitals, 1973–1982," *Inquiry* 21 (Summer 1984): 144–151. Marmor, Schlesinger, and Smithey show similar patterns among other types of for-profits. Thus, for-profit psychiatric hospitals are disproportionately found in states whose laws mandate coverage of inpatient psychiatric services by private insurance; for-profit home health agencies are found in disproportionate numbers in states with relatively generous Medicaid programs; and for-profit dialysis centers are slightly more common in states that have special Medicaid coverage for end-stage renal disease patients. Theodore R. Marmor, Mark Schlesinger, and Richard W. Smithey, "Nonprofit Organizations and Health Care," in Walter W. Powell, ed., *The Nonprofit Sector: A Research Handbook* (New Haven: Yale University Press, 1987), p. 231.

9. Elizabeth W. Hoy and Bradford H. Gray, "Growth Trends of the Major Hospital Companies," pp. 250–259 in Gray, *For-Profit Enterprise in Health Care*, Table 5.

10. Steinwald and Neuhauser, "Role of the Proprietary Hospital," for example, found that proprietary hospitals, which represented 13 percent of community hospitals in 1968, accounted for 59 percent of hospital closures and 37 percent of openings between 1960 and 1986. One-third of all proprietary hospitals closed during that period (p. 825).

11. Hoy and Gray, "Growth Trends," p. 253.

12. Jessica Townsend, "Hospitals and Their Communities: A Report on Three Case Studies," pp. 458–473 in Gray, *For-Profit Enterprise in Health Care*.

13. During this period the forty-six hospitals built by the companies studied by Hoy and Gray, "Growth Trends," accounted for 35 percent of their growth; by the period 1980–1984 the twenty-seven hospitals built accounted for 11 percent of the six largest companies' growth.

14. Hoy and Gray, "Growth Trends," p. 255.

15. Examples include Wesley Medical Center in Wichita, Presbyterian Hospital in Oklahoma City, Presbyterian–Saint Luke's in Denver, Saint Joseph's Hospital in Omaha, University of Louisville Hospital, and Scripps Memorial Hospital in La Jolla, California.

16. *1985 Directory of the Federation of American Hospitals* (Little Rock: Federation of American Hospitals, 1984); and American Hospital Association, *Hospital Statistics* (Chicago: American Hospital Association, 1985).

17. Data come from the American Hospital Association, as reported in Gray, *For-Profit Enterprise in Health Care*, p. 99.

18. This does not necessarily mean that the average hospital was insolvent during this period. Many hospitals that had the ability to generate

enough revenue to cover expenses tended to spend slightly beyond those revenues.

19. Comptroller General, *Hospital Merger Increased Medicare and Medicaid Payments for Capital Costs* (Washington, D.C.: General Accounting Office, 1983).

20. "Hospital Corp. Says GAO Report Assails Its 1981 Purchase of Health-Care Concern," *Wall Street Journal*, November 2, 1983, p. 12.

21. "HCA Comments on GAO Study," press release, Hospital Corporation of America, Nashville, January 18, 1984. Among other things, HCA pointed to the capital gains taxes generated by the sale of HAI's assets.

22. Section 2314 of the Deficit Reduction Act of 1984, Public Law 98-369.

23. It should be noted that this change in policy did not address the largest source of costs in transactions such as the HCA-HAI example: interest expenses for the borrowed money. This use of Medicare money to help finance acquisition activity in health care seems likely to be addressed only when the decision is made on how to incorporate capital expenses into the rates that Medicare pays hospitals.

24. Hospital Research and Educational Trust, *Economic Trends* 2 (Spring 1986): 11. In a series of reports the Inspector General's Office in the Department of Health and Human Services called attention to the fact that the cost reports filed by hospitals showed that their profit margins on Medicare patients during the early experience with the prospective payment system (PPS) were in the vigorously healthy range of 14 to 18 percent of revenues, instead of being zero, as they supposedly had been under the cost-based reimbursement system. A later analysis by the Congressional Budget Office reported that 1984 hospital operating margins on Medicare PPS payments were 13.1 percent for urban hospitals and 6.6 percent for rural hospitals. From U.S. Congress, Senate Finance Committee, testimony by Nancy M. Gordon, Congressional Budget Office, 100th Cong., 1st sess., April 7, 1987. Total hospital margins (that is, not just on Medicare patients) were much lower (averaging approximately 5 to 6 percent) during this period.

25. Senate Finance Committee, Gordon testimony, April 7, 1987.

26. "Net patient margin dropped by more than half, from 1.5 percent in 1985 to 0.7 percent in 1986, while total net margin fell from 6 percent to 5.1 percent." Mary Gallivan, "Margins Fall Despite Slower Inpatient Declines," *Hospitals*, May 5, 1987, p. 42. Hospital margins continued to fall, and by late in the 1980s the American Hospital Association reported that the average hospital was losing money on Medicare patients.

27. *Hospitals*, May 5, 1987, p. 38.

28. The 1986 and 1987 directories of the Federation of American Hospitals—which changed its name to the Federation of American Health Systems in 1987—showed that the number of U.S. hospitals owned by HCA declined from 230 in 1985 to 224 in 1986; AMI's ownership declined from 116 to 101; NME dropped from 50 to 41.

29. The 1984 figure comes from *Statistical Profile of the Investor-Owned Hospital Industry, 1984* (n.p.: Federation of American Hospitals, n.d.), which shows a total of 1,174 hospitals (p. 2), of which 853 were of the acute care variety (p. 15). The 1989 figure comes from the same organization's *1990 Directory of Investor-Owned Hospitals, Hospital Management Companies, and Health Systems* (Little Rock: FAHS Review, 1989), pp. 10, 12.

30. "Psyc Hospitals See Admissions Slowing as Fees Keep Growing," *Wall Street Journal,* March 8, 1990, p. 1.

31. David Starkweather, *Hospital Mergers in the Making* (Ann Arbor: Health Administration Press, 1981), p. 35.

32. Commission on Hospital Care, *Hospital Care in the United States* (New York: Commonwealth Fund, 1947), p. 18.

33. Committee on the Costs of Medical Care, *Medical Care for the American People* (Chicago: University of Chicago Press, 1932), p. xvi.

34. "It is the Foundation's hope that these [hospital-based or affiliated] groups may serve as a single identifiable source of continuing care for the whole family, with around-the-clock, front-line coverage and an integrated and coordinated referral system." Quoted in Stephen M. Shortell, Thomas M. Wickizer, and John R. C. Wheeler, *Hospital-Physician Joint Ventures: Results and Lessons from a National Demonstration in Primary Care* (Ann Arbor: Health Administration Press, 1984), p. 1.

35. James E. Schutte, "The Shoot-Out Between Texas Doctors and Corporate Medicine," *Medical Economics,* March 17, 1986, pp. 21–30.

36. Cynthia Wallace, "Investor-Owned Hospitals Claim Streamlining Existing Operations," *Modern Healthcare,* January 2, 1987, p. 48.

37. The most notable example involving nonprofit hospitals was "Partners, National Health Plans," a joint venture between the Aetna Life and Casualty Company and the Voluntary Hospitals of America.

38. Cynthia Wallace, "AMI Closing Insurance Subsidiary as Part of Its Massive Restructuring," *Modern Healthcare,* September 12, 1986, p. 35; Neil McLaughlin, "Experts Say It's Too Early to Predict Fate of Chain-Insurer Managed Care," *Modern Healthcare,* January 16, 1987, p. 40.

39. Sandy Lutz, "Partners Expansion Caused 1986 Losses to Reach $24 Million at VHA Enterprises," *Modern Healthcare,* April 24, 1987, p. 74.

40. Westworld and American Healthcare Management (which between them owned sixty-six hospitals) filed for bankruptcy in 1987 and 1988, respectively. International Medical Centers, the largest Medicare HMO, was saved from bankruptcy by its acquisition by Humana in 1987. Maxicare, the largest HMO company, ceased operations in 1988. Republic Health Corporation, which had been the fifth-largest chain (thirty-one hospitals) in 1984, before being taken private by its management, filed for bankruptcy in 1989. It owned eighteen hospitals at the time. Other health care companies that filed for bankruptcy in 1988 include Americare, Columbia Corporation, and American

Health Care. *Predicasts F&S Index of Corporate Change,* 1987 and 1988 annual editions (Cleveland: Predicasts, 1988, 1989).

41. Seth H. Shaw and Mark G. Banta, Prudential-Bache research report, November 16, 1989, p. 1.

42. Richard W. Foster, "Hospitals and the Choice of Organizational Form," *Financial Accountability and Management* 3 (Winter 1987): 356.

### 4 · Accountability in Nonprofit Hospitals

1. David Rosner, *A Once Charitable Enterprise: Hospitals and Health Care in Brooklyn and New York, 1885–1915* (Cambridge: Cambridge University Press, 1982); Morris J. Vogel, *The Invention of the Modern Hospitals: Boston, 1879–1930* (Chicago: University of Chicago Press, 1980); Rosemary Stevens, *In Sickness and in Wealth: The American Hospital in the Twentieth Century* (New York: Basic Books, 1989).

2. Contrary to commonplace assumptions, nonprofit organizations are not precluded from generating operating surpluses. The total net margin of nonprofit hospitals has been similar to or higher than the after-tax profits of investor-owned hospitals in recent years. In every year since the AHA began compiling such data in 1963, the average community hospital in the United States has had a surplus of revenues over expenses. During that period the total net margin (revenues less expenses as a percentage of revenues) ranged from a low of 1.2 percent in 1973 to 6.2 percent in 1984. Data are taken from the American Hospital Association's National Hospital Panel Survey, published in Bradford H. Gray, ed., *For-Profit Enterprise in Health Care* (Washington, D.C.: National Academy Press), p. 99.

3. William H. Hranchak, "Incentive Compensation and Benefits of Profit-Sharing Plans," *Topics in Health Care Financing* 12 (1985): 34.

4. Henry B. Hansmann, "The Role of Nonprofit Enterprise," *Yale Law Journal* 89 (April 1980): 835–901. See also Burton A. Weisbrod, *The Voluntary Non-Profit Sector: An Economic Analysis* (Lexington, Mass.: Lexington Books, 1977).

5. Edith L. Fisch, Doris Jonas Freed, and Esther R. Schachter, *Charities and Charitable Foundations* (Pomona, N.Y.: Lond Publications, 1974), chap. 25. An updating is contained on pp. 121–130 in the *1986–1987 Cumulative Pocket Supplement* (Pomona, N.Y.: Lond Publications, 1986) to the Fisch, Freed, and Schachter volume. In the twelve years between those publications, the number of states with "complete charitable tort immunity" declined from four to two (Arkansas and Maine), and the number of states that "enforce full liability" increased from thirty to thirty-two. The remaining states have various forms of partial immunity.

6. Ironically, the Massachusetts court that originally adopted the doctrine was apparently unaware that the British decision on which it was based had already been overturned. Fisch, Freed, and Schachter, *Charities,* pp. 471–472.

7. Ibid., p. 472.
8. Judge Michael A. Musmanno, in *Michael v. Hahnemann Medical College and Hospital,* quoted ibid., p. 494.
9. Ibid., p. 495.
10. Stevens, *In Sickness and in Wealth,* p. 20.
11. Ibid., pp. 23–24, 25.
12. Eli Ginzberg, "The Monetarization of Medical Care," *New England Journal of Medicine,* May 3, 1984, pp. 1162–65.
13. Paul Teslow, president of HealthWest, quoted in Kelly Guncheon, "Not-For-Profits Expected to Simulate IOs' Strategies," *Hospitals,* January 1, 1983, p. 38.
14. Tamar Lewin, "Hospitals Pitch Harder for Patients," *New York Times,* May 10, 1987, pp. F1, F28.
15. Kari E. Super, "Hospitals Need Physicians' Help to Capture Market," *Modern Healthcare,* April 11, 1986, p. 73.
16. Lewin and Associates, *Studies in the Comparative Performance of Investor-Owned and Not-For-Profit Hospitals,* vol. 1, *Industry Analysis* (Washington, D.C.: Lewin and Associates, 1981), p. 114.
17. Joyce Bermal, "Hospitals Join the Ad Game, With Mixed Results," *Hastings Center Report* 16 (August 1986): 2–3; N. R. Kleinfield, "A Push to Market Health Care," *New York Times,* April 16, 1984, pp. D8–D9.
18. Standard & Poor's, *Health-Care Finance Credit Review,* March 31, 1986, p. 1.
19. Brian Kinkead, *Historical Trends in Hospital Capital Investment* (Washington, D.C.: Department of Health and Human Services, 1984); this is one of a series of Hospital Capital Finance background papers. See also Ross Mullner et al., "Debt Financing: An Alternative for Hospital Construction Funding," *Healthcare Financial Management* 13 (April 1983): 19.
20. Kinkead, *Historical Trends.*
21. Maureen Metz, "Trends in Sources of Capital in the Hospital Industry," Appendix D to the *Report of the Special Committee on Equity of Payment for Not-For-Profit Hospitals and Investor-Owned Hospitals* (Chicago: American Hospital Association, 1983).
22. Although enforcement of these obligations was long a matter of controversy and lawsuits, it is clear that Hill-Burton funds—like charitable contributions—came with expectations attached that the institution would behave in some ways that might not contribute to a healthy bottom line.
23. Under the use of industrial development bonds, some of the for-profits gained access to tax-exempt debt too, but this was not the dominant pattern.
24. William O. Cleverley and Willard H. Rosegay, "Factors Affecting the Cost of Hospital Tax-Exempt Revenue Bonds," *Inquiry* 19 (Winter 1982): 318.
25. Rating agencies do not find all hospitals to be creditworthy at all. Of

the approximately 7,000 U.S. hospitals, Standard & Poor's rates only about 1,600 to 1,700 hospitals and hospital systems in the United States. Edward F. Appel, assistant vice president, Municipal Finance Department, Standard & Poor's Corporation, New York, personal communication, September 16, 1986.

26. Standard & Poor's *Health-Care Finance Credit Review,* March 31, 1986, p. 4. The institutional characteristics that Standard & Poor's considers in rating a hospital all pertain directly to its economic soundness and prospects. They include the institution's type and level of services; its competitive position and market share; its size and membership in a multihospital system; its "performance history" and "responsiveness to competitive challenges"; utilization statistics for five years; the competitive environment; the depth and experience of the management team; the board's composition, mechanisms for obtaining physician participation in policy making, and role in setting financial policies; the "management team's" budgeting procedures, monitoring reports, and cash management systems and credit policies; data-processing capabilities; staffing patterns; risk management and history of malpractice claims; number, specialties, and average age of active staff members and percentage who are board certified and board eligible; a list of the top ten admitting physicians by age, specialty, and percentage of total hospital admissions; profitability over the previous five years ("of particular concern"); extent of reliance on nonoperating income; liquidity (cash balances and ratio of current assets to current liabilities); borrowing for cash-flow purposes and levels of accounts receivable ("accounts receivable exceeding 60 days [are a] particular concern"); and various capital structure ratios (e.g., cash flow to total debt) and ratio analysis of income and expense statements.

The result of this analysis goes into an evaluation of the following sort, taken from a 1985 Standard & Poor's rating of a nonprofit multihospital system: "S&P rates as 'AA' the $103 million revenue bonds issued by the municipality of Anchorage, Alaska, for the Sisters of Providence . . . [which] owns and operates 13 hospitals in Alaska, California, Oregon and Washington. Proceeds will be used for expansion at the Anchorage facility . . . The rating reflects the strong revenue base, impressive profitability, stable utilization, and geographic dispersion of this group. In 1984, gross revenues approximated $750 million and bottom line excess was over $70 million. The system has generated substantial cash flow, enabling it to meet capital needs primarily with internal funds, keep debt financing minimal, and retain ample cash reserves. Cash and board-designated funds in 1984 of $83 million, and debt less than one-third of total capitalization reflect this strength. After issuance of [four planned subsequent series of bonds], leverage remains low with debt to capitalization of 40% in 1986. Depth and quality of corporate level management is excellent, and strong administration at the respective institutions completes an effective management team. Most service areas served by system hospitals exhibit favorable economics and population growth. The positive consolidated admissions trend is indicative of the healthy market share the majority of system hospitals enjoy. In the more competitive markets of Burbank and Oakland, Calif.; Portland, Oreg.; and Seattle, Wash., system hospitals compete effectively to retain and increase market penetration" (p. 19).

27. This account is based on a description of several bond issues by Glenn Wilson, Cecil G. Sheps, and Thomas R. Oliver, "Effects of Hospital Revenue Bonds on Hospital Planning and Operations," *New England Journal of Medicine* 307 (December 2, 1982): 1426–30.

28. Ibid., p. 1428.

29. Gray, *For-Profit Enterprise in Health Care*, p. 29.

30. As the president of the AHA put it: "A host of environmental changes—including more limited resources; increased regulation; advances in medical technology and greater diversity of services; and growing public awareness and demand for health services—have made it increasingly difficult for the freestanding, local hospital to deliver effective community health services." J. Alexander McMahon, "Foreword," in Gerald E. Bisbee, ed., *Multihospital Systems: Policy Issues for the Future* (Chicago: Hospital Research and Educational Trust, 1980), p. i.

31. Dan Ermann and Jon Gabel, "Multihospital Systems: Issues and Empirical Findings," *Health Affairs* 3 (September 1984): 52.

32. Bernard Friedman, "The Changing Structure of the Health Care Industry and the Influence of Medicare Prospective Payments," paper prepared for the Prospective Payment Advisory Commission, Washington, D.C., 1988.

33. Gray, *For-Profit Enterprise in Health Care*, p. 30.

34. Laura L. Morlock and Jeffrey A. Alexander, "Models of Governance in Multihospital Systems: Implications for Hospital and System-Level Decision-Making," *Medical Care* 24 (December 1986): 1118–35.

35. According to empirical work by the American College of Hospital Administrators, the major responsibilities of the "hospital chief executive officer" include planning and organizing, achieving hospital objectives, maintaining quality of medical services, allocating resources, resolving crises, complying with regulations, and promoting the hospital. *Modern Healthcare*, June 6, 1986, p. 136.

36. Informal accountability—especially to the medical staff—has also traditionally been critical to administrators' institutional survival, and may remain so, even in multihospital systems. For example, even in a highly centralized multihospital system a deeply dissatisfied medical staff can spell doom for a hospital administrator. Jessica Townsend, "Hospitals and Their Communities: A Report on Three Case Studies," in Gray, *For-Profit Enterprise in Health Care*, pp. 470–471.

37. Lynn Kahn and Mark Harju, "Contract Management: More Buyers, Smarter Shoppers," *Hospitals*, February 1, 1984, p. 56.

38. According to the Federation of American Hospitals, investor-owned hospital companies managed 330 nonprofit hospitals in 1985. Federation of American Hospitals, *1986 Directory of Investor-Owned Hospitals* (Little Rock: Federation of American Hospitals, 1985), p. 14. (This figure apparently includes both nonprofit and public hospitals; AHA data suggest that approximately 60 percent of managed hospitals are nonprofit.) See also Kahn and Harju, "Contract Management." An unknown additional number of nonprofit hospitals are managed by other for-profit management companies or by for-profit subsidiaries of nonprofit hospitals or hospital systems.

39. A physician-trustee of a nonprofit hospital described the problems that led his hospital to seek help from a management company: "The [80-bed] hospital was down to three physicians on staff, census was low, expenses were up, and we had no reserves. The hospital had gradually slipped sideways in time with an administrative capability that dated back to early Medicare days. [After two administrators] resigned, several board members began to push not for a new administrator, but for a system to manage the chaos . . . We had already seen that having a very competent administrator, but no back-up support for him, would not work in our situation . . . We could not handle such areas as accounting, reimbursement, and purchasing on a local basis, [and] could not deal with federal rules and regulations for medical reimbursement or state regulatory laws, which often were conflicting and capricious." Glenn R. Womack, "A Trustee Views the Pros and Cons of a Hospital Management Contract," *Trustee* 37 (August 1984): 33.

40. Such problems echo in a California study of county hospitals that signed management contracts: "Billing and collection were often vestigial systems inherited from a previous era when they could be loosely operated without serious loss . . . Low income patients were often admitted with only cursory investigation of their eligibility for Medi-Cal . . . New mechanisms had to be developed for meticulously capturing charges, by personnel to whom such procedures were strange and even abhorrent." William Shonick and Ruth Roemer, *Public Hospitals under Private Management: The California Experience* (Berkeley: University of California Institute of Governmental Studies, 1983), p. 20.

   Some hospitals that sign a management contract as a way of modernizing many of its managerial functions end the contract after several years when new systems are in place.

41. Robert A. Derzon, Roger B. LeCompte, and Lawrence S. Lewin, "Hospitals Say Yes to Contract Management," *Trustee* 34 (July 1981): 36.

42. For a cross-sectional study of contract management in nonprofit hospitals, which found few differences, see Errol L. Biggs, John E. Kralewski, and Gordon D. Brown, "A Comparison of Contract-Managed and Traditionally Managed Nonprofit Hospitals," *Medical Care* 18 (June 1980): 585–596. Cross-sectional studies of contract management of

public hospitals include Shonick and Roemer, *Public Hospitals*, and Jeffrey A. Alexander and Thomas G. Rundall, "Public Hospitals under Contract Management," *Medical Care* 23 (March 1985): 209–219.

43. John E. Kralewski, "The Effects of Contract Management on Hospital Performance," University of Minnesota School of Public Health, 1986.

44. Derzon, LeCompte, and Lewin, "Hospitals Say Yes to Contract Management."

45. Shonick and Roemer, *Public Hospitals*, pp. 197–198. The Shonick-Roemer study identified several other attractions contract management has for public hospitals, including offering an escape from (1) government-imposed salary restrictions, (2) constraints of civil service hiring requirements, and (3) government purchasing procedures and requirements. Contract management is sometimes part of an effort to make county hospitals economically self-sufficient. Indeed, it is sometimes hoped that the management firm can achieve such positive economic results that it will pay for itself. Although this result has been reported in the early years of a contract—when new procedures are introduced for billing and collection, purchasing, and personnel—it is difficult for a management contract to continue paying for itself after these procedures are put into effect.

46. Lynn Kahn, "Departmental Contract Management Up as Much as 162 Percent," *Hospitals*, February 1, 1984, p. 62; Howard J. Anderson, "Large Hospitals Hiring Contract Managers to Reduce Expenses," *Modern Healthcare*, August 29, 1986, pp. 49–59.

47. Martin Paris, "Hospital-Physician Joint Ventures," in Jesus J. Penn and Valerie A. Glesnes-Anderson, eds., *Hospital Management: Winning Strategies for the '80s* (Rockville, Md.: Aspen, 1985), p. 287.

48. A 1983 survey reported that one-third of all hospitals had equipment-sharing arrangements with other hospitals, although only about half of these were in the form of a joint venture. Bill Jackson and Joyce Jensen, "Hospitals Turning to Joint Ventures to Gain Access to Costly Equipment," *Modern Healthcare* 14 (October 1984): 108, 110.

49. Michael A. Morrisey and Deal Chandler Brooks, "Hospital-Physician Joint Ventures: Who's Doing What?" *Hospitals*, May 1, 1985, p. 74.

50. Paris, "Hospital-Physician Joint Ventures," p. 287.

51. Another category of joint venture, of less relevance to concerns about accountability, includes construction, real estate, and equipment-leasing deals in which physicians make the capital investments, thereby benefiting from tax credits and depreciation allowances, and then lease to the hospital.

52. Paris, "Hospital-Physician Joint Ventures," p. 298.

53. Ibid., p. 297.

54. Voluntary Hospitals of America, "Building America's Preeminent Health Care System" (Irving, Texas: VHA, 1986), p. 2.

55. Ibid.

56. American Healthcare Systems descriptive brochure.

57. Judith Graham, "Alliances Look to Innovative Ways to Meet Members' Capital Needs," *Modern Healthcare*, March 28, 1986, p. 118.
58. Voluntary Hospitals of America, "Building America's Preeminent Health Care System," p. 3.
59. Ibid., p. 8.
60. Jennifer Fine, "VHA Regional Systems Developing Their Own Financing, Venture Options," *Modern Healthcare*, September 26, 1986, p. 88.
61. Charles M. Ewell, quoted in press release from Hill and Knowlton, Los Angeles, August 15, 1984.
62. Samuel J. Tibbits, quoted ibid.
63. Ibid.
64. Ibid.
65. Donald E. L. Johnson, "American Healthcare Systems: Can It Be an Old Boys' Club and Play with the Fortune 500?" *Modern Healthcare*, March 28, 1986, p. 78.
66. Leon Eisenberg, "Health Care: For Patients or For Profits?" *American Journal of Psychiatry* 143 (August 1986): 1017.
67. See, for example, the United Hospital Fund (New York) publication *Mission Matters*, by J. David Seay and Bruce C. Vladeck (1987), and the Catholic Health Association (CHA) project to develop a "social accountability budget," a process approved by the CHA board of trustees in April 1989. Catholic Health Association, *Social Accountability Budget: A Process for Planning and Reporting Community Service in a Time of Fiscal Restraint* (St. Louis: Catholic Health Association of the United States, 1989).

## 5 · The Performance of For-Profit and Nonprofit Health Care Organizations

1. The most influential and persistent critic of for-profit health care has been Arnold S. Relman, editor of the *New England Journal of Medicine*. See Arnold S. Relman, "The New Medical-Industrial Complex," *New England Journal of Medicine*, October 23, 1980, pp. 963–969; and Arnold S. Relman and Uwe Reinhardt, "An Exchange on For-Profit Health Care," in Bradford H. Gray, ed. *For-Profit Enterprise in Health Care* (Washington, D.C.: National Academy Press, 1986), pp. 209–223.
2. Michael Bromberg, "The Medical-Industrial Complex: Our National Defense," *New England Journal of Medicine*, November 24, 1983, pp. 1314–15.
3. See, for example, Frank A. Sloan, "Property Rights in the Hospital Industry," pp. 103–141 in H. E. Frech III, *Health Care in America* (San Francisco: Pacific Research Institute for Public Policy, 1988); and Regina Herzlinger and William S. Krasker, "Who Profits from Nonprofits?" *Harvard Business Review* 65 (January–February 1987): 93–105. Of course, there are difficulties in knowing what efficiency means in health care, where products are far from standardized. For example,

hospitals may differ in their costs of caring for particular kinds of patients because patients are discharged earlier in the course of their recovery from one hospital than from another. Family members may provide care in one instance that is provided in the hospital in another. From the standpoint of the purchaser, one hospital might be less costly than the other; but because the two hospitals are not providing identical sets of services, it is difficult to reach conclusions about efficiency. Comparisons of the costliness of services provided by different hospitals may be influenced by such factors as differences in the severity of illness of patients, recent renovations or major capital expenditures, or location in an area where wages are comparatively high. These are all factors that researchers attempt to adjust for, with varying degrees of success, in comparing the costliness or efficiency of the services provided by different types of hospitals.

4. Paul DiMaggio and Walter W. Powell, "The Iron Cage Revisited: Institutional Isomorphism and Collective Rationality in Organizational Fields," *American Sociological Review* 82 (1983): 147–160.

5. Gray, *For-Profit Enterprise in Health Care,* pp. 78–79. The one study that did not reach such findings was coauthored by a researcher-executive from the Hospital Corporation of America and attracted serious methodological criticism (see note 12). Frank A. Sloan and Robert A. Vraciu, "Investor-Owned and Not-For-Profit Hospitals," *Health Affairs* 2 (1983): 25–37.

6. This pattern, which does not comport with obvious economic incentives under cost-based reimbursement, has never been adequately explained. One hypothesis is that the patients admitted to nonprofit hospitals are, on average, sicker because there are so many more referral centers among nonprofit hospitals. Although this seems plausible, studies that have examined case mix have found little difference in this regard between investor-owned and nonprofit hospitals. The other likely explanatory factor concerns geographic variations in length of hospital stay. For example, it has long been known that diagnosis-specific lengths of stay are about two days shorter, on average, on the West Coast than on the East Coast. Unfortunately, the studies that have controlled for geographic variations by matching hospitals have included lengths of stay among the variables on which hospitals are matched, thereby making it impossible to make comparisons on that dimension. See, for example, J. Michael Watt et al., "The Comparative Economic Performance of Investor-Owned Chain and Not-For-Profit Hospitals," *New England Journal of Medicine,* January 9, 1986, pp. 89–96.

7. Elizabeth W. Hoy and Bradford H. Gray, "Trends in the Growth of the Major Investor-Owned Hospital Companies," in Gray, *For-Profit Enterprise in Health Care,* pp. 250–259.

8. Robert V. Pattison and Hallie M. Katz, "Investor-Owned and Not-for-Profit Hospitals," *New England Journal of Medicine,* August 11, 1983, pp. 347–353.

9. The economist Frank Sloan has identified the factors that should be adjusted for or otherwise included in a data analysis to examine the question of efficiency: (1) economic costs, not accounting costs, should be measured; (2) adjustments should be made for systematic differences between the for-profit and nonprofit sectors in accounting practices (for example, the for-profit organization has a greater incentive to account for depreciation on an accelerated basis); (3) the likelihood that acquired hospitals were previously mismanaged must be controlled for; (4) taxes paid by for-profits but not by nonprofits should be removed from the analysis; (5) "some weight" should be given to "taxes" that an institution "voluntarily" imposes on itself by providing services whose revenues fall short of costs; and (6) variables such as case mix, quality, and location should be controlled for, since they may affect costs. Frank Sloan, "Property Rights in the Hospital Industry," in Frech, *Health Care in America*, pp. 130–131.

10. Watt et al., "Comparative Economic Performance," pp. 89–96; see also Lawrence S. Lewin, Robert A. Derzon, and Rhea Margulies, "Investor-Owned and Nonprofits Differ in Economic Performance," *Hospitals* 55 (July 1, 1981): 52–58.

11. Sloan and Vraciu, "Investor-Owned and Not-For-Profit Hospitals," pp. 25–37.

12. For example, Florida appears to be unusual with regard to the relative costliness of for-profit and nonprofit hospitals. Also, the authors' decision to exclude hospitals with more than four hundred beds had the effect of narrowing the cost differences between the two types. See letters to the editor, *Health Affairs* 2 (Fall 1983): 132–144.

13. Herzlinger and Krasker, "Who Profits from Nonprofits?" pp. 93–105.

14. The tone, the publication of the study in the *Harvard Business Review* (rather than a health services research journal), and the publicity that ensued from a prepublication press conference and a *Wall Street Journal* article (Regina E. Herzlinger, "Nonprofit Hospitals Seldom Profit the Needy," March 23, 1987), all attracted attention. The fact that the sweeping conclusions about the superiority of for-profit hospitals in virtually all respects were strikingly at variance with most other empirical work led a number of critics, including myself, to examine the evidence closely. The length of the inferential leaps between the evidence and the conclusions and policy recommendations were suggestive of a strong bias. In addition, although methodological innovations were offered as a prominent component of the article, these and other aspects of the methodology were not described clearly enough to allow readers to understand just what steps the researchers had followed. It was apparent, however, that the sample of hospitals that was used for the analysis had significant flaws: the for-profits and nonprofits were mostly located in different states (with different payment environments and populations of uninsured patients), and hospitals belonging to the Kaiser HMO were included in the nonprofit sample. For a more detailed critique of the Herzlinger-Krasker study, see Brad-

ford H. Gray, "Shaky Basis for Report's Sweeping Recommendations," *Health Progress* 68 (April 1987): 38–41; Jeanne Fitzgerald and Brent Jacobsen, "Study Fails to Prove For-Profits' Superiority," *Health Progress* 68 (April 1987): 42–45; and various letters to the editor in the March–April and May–June 1987 issues of the *Harvard Business Review* and the *Wall Street Journal* on April 7, 1987. See also Tamar Lewin, "A Sharp Debate on Hospitals," *New York Times*, April 2, 1987, pp. D1, D5.

15. Memorandum dated March 16, 1983, from Paul Ginsburg of Congressional Budget Office to John Kern, staff of House Ways and Means Committee.

16. This was documented in a study by the Office of the Inspector General, Department of Health and Human Services; see also Bernard Friedman and Stephen Shortell, "The Financial Performance of Selected Investor-Owned and Not-For-Profit System Hospitals before and after Medicare Prospective Payment," *Health Services Research* 23 (June 1988): 237–267.

17. Gray, *For-Profit Enterprise in Health Care*, p. 81. See also Thomas G. Rundall, Shoshanna Sofaer, and Wendy Lambert, "Uncompensated Hospital Care in California: Private and Public Hospital Responses to Competitive Market Forces," *Advances in Health Economics and Health Services Research* 9 (1988): 113–133, particularly Table 5.

18. Gray, *For-Profit Enterprise in Health Care*, p. 80.

19. Ibid.

20. Mark Schlesinger, David Blumenthal, and Eric Schlesinger, "Profits under Pressure: The Economic Performance of Investor-Owned and Nonprofit Health Maintenance Organizations," *Medical Care* 24 (July 1986): 615–627.

21. See studies cited by Catherine Hawes and Charles D. Phillips, "The Changing Structure of the Nursing Home Industry and the Impact of Ownership on Quality, Cost, and Access," in Gray, *For-Profit Enterprise in Health Care*, pp. 521–525; and Sloan, "Property Rights in the Hospital Industry," p. 132.

22. Burton A. Weisbrod and Mark Schlesinger, "Public, Private, Nonprofit Ownership and the Response to Asymmetric Information: The Case of Nursing Homes," Discussion Paper no. 209, University of Wisconsin Center for Health Economics and Law, Madison, 1983.

23. Lewin and Associates examined data from Jury Verdict Research, Inc., on malpractice convictions against a sample of 345 hospitals between 1970 and 1974 and found that in the 23 cases, the percentages of nonprofit, proprietary, and investor-owned chain hospitals "approximately match[ed] the proportion of hospitals in each category in the sample as a whole." Health Services Foundation (Blue Cross), *Investor Owned Hospitals: An Examination of Performance* (Chicago: Health Services Foundation, 1976). The National Association of Insurance Commissioners (NAIC) published data from 128 insurers on 71,782 malpractice claims closed between July 1, 1975, and December 31,

1978. *NAIC Malpractice Claims, 1975–1978* 2, no. 2 (1980). Approximately one-third of those were against hospitals. Of the 8,042 closed malpractice claims against hospitals whose ownership type was known, 11.5 percent were against for-profit hospitals, 76.9 percent were against nonprofit hospitals, and 11.6 percent were against nonfederal public hospitals. During that period approximately 8.3 percent of admissions to community hospitals were to for-profit institutions, 70.6 percent were to nonprofit hospitals, and 21.1 percent were to public hospitals. Data calculated for 1978 from American Hospital Association, *Hospital Statistics* (Chicago: American Hospital Association, 1980), p. 6, Table 1. (The NAIC data were not limited to community hospitals.) Thus, although public hospitals were sued at a rate somewhat lower than expected, there was only a slight difference between for-profit and nonprofit hospitals.

24. Bradford H. Gray and Walter J. McNerney, "For-Profit Enterprise in Health Care," *New England Journal of Medicine*, June 5, 1986, p. 1526.

25. Robert V. Pattison, "Response to Financial Incentives among Investor-Owned and Not-For-Profit Hospitals: An Analysis Based on California Data, 1978–82," in Gray, *For-Profit Enterprise in Health Care*, p. 301. A further clue about the comparatively poor economic health of acquired institutions is the finding that acquired hospitals had comparatively low occupancy rates. Ross M. Mullner and Ronald M. Andersen, "A Descriptive and Financial Ratio Analysis of Merged and Consolidated Hospitals: United States, 1980–1985," *Advances in Health Economics and Health Services Research* 7 (1987): 41–58.

26. Hoy and Gray, "Trends in Growth," pp. 250–259.

27. Gray, *For-Profit Enterprise in Health Care*, p. 129.

28. Stephen M. Shortell and Edward F. X. Hughes, "The Effects of Regulation, Competition, and Ownership on Mortality Rates among Hospital Inpatients," *New England Journal of Medicine*, April 28, 1988, pp. 1100–7. See also Friedman and Shortell, "Financial Performance," pp. 237–267.

29. Arthur J. Hartz et al., "Hospital Characteristics and Mortality Rates," *New England Journal of Medicine*, December 21, 1989, pp. 1720–25.

30. The relationship to occupancy rates may be due to the comparative economic well-being of hospitals that are relatively full and may be peculiar to circumstances (existing in 1986) in which most hospitals were operating far from capacity. The association with payroll expenses per bed could also be an effect of the hospital's economic status, or perhaps to priorities regarding where expenditures were made.

31. Gary Gaumer, "Medicare Patient Outcomes and Hospital Organizational Mission," pp. 354–374 in Gray, *For-Profit Enterprise in Health Care*; Shortell and Hughes, "Effects of Regulation."

32. Hawes and Phillips, "Changing Structure of the Nursing Home Industry," pp. 510–520.

33. Frank A. Sloan, Joseph Valvona, and Ross Mullner, "Identifying the Issues: A Statistical Profile," in Frank A. Sloan, James F. Blumstein,

and James J. Perrin, eds., *Uncompensated Hospital Care: Rights and Responsibilities* (Baltimore: Johns Hopkins University Press, 1986); Gray, *For-Profit Enterprise in Health Care*, p. 102.

34. Data from an unpublished paper by Diane Rowland based on 1981 survey by the Office for Civil Rights in the Department of Health and Human Services. See Gray, *For-Profit Enterprise in Health Care*, p. 101.

35. Ibid.

36. Office of Inspector General, *Semi-Annual Report to the Congress, October 1, 1987–March 31, 1988* (Washington, D.C.: Department of Health and Human Services, 1988), pp. 30–31. The handful of hospitals that have been publicly identified include both nonprofit and investor-owned institutions. See, for example, Sandy Lutz, "Texas Attorney General Files 'Patient Dumping' Lawsuit," *Modern Healthcare*, February 12, 1988, p. 4.

37. See Gray, *For-Profit Enterprise in Health Care*, pp. 121–126.

38. See ibid., chap. 7; Richard McK. F. Southby and Warren Greenberg, eds., *The For-Profit Hospital* (Columbus, Ohio: Battelle Press, 1986); and American Medical Association, *The Investor-Related Academic Health Center and Medical Education: An Uncertain Courtship* (Chicago: American Medical Association, 1986).

39. Comparisons with publicly owned facilities may also seem warranted because all sources of data show that they provide much higher levels of uncompensated care than do either for-profit or nonprofit hospitals. Because public hospitals are financed in part by government appropriations, however, and those appropriations depend in part on the organization's financial circumstances, it is difficult to compare the behavior of public and private institutions, and even more difficult to interpret it.

40. Gray, *For-Profit Enterprise in Health Care*, pp. 101–102.

41. Not all uninsured patients lack the means to pay. Bad debt may not reflect volition on the hospital's part and may represent only a share (the deductibles remaining after insurance coverage) of a given patient's bill. "Charity care" figures are notoriously subject to manipulation by nonprofit hospitals seeking to discharge the "free care" obligations that came with grants under the Hill-Burton program.

42. Richard G. Frank, David S. Salkever, and Fitzhugh Mullan, "Hospital Ownership and the Care of Uninsured and Medicaid Patients: Findings from the National Hospital Discharge Survey 1979–1984," *Health Policy* 14 (1990): 1–11.

43. Lawrence S. Lewin, Timothy J. Eckels, and Dale Roenigk, *Setting the Record Straight: The Provision of Uncompensated Care by Not-For-Profit Hospitals* (Washington, D.C.: Lewin and Associates, 1988).

44. State of Florida Hospital Cost Containment Board, "Hospital Financial Data, 1980–1985." For data showing a similar, though less dramatic, trend in California, see Rundall, Sofaer, and Lambert, "Uncompensated Hospital Care in California." It should be noted that this pattern

did not appear in the national data for 1979–1984, as reported by Frank, Salkever, and Mullan, "Hospital Ownership."

45. Mark Schlesinger et al., "The Privatization of Health Care and Physicians' Perceptions of Access to Hospital Services," *Milbank Quarterly* 65 (1987): 33.

46. Samuel Mitchell, director of research, Federation of American Health Systems, personal communications.

47. Gray, *For-Profit Enterprise in Health Care*, p. 142.

48. Ibid., pp. 121–126.

49. Stephen M. Shortell et al., "Diversification of Health Care Services: The Effects of Ownership, Environment, and Strategy," *Advances in Health Economics and Health Services Research* 7 (1987): 22–23.

50. Mark Schlesinger, Theodore R. Marmor, and Richard Smithey, "Nonprofit and For-Profit Medical Care: Shifting Roles and Implications for Health Policy," *Journal of Health Politics, Policy, and Law* 12 (Fall 1987): 427–457; Theodore R. Marmor, Mark Schlesinger, and Richard Smithey, "Nonprofit Organizations and Health Care," pp. 221–239 in Walter Powell, ed., *The Nonprofit Sector: A Research Handbook* (New Haven: Yale University Press, 1967).

51. See also Hawes and Phillips, "Changing Structure of the Nursing Home Industry."

52. See Schlesinger, Marmor, and Smithey, "Nonprofit and For-Profit Medical Care."

53. Hawes and Phillips, "Changing Structure of the Nursing Home Industry," p. 512.

54. Mark Schlesinger and Robert Dorwart, "Ownership and Mental Health Services: A Reappraisal of the Shift toward Privately Owned Facilities," *New England Journal of Medicine* 311 (1984): 959–965.

55. Schlesinger et al., "Privatization of Health Care."

56. Marmor, Schlesinger, and Smithey, "Nonprofit Organizations and Health Care."

57. Hawes and Phillips, "Changing Structure of the Nursing Home Industry." Burton Weisbrod, in *The Nonprofit Economy* (Cambridge, Mass.: Harvard University Press, 1988), shows that nonprofit nursing homes have longer waiting lists, an indication that they have more choices in selecting clients.

58. Schlesinger, Marmor, and Smithey, "Nonprofit and For-Profit Medical Care," p. 450.

### 6 · External Accountability and Problems of Fraud and Abuse

1. This topic has been written about in many places. See, for example, the New York State Moreland Act Commission report, published in seven volumes between October 1975 and February 1976; Frank Moss and Val Halamandaris, *Too Old, Too Sick, Too Bad: Nursing Homes in*

*America* (Germantown, Md.: Aspen Systems, 1978); Bruce Vladeck, *Unloving Care: The Nursing Home Tragedy* (New York: Basic Books, 1980).

2. "There are many reasons that government might wish to survey and regulate health care institutions. These include protecting the public from unsafe or unsanitary conditions and incompetent care, establishing standards of performance where the public is unable to make its own judgments, encouraging high quality care practices, rationalizing the system, conserving limited health resources, and assuring the provision of adequate health services. And as government is paying for a larger and larger portion of hospital care, there has been a growing interest in evaluating that which is being paid for . . . Many other regulatory goals could be listed, but all would fall under one of three broad headings: assuring quality, controlling costs, and providing for equity of access." Tom Christoffel, *Health and the Law: A Handbook for Health Professionals* (New York: Free Press, 1982), pp. 111–112.

3. Some basic questions about the constitutional limits of the government's authority to regulate health care providers have never been resolved through litigation. Kenneth R. Wing, *The Law and the Public's Health*, 2nd ed. (Ann Arbor: Health Administration Press, 1985), pp. 119–143. In many instances, however, the courts have found a public interest in the activities of hospitals, as in this 1972 decision by the Supreme Court of Hawaii: "If the proposition that any hospital occupies a fiduciary trust relationship between itself, its staff and the public it seeks to serve is accepted, then the rationale for any distinction between public, 'quasi public' and truly private breaks down and becomes meaningless, especially if the hospital's patients are considered to be of primary concern." *Silver v. Castle Memorial Hospital*, 53 Hawaii 475, 497 P.2d 564 (1972), quoted in Christoffel, *Health and the Law*, p. 110. This view, Christoffel notes, "provides a rationale for public accountability, without which hospital decisions to deny a physician or podiatrist staff privileges or to bar husbands from delivery rooms would be entirely private matters impervious to court challenge by affected individuals" (pp. 110–111).

4. Hospital Association of New York, *Report of the Task Force on Regulation* (Albany: Hospital Association of New York, 1976).

5. Comptroller General, *Information on Hospital Inspection Reporting Requirements and Life Safety Code Enforcement*, HRD-80 (Washington, D.C.: General Accounting Office, July 2, 1980).

6. Christoffel, *Health and the Law*, p. 113.

7. Daniel M. Mulholland III, "The Corporate Responsibility of the Community Hospital," *University of Toledo Law Review* 17 (Winter 1986): 344.

8. Until the early 1980s, if a nonprofit or public hospital that had an undischarged Hill-Burton obligation was purchased by a for-profit organization, the new owner had to pay back the federal government. Subsequently, new owners were given the alternative of establishing

an indigent care fund rather than making a payment to the federal government. Because few nonprofit and public hospitals have been acquired by investment-owned companies since the new regulations were issued, however, few hospitals have been affected.

9. Institute of Medicine, *Health Care in a Civil Rights Context* (Washington, D.C.: National Academy Press, 1981), pp. 148–153; Marcia Rose, "Federal Regulation of Services to the Poor under the Hill-Burton Act: Realities and Pitfalls," *Northwestern University Law Review* 70 (1975): 168.

10. Wing, *Law and the Public's Health,* pp. 234–237.

11. Sandy Lutz, "Texas Attorney General Files 'Patient Dumping' Lawsuit," *Modern Healthcare* 18 (February 12, 1988): 4.

12. Ibid.

13. U.S. Congress, "Legislative History PL 95-142," in *U.S. Code Congressional and Administrative News.* 95th Cong., 1st sess., 1977, p. 3050.

14. Ibid.

15. U.S. Congress, House Select Committee on Aging, *Medicaid Fraud: A Case History in the Failure of State Enforcement,* 97th Cong., 2d sess., 1982.

16. Carey M. Adams and S. Lynne Klein, "Medicare and Medicaid Anti-Fraud and Abuse Law: The Need for Legislative Change," *Healthspan* 2, no. 1 (January 1985): 19–24. Also included in the 1972 legislation was the establishment of professional standards review organizations (PSROs) which replaced provider-based utilization review requirements. Although these were not fraud and abuse agencies, the PSROs were meant to review the appropriateness, necessity, and quality of care received by Medicare patients. PSROs were replaced by new peer review organizations (PROs) in 1982 legislation.

17. House Select Committee on Aging, *Medicaid Fraud,* p. 1.

18. Office of the Inspector General, *Semi-Annual Report, April 1983–September 1983* (Washington, D.C.: Department of Health and Human Services, 1983); Office of Inspector General, *Semi-Annual Report, April 1984–September 1984* (Washington, D.C.: Department of Health and Human Services, 1984), p. 1.

19. Office of the Inspector General, *Semi-Annual Report, April 1984–September 1984.*

20. Adams and Klein, "Medicare and Medicaid Anti-Fraud and Abuse Law," pp. 19–24.

21. House Select Committee on Aging, *Medicaid Fraud.*

22. General Accounting Office, *Hospital Links with Related Firms Can Conceal Unreasonable Costs and Increase Administrative Burden, Thus Inflating Health Care Expenditures,* HRD 83.18 (Washington, D.C.: General Accounting Office, January 19, 1983).

23. Dennis Barry, "Medicare and Medicaid Sanctions," pp. 67–71, in Jeannie M. Johnson and Janet Siefert, eds., *Medicare Fraud and Abuse* (Washington, D.C.: Health Lawyers Association, 1986). The Civil Monetary Penalties Law (CMPL) provides for civil penalties on false

claims in an amount up to $2,000 for each item or service falsely claimed, whereas previous law—the False Claims Act of 1863—allowed fines and penalties for each false claim rather than for each item or service. CMPL also allows fraud and abuse to be prosecuted in a civil context by an administrative law judge. John Meyer, "Update," in Johnson and Siefert, *Medicare Fraud and Abuse*, pp. 136–139.

24. Dianna Soli, "Hermann Hospital Estate, Founded for the Poor, Has Benefited the Wealthy, Investigators Allege," *Wall Street Journal*, March 13, 1985, p. 4.

25. Deputy Attorney General (New York) for Medicaid Fraud Control, "Special Prosecutor Arrests 6 in $1,800,000 Medicaid Fraud and Cover-Up by Long Island Based National Home Health Care Firm," news release, August 7, 1986; "Professional Care, Inc.: Five Persons Indicted for Medicaid Fraud," *Wall Street Journal*, August 8, 1986, p. 3.

26. Marshall Clinard, *Corporate Ethics and Crime* (Beverly Hills: Sage, 1983).

27. Henry N. Pontell et al., "A Demographic Portrait of Physicians Sanctioned by the Federal Government for Fraud and Abuse against Medicare and Medicaid," *Medical Care* 23 (August 1985): 1028–31; John A. Gardner and Theodore R. Lyman, *The Fraud Control Game: State Responses to Fraud and Abuse in AFDC and Medicaid Programs* (Bloomington: Indiana University Press, 1984).

28. Some nursing home companies have had a history of conflict with regulatory authorities. See, for example, Phyllis Gaspen, "Beverly Loses $30 Million—Despite Shift in Tough Image," *American Medical News*, February 19, 1988, pp. 3, 44–45. For a broad review of fraud and abuse in the nursing home field, see Vladeck, *Unloving Care*, chap. 8.

29. The data are for 1987 and come from the Office of the Actuary, Health Care Financing Administration. See *Health Care Financing Review* 11 (Fall 1989): 167.

30. For example, in the data on cases pending before Medicaid fraud units in 1981, nursing homes and medical clinics, both of which tend to be proprietary in ownership, accounted for 84 percent and 16 percent, respectively, of the cases involving "other facilities." In most cases involving "other facilities" listed as sanctioned by OIG, the actual sanction was directed against an individual.

31. I determined the ownership status of these hospitals (nonprofit, proprietary, multi-institutional) by reference to directories published by the American Hospital Association and the Federation of American Hospitals.

32. The multi-institutional systems involved were Hospital Affiliates International (now merged with Hospital Corporation of America), Westworld, and Comprehensive Care Corporation.

33. Such surveys are conducted by state agencies under procedures defined in HCFA's *State Operations Manual*, HIM.7, sec. 3010. The substantial allegation surveys focus on "key standards" that are part of the regula-

tions that define the requirements of Section 1861(c) of Title XVIII of the Social Security Act. These standards pertain to such topics as the governing body, conformity with state and local laws, physical environment, medical records, dietary department, nursing department, medical staff, medical records, pharmacy, laboratories, radiology department, complementary departments, medical library, emergency room service, social work department, and outpatient department. *Medicare and Medicaid Guide* (Chicago: Commerce Clearing House, 1976), pp. 5059–61.

34. American Society of Hospital Attorneys, *Federal Regulation: Hospital Attorney's Desk Reference* (Chicago: American Hospital Association, 1980).
35. "CONs and the Louisiana 'Purchase,'" *Medical World News*, July 8, 1985, pp. 332–335.
36. Telephone interview, July 21, 1986. Westworld's other Arkansas hospital, the fifty-nine-bed Central Ozarks Medical Center in Yellville, had undergone extensive renovation by its former owner, another small investor-owned company.
37. Telephone interview, July 28, 1986.
38. My discussion of Westworld's legal difficulties rests heavily on articles by Audrey Kraus that were published in the *Fresno Bee* on December 22, 1985, and August 4 and 31, 1986. My other sources are cited separately.
39. Press release from the Missouri attorney general's office, June 27, 1986.
40. Frank Sokilick, Health Care Financing Administration, telephone interview, October 17, 1986.
41. March 4, 5, and 27, 1986.
42. As has been noted, treatment for alcoholism and drug abuse as well as psychiatric services present payers with particularly difficult utilization control problems because of the limited amount of scientific evidence and the lack of a strong professional consensus regarding criteria for and modes of treatment. Leonard Saxe et al., *The Effectiveness and Costs of Alcoholism Treatment*, Health Technology Case Study 22 (Washington, D.C.: Office of Technology Assessment, 1983).
43. Maria Henson, "Clark's Office Gets Complaints about Intercept Fees, Actions," *Arkansas Gazette*, March 5, 1986, p. 7A.
44. Maria M. Rullo, personal interview, September 18, 1986.
45. Cynthia Wallace, "Westworld Cuts Back to 18 Facilities, Restructures as It Struggles to Survive," *Modern Healthcare*, January 16, 1987, p. 50.
46. Cynthia Wallace, "Some of Westworld's Rural Hospitals Finding Ways to Remain in Business," *Modern Healthcare*, February 12, 1988, p. 35.
47. To evaluate the potential savings to Medicare of a program that contracted with HMOs for services, a pilot program was established by HCFA in 1982. The "risk contracts" between Medicare and HMOs were based on Medicare's paying capitation rates equivalent to 95 percent of its average costs per patient in exchange for the HMOs' providing all the Medicare-covered services needed by beneficiaries, theoretically

saving the program 5 percent. IMC was selected as one of the HMOs that would participate in the demonstration project.

48. Federal regulations are set forth under the Public Health Service Act of 1973 and the Tax Equity and Fiscal Responsibility Act of 1982 (TEFRA), which provided for the enrollment of Medicare patients under risk contracts in HMOs and other competitive medical plans. TEFRA provisions implemented in 1985 made risk contracts more feasible and appealing to HMOs by reducing the beneficiary enrollment requirements from 25,000 to 5,000 people, so long as no more than 50 percent of the enrollees were Medicare or Medicaid beneficiaries. TEFRA also increased the financial incentives to HMOs: "Instead of sharing profits with Medicare, HMOs could retain all profits up to the level of profits earned on non-Medicare enrollment." General Accounting Office, *Medicare: Issues Raised by Florida Health Maintenance Organization Demonstrations,* HRD 86.97 (Washington, D.C.: General Accounting Office, July 1986), p. 17.

49. Ibid., p. 3.

50. Florida requires that HMOs deposit a substantial sum with the state as protection against insolvency. Jeannie M. Johnson, *Introduction to Alternative Delivery Mechanisms; HMOs, PPOs, and CMPs* (Washington, D.C.: National Health Lawyers Association, 1986), p. 34. The financial solvency standards for a federally qualified HMO require that "the HMO maintain assets greater than its subordinated liabilities; 2) sufficient cash flow and adequate liability to meet its obligations as they became due; and 3) a net equity surplus." GAO, *Medicare,* p. 19.

51. GAO, *Medicare,* pp. 35–38; "Florida Health Empire Facing Tough Scrutiny," *Miami Herald,* May 11, 1986, p. 1A; Jorge Aquino, "Despite Deficits, IMC Lending to Sister Units," *South Florida Medical Review,* April 22, 1986, p. 1.

52. GAO, *Medicare,* p. 46.

53. Letter to Miguel Recarey, president of IMC, from William Roper, administrator of HCFA, May 30, 1986.

54. Ibid.

55. GAO, *Medicare,* p. 26.

56. Ibid., p. 32; John K. Iglehart, "Second Thoughts about HMOs for Medicare Patients," *New England Journal of Medicine,* June 4, 1987, p. 487.

57. "State Fines IMC $5,000 for Misleading Ads," *Florida Medical Association Today* (April 1986): 3.

58. Gregory Spears and David Lyons, "IMC Vows to Prove Solvency," *Miami Herald,* April 17, 1986, p. 1PB.

59. Alan Bavley, "HMO a 'Disgrace in Serving Elderly,' Mica Hearing Told," *Palm Beach Post,* April 2, 1986.

60. Ken Cummins, "Top HMO Is Target of Probe," *Fort Lauderdale Sun-Sentinel,* April 11, 1986, p. 1A.

61. Fred Schulte and Ken Cummins, "IMC Given Contract Despite U.S. Probe," *Fort Lauderdale Sun-Sentinel,* May 11, 1986, p. 1A.

62. Michael Abramowitz, "Sticky 'Revolving Door' at Bankrupt Health Plan," *Washington Post,* December 10, 1987, p. A-25; see also "IMC Paid Lobbyist Large Fees," *St. Petersburg Times,* May 27, 1987, p. 1.

63. Stephen Nohlgren, "IMC Paid Its Owners Millions," *St. Petersburg Times,* May 29, 1987, p. 1.

64. Ibid.; Abramowitz, "Sticky 'Revolving Door.'"

65. Iglehart, "Second Thoughts about HMOs."

66. General Accounting Office, *Medicare: Physician Incentive Payments by Hospitals Could Lead to Abuse,* GAO/HRD 86.103 (Washington, D.C.: General Accounting Office, July 1986).

67. Paul Ellwood, *The MESH Method for Helping Doctors and Hospitals Work Together* (Excelsior, Minn.: InterStudy, 1985); Marion Elmquist, "Incentive Plan Can Add Doctors to Savings Team," *Modern Healthcare,* January 4, 1985, p. 24.

68. "Kickback Plan by Hospital Hit," *American Medical News,* June 28–July 5, 1986, pp. 1, 34.

69. According to the OIG, the Paracelsus investigation is the first criminal case against a hospital since the 1979 case involving a proprietary hospital in Puerto Rico.

70. Office of the Inspector General, *Fact Sheet on the Paracelsus Investigation* (Washington, D.C.: Department of Health and Human Services, 1986).

71. *United States of America v. Paracelsus Healthcare Corporation,* U.S. District Court, Central District of California, no. 86-1065 (1986). See also "Firm Admits Fraud Guilt," *Los Angeles Times,* December 2, 1986, p. 2.

72. Office of the Inspector General, *Fact Sheet on Paracelsus.*

73. For example, the development in the late 1970s of hospice care for terminally ill patients helped to bring about more humane approaches to care. But the institutionalization of the hospice concept of care was not just a simple matter of an organization's deciding to offer a new service to the public, which either would or would not accept and use it. On the contrary, giving institutional form to the hospice concept raised many questions, beginning with ethical issues of patients' rights and professionals' responsibilities that had to be dealt with by numerous organizations involved in the regulation and financing of health care: What constitutes hospice care; who should provide it; how should they be trained; in what kinds of settings should it be provided; should facilities be licensed; what criteria should they have to meet; how much should be paid; and so forth. The proposal to use heroin for the relief of intractable pain raised its own set of issues and complications, which have yet to be resolved.

74. Vladeck, *Unloving Care,* p. 174.

75. U.S. Congress, Senate Select Committee on Aging, *Problems Associated with the Medicare Reimbursement System for Hospitals,* 97th Cong., 2d sess., 1982, p. 13.

76. Office of the Inspector General, *Chain-Operated Health Care Organi-*

*zations* (Washington, D.C.: Department of Health, Education and Welfare, August 4, 1978).

77. Ibid.

78. Amitai Etzioni and Pamela Doty, "Profit in Not-for-Profit Corporations: The Example of Health Care," *Political Science Quarterly* 91 (Fall 1976): 433–453.

79. U.S. Congress, Senate Permanent Subcommittee on Investigations, *Prepaid Health Plans and Health Maintenance Organizations*, 95th Cong., 2d sess., April 20, 1978, p. 9.

80. Ibid.

81. General Accounting Office, *Relationships between Nonprofit Prepaid Health Plans with California Medicaid Contracts and For-Profit Entities Affiliated with Them*, HRD 77.4, November 1, 1976.

82. The Internal Revenue Service questioned the tax-exempt status of this hospital but did not pursue the case beyond an initial letter of inquiry.

83. Senate Select Committee on Aging, *Problems Associated with Medicare Reimbursement System*, p. 17.

84. Ibid., p. 19.

85. Ibid.

86. GAO, *Hospital Links with Related Firms Can Conceal Unreasonable Costs*, p. 38.

87. Office of the Inspector General, *Chain-Operated Health Care Organizations*.

88. Ibid.

89. "It is the intent of the program that providers will be reimbursed for the actual costs of providing high quality care, regardless of how widely they may vary from provider to provider, except where a particular institution's costs are found to be substantially out of line with other institutions in the same area which are similar in size, scope of services, utilization, and other relevant factors." Excerpt from Health Care Financing Administration, "Provider Reimbursement Manual," sec. 5858, in *Medicare and Medicaid Guide* (Chicago: Commerce Clearing House, 1987), p. 1943.10.

90. General Accounting Office, *Problems in Auditing Medicaid Nursing Home Chains*, HRD 78.155 (Washington, D.C.: General Accounting Office, January 9, 1979).

91. General Accounting Office, letter to Health Care Financing Administration, June 30, 1980, in sec. 30,655, *Medicare and Medicaid Guide: New Developments* (Chicago: Commerce Clearing House, 1980), pp. 10, 674–684.

92. For management fees to be reimbursed by Medicare, the management contract must be the result of a competitive bidding process, the contract must be between unrelated parties, and the provider must maintain adequate documentation of the services provided.

93. "Hospital Target of Grand Jury" and "Grand Jury Presentments," *Northwest Georgian* (Cordelia), July 31, 1984, pp. 1, 4.

94. "Home Office Costs—Chain Operations," excerpt from "Health Care Financing Manual," sec. 9901–9916, in *Medicare and Medicaid Guide* (Chicago: Commerce Clearing House, 1984), pp. 3841–50. The calculation of the home office costs occurs in three stages. The first step involves the determination of home office costs that are allowable and are related to patient care. Following this step, costs are assigned to providers as they are incurred. Functional costs are allocated to the facilities on the basis of function. For example, interest expense is allocated to the facility for which the loan was made. The remaining pooled costs—that is, administrative or management services—are allocated among the providers on a reasonable basis such as number of beds. The home office is not supposed to use creative accounting to transfer pooled costs from facilities in which a low percentage of costs is attributable to Medicare patients to facilities in which Medicare pays a comparative high percentage of costs. GAO, *Problems in Auditing Medicaid Nursing Home Chains.*

95. Office of the Inspector General, *Chain-Operated Health Care Organizations*, p. 29.

96. GAO, *Problems in Auditing Medicaid Nursing Home Chains.*

97. *Medicare and Medicaid Guide: New Developments, May–December 1984* (Chicago: Commerce Clearing House, 1984), p. 9359.

98. Senate Select Committee on Aging, *Problems Associated with Medicare Reimbursement System*, p. 36.

99. Richard Kusserow, "Keynote Address," in Johnson and Siefert, *Medicare Fraud and Abuse*, pp. 41–59.

100. Sanford Tepliztky and Eugene Tillman, "Introduction," in Johnson and Siefert, *Medicare Fraud and Abuse*, pp. 1–4.

101. Senate Select Committee on Aging, *Problems Associated with Medicare Reimbursement System*, p. 40.

102. House Select Committee on Aging, *Medicaid Fraud.*

103. These limitations of state agencies were stressed in a 1979 General Accounting Office study of auditing problems involving nine nursing home chains. The study found that because the states were not effectively auditing payments to these chains, states were improperly reimbursing nursing homes for services provided by the headquarters that exceeded the allowable cost, interest on intercompany loans, and charges associated with various property transactions among related parties. In most cases the state agency had conducted a desk audit but not a field audit of the headquarters office. Typically headquarters were audited only if they were located within the state. Interstate investigations were rare, even though certain problems—such as less-than-arm's-length transactions—cannot usually be identified unless the headquarters are field audited and cost reports from related organizations are examined. "GAO Study of Medicaid Nursing Home Chains," sec. 29,485, in *Medicare and Medicaid Guide: New Developments* (Chicago: Commerce Clearing House, 1979), pp. 9378–92.

104. Excerpt from the "Health Care Financing Administration's Provider Reimbursement Manual," sec. 5868, in *Medicare and Medicaid Guide* (Chicago: Commerce Clearing House, 1987), p. 1943.39.

105. National Association of Attorneys General, *Medicaid Fraud Report* (June 1981): 5.

106. Ibid.

107. Ted Rohrlich, "Theft Counts Dismissed against LA Doctor in Medi-Cal Fraud," *Los Angeles Times*, August 6, 1983, p. 22.

108. National Association of Attorneys General, *Medicaid Fraud Report*, p. 5.

109. Telephone conversation with L. Lisa Witten, program analyst at Medi-Cal, Sacramento, June 1986.

110. Office of the Inspector General, *Semi-Annual Report, April 1984–September 1984*, p. 3. Within Florida, IMC is subject to regulations of the Department of Health and Rehabilitative Services and the Department of Insurance.

111. It can be argued that the return-on-equity (ROE) payments received by for-profit providers constitute a payment of profits. Such providers argued with some justification that this was nothing more than a fair reimbursement for the cost of equity capital, which was otherwise not provided for in a cost-based payment system. At most, however, ROE payments constitute a limited exception to the statement that providers were supposedly reimbursed only for costs under cost-based methods, and because of the way it was figured, it is not relevant to the present discussion.

7 · *Provider Efforts to Shape the Reimbursement and Regulatory Environment*

1. Paul Starr, *The Social Transformation of American Medicine* (New York: Basic Books, 1982), p. 448.

2. I heard this striking characterization in the early 1980s in a speech by Samuel Mitchell, director of research for the Federation of American Hospitals.

3. Robert A. Klein and Kathleen Drummy, "The PRRB: Its Past, Present, and Future," *Topics in Health Care Financing* 5:3 (1979): 7–16.

4. J. D. Epstein, "Significant PRRB Decisions," *Topics in Health Care Financing* 5:3 (1979): 17–61.

5. Other cases involved home health agencies, nursing homes, and other types of providers. In twenty-one cases the type of provider could not be determined. Data were compiled from the "Provider Reimbursement Review Board" section of *Medicare and Medicaid Guide* (Chicago: Commerce Clearing House, 1986).

6. Ownership status for each hospital was obtained from the appropriate year's edition of the American Hospital Association's *Guide to the*

*Health Care Field* and the Federation of American Hospitals' *Directory of Investor-Owned Hospitals.*

7. Another major decision involving stock issues came in 1985. The Hospital Corporation of America (HCA) appealed the decision of the intermediary regarding stock option plans. The issue involved whether or not the costs of employee stock options and stock purchase plans were reimbursable. Medicare laws and regulations did not specifically address the matter. HCA wanted reimbursement for costs incurred when the plans were exercised. The PRRB found that the cost of stock options must be recognized in the years in which the options were granted to the employees, not in the years in which the options were exercised. HCA appealed the ruling.

8. Epstein, "Significant PRRB Decisions," pp. 53–60.

9. "PRRB Decisions," *Medicare and Medicaid Guide* (Chicago: Commerce Clearing House, 1986).

10. In Table 7.1 an *affirmed* PRRB decision means that the position of the intermediary in disallowing costs was upheld. A *reversed* outcome means that the determination of the intermediary was deemed incorrect and that the decisions on the various issues were reversed to support the provider's position. Because many cases involved multiple issues that might produce a variety of outcomes, a *mixed* outcome indicates that some issues were decided in favor of the intermediary and some in favor of the provider. All decisions by the PRRB can be *appealed.* Decisions by the PRRB that were appealed are indicated as such. If the intermediary's determination was altered but not changed to support the position of the provider, the decision is referred to as *modified.*

11. As categorized by the Western Center for Health Planning, the issues in these cases involved, in ascending order, constitutionality of CON/1122 statutes; project coverage issues; grandfather exemption and/or effective date issues; validity of agency review procedures; general administrative and/or civil procedure issues; and substantive validity of agency CON/1122 decisions. On the last matter, the health planning agencies were supported by the courts about two-thirds of the time.

12. James B. Simpson and Ted Bogue, *The Guide to Health Planning Law: A Topical Digest of Health Planning and Certificate of Need Case Law,* 4th ed. (San Francisco: Western Center for Health Planning, 1986). In a small number of cases planning agencies were plaintiffs, but these cases generally dealt with internal agency matters, not with the activities of providers. Two cases brought by the Federal Trade Commission were included because they were a response to provider activities. In some instances several cases developed from a single set of circumstances (for example, cases that went through more than one court). These were counted as one case, and the most recent decision was treated as the outcome. Ownership of hospitals was determined

from the appropriate year's directories of the American Hospital Association and the Federation of American Hospitals.

13. The eleven states are Alabama, Arkansas, California, Florida, Georgia, Kentucky, Louisiana, Nevada, Tennessee, Texas, and Virginia.

14. Nonetheless, the presence of large numbers of investor-owned hospitals does not appear to have increased the overall level of litigation over health planning. Thirty-four percent of U.S. hospitals are in the eleven states with comparatively high percentages of for-profit hospitals; 34.4 percent of all lawsuits (including those that did not involve hospitals) took place in those states. Of the cases in which a provider was the plaintiff, 36 percent of the cases were in those states, and of the cases in which the plaintiff-provider was a hospital, 41 percent were in those states. These differences are not statistically significant.

15. Overall, 21.5 percent of protective litigation was brought to resist competition from for-profit hospitals.

16. Paul Feldstein and Glenn Melnick, "Political Contributions by Health PACs to the 96th Congress," *Inquiry* 19 (1982): 283–294.

17. From January 1, 1985, to June 30, 1986, the AMA contributed $1,052,202 to candidates for federal office and was reported to have raised $4.5 million to support its political activities. "Full Speed Ahead," press release from Common Cause, August 1, 1986; Mark Baldwin, "Industry PACs Donate Thousands to 'Maintain Access' to Legislators," *Modern Healthcare*, October 24, 1986, p. 35.

18. During the process for which data were collected, the Catholic Hospital Association (now the Catholic Health Association) did not consider itself to be a lobbying organization—its Washington office notwithstanding—and did not file the information on which my analysis is based.

19. A complication with using these data is that organizations that are tax exempt under Section 501(c)(3) of the Tax Code are not allowed to engage in any activities on behalf of a candidate for public office. Tax-exempt organizations engage in nonpartisan activities such as voter registration and the sponsoring of candidate forums. Nonprofit organizations, however, can engage indirectly in partisan activities through for-profit subsidiaries, and/or through affiliated organizations exempt under another section of the code. Douglas Hastings, William Ordaker, and Leslie Kerman, "Tax-Exempt Hospitals and Electoral Politics," *Hospitals*, August 1, 1984, p. 80. Thus, in some cases information about these affiliated organizations is used in the analyses.

20. Percentages are based on the total number of nonfederal short-term general hospitals, published in the American Hospital Association's *Hospital Statistics* (Chicago: American Hospital Association, 1986), Table 1.

21. Mark Tatge, "NME Political Donation Is Subject of FBI Probe," *Modern Healthcare*, February 1, 1985, p. 16.

22. John Harwood, "Health Firm Wields Heavy Political Clout," *St. Petersburg Times*, May 4, 1986, p. 1B.

23. "Gunter: No Conflict in Contribution from Troubled Firm," *Fort Lauderdale Sun-Sentinel,* May 5, 1986, p. 6A.

24. Harwood, "Health Firm Wields Heavy Political Clout"; "Gunter: No Conflict in Contribution."

25. "HMO under Investigation," *Key West Citizen,* May 5, 1986. Within the state, campaign contributions totaling $26,000 were given to the Insurance Commissioner by IMC affiliates and from various lawyers and consultants hired by IMC to negotiate with the Department of Insurance. "Gunter: No Conflict in Contribution."

26. Richard Harris, *A Sacred Trust* (New York: New American Library, 1966); Elton Rayack, *Professional Power and American Medicine* (Cleveland: World, 1968).

27. Beverly Enterprises, the largest nursing home chain in the nation, provides an example. Reviewing the company's history of conflict with regulatory agencies over the past several years, a journalist observed in early 1988 that the company was trying to change an image that was "tough, even callous." "Health officials from California to Florida felt the heat from Beverly's lawyers every time serious violations were cited in the nursing homes the corporation operated. Beverly attorneys filed countless appeals of citations issued by inspectors who saw the company's U.S. homes firsthand. The more appeals, the longer monetary fines and operating penalties were delayed for the violations that allegedly sometimes risked the lives of some Beverly patients." Phyllis Gapen, "Beverly Loses $30 Million—Despite Shift in Tough Image," *American Medical News,* February 19, 1988, p. 3. It was that image, earned over many years, that Beverly was seeking to change: "Officials are consciously marketing Beverly Enterprises as an enterprise focused on the provision of quality of care" (ibid.). Whether the change in behavior will go beyond marketing efforts remains to be seen. Beverly's past strategy of taking on the regulatory agencies has been there for all to see.

## 8 · For-Profit Health Care and the Accountability of Physicians

1. Mark Blumberg, "Provider Price Changes for Improved Health Care Use," in George Chacko, ed., *Health Handbook: An International Reference on Care and Cure* (Amsterdam: North Holland, 1979), p. 1060. Blumberg's number, or approximations of it, is often used without attribution in the health services research literature. It has become a part of the culture—passed along like folk wisdom. It is actually based, however, on a careful data analysis in which he distinguished patient-initiated health care utilization from utilization initiated by physicians or for which physicians act as gatekeepers (for example, admission to a hospital). The estimate excludes dental care.

2. Robert M. Veatch, "Ethical Dilemmas of For-Profit Enterprise in

Health Care," in Bradford H. Gray, ed., *The New Health Care for Profit* (Washington, D.C.: National Academy Press, 1983), p. 132.

3. American Medical Association, *Current Opinions of the Council on Ethical and Judicial Affairs of the American Medical Association, 1986* (Chicago: American Medical Association, 1986), p. 16.

4. Frances H. Miller, "Secondary Income from Recommended Treatment: Should Fiduciary Principles Constrain Physician Behavior," pp. 153–169 in Gray, *The New Health Care for Profit*, p. 154. In defining *fiduciary* she quotes from a 1928 decision by Justice Benjamin Cardozo (*Meinhard v. Salmon*) as follows: "Many forms of conduct permissible in a workaday world for those acting at arm's length, are forbidden to those bound by fiduciary ties. A fiduciary is held to something stricter than the morals of the market place. Not honesty alone, but the punctilio of an honor the most sensitive, is then the standard of behavior" (p. 154).

5. See R. Crawford Morris and Alan R. Moritz, *Doctor and Patient and the Law*, 5th ed. (St. Louis: Mosby, 1972); Angela Roddey Holder, *Medical Malpractice Law*, 2nd ed. (New York: John Wiley & Sons, 1978); Miller, "Secondary Income from Recommended Treatment." Cases in which patients have alleged fraud involve such matters as the physician's failing to be truthful about untoward events that occurred during treatment.

6. Some physicians see in the doctrine of informed consent an assumption that the physician cannot be trusted to adhere to the patient's best interests. This view helps explain why informed-consent requirements are often resented by physicians. It seems likely, however, that few physicians see informed consent as a genuine substitute for reliance on trust in the physician because they commonly believe that most patients in most circumstances make decisions based as much (or more) on trust in the physician as on the basis of an informed consent process.

7. Eric J. Cassell, "The Changing Concept of the Ideal Physician," *Daedalus* 115 (Spring 1986): 202.

8. As Bernard Barber notes, two forms of trust are involved in the doctor-patient relationship: trust in the technical competence of the professional and trust in the ethical capacity of that professional to make decisions that reflect the patient's needs and desires rather than the physician's personal interests. Bernard Barber, *The Logic and Limits of Trust* (New Brunswick, N.J.: Rutgers University Press, 1983).

9. Michael P. Powell, "Developments in the Regulation of Lawyers: Competing Segments and Market, Client, and Government Controls," *Social Forces* 64 (December 1985): 282.

10. Barber, *Logic and Limits of Trust*, p. 140.

11. Jeffrey L. Berlant, *Profession and Monopoly: A Study of Medicine in the United States and Great Britain* (Berkeley: University of California Press, 1975), p. 70.

12. Eliot Freidson, *Professional Powers: A Study of the Institutionaliza-*

*tion of Formal Knowledge* (Chicago: University of Chicago Press, 1986).

13. Talcott Parsons, *The Social System* (New York: Free Press, 1951).

14. Freidson, *Professional Powers*, p. 290.

15. Barber, *Logic and Limits of Trust*, p. 136.

16. David Mechanic, *Medical Sociology*, 2nd ed. (New York: Free Press, 1978), p. 117.

17. Medical commentators who make this point probably give insufficient recognition to the circumstances in business in which a fiduciary ethic *does* apply, as in the responsibilities of corporate directors.

18. Arnold S. Relman, "The Doctor-Patient Relationship," letter to the editor, *Wall Street Journal*, July 2, 1986, p. 27: "The doctor-patient relationship [cannot] be adequately described in purely business terms. It is not that doctors are inherently more virtuous than businessmen. They aren't. It is simply that patients have to depend on doctors to take care of them, and this trust places legal and ethical obligations on doctors that do not apply to businessmen."

19. Paul Starr, *The Social Transformation of American Medicine* (New York: Basic Books, 1982), p. 23. In a similar vein the economist Robert Evans observes that the asymmetry of information between doctor and patient "leaves open the possibility (or certainty) of severe exploitation of buyers by sellers in an arms-length, *caveat emptor* market environment." Robert G. Evans, *Strained Mercy: The Economics of Canadian Health Care* (Toronto: Butterworths, 1984), p. 71.

20. The contrast between the ethic of business and the fiduciary ethic of the professions should not, of course, be interpreted to suggest that ethics have no place in business or that businesses cannot be held accountable under some circumstances for breaches of fiduciary obligations to customers.

21. Mark Schlesinger et al., "The Privatization of Health Care and Physicians' Perceptions of Access to Hospital Services," *Milbank Quarterly* 65 (November 1, 1987): 33.

22. Site visits to investor-owned, nonprofit, and public hospitals in three cities during the Institute of Medicine's study of for-profit health care revealed perceptible differences among institutions. Relationships between medical staff and administration ranged from cooperative to contentious. Both high and low staff morale were seen, as were effects of how well the institution was doing financially; some hospitals were bustling with activity, but one was virtually deserted. Nonetheless, these matters all seemed to be independent of type of ownership. Furthermore, no matter what a hospital's ownership type, if it is located in an urban area it is likely to be in aggressive competition with other health care facilities.

23. Robert V. Pattison and Hallie M. Katz, "Investor-Owned and Not-For-Profit Hospitals," *New England Journal of Medicine*, August 11, 1983, p. 350.

24. Higher rates of ancillary service use could result, for example, from a

hospital's having more and better equipment or being more rapidly responsive to physicians' orders.

25. Ernest W. Saward, "Institutional Organization, Incentives, and Change," *Daedalus* 106 (Winter 1977): 195.

26. Starr, *Social Transformation of American Medicine,* pp. 420–449.

27. American Medical Association, *SMS Report* 2, no. 8 (November 1983).

28. American Hospital Association data from 1982 showed an average of only 0.28 physicians or dentists on the payroll of investor-owned hospitals, compared with 6 to 8 in nonprofit hospitals and 80 in hospitals in public multihospital systems. Michael A. Morrisey, Jeffrey A. Alexander, and Stephen M. Shortell, "Medical Staff Size, Hospital Privileges, and Compensation Arrangements: A Comparison of System Hospitals," in Bradford H. Gray, ed., *For-Profit Enterprise in Health Care* (Washington, D.C.: National Academy Press, 1986), p. 429.

29. Robert A. Musacchio et al., "Hospital Ownership and the Practice of Medicine: Evidence from the Physician's Perspective," in Gray, *For-Profit Enterprise in Health Care,* p. 391.

30. Jeffrey A. Alexander, Michael A. Morrisey, and Stephen M. Shortell, "Physician Participation in the Administration and Governance of System and Freestanding Hospitals: A Comparison by Type of Ownership," in Gray, *For-Profit Enterprise in Health Care,* pp. 402–421; Arthur Young and Company, *The Hospital Governing Board Chairman* (Los Angeles: Arthur Young, 1983).

31. Musacchio et al., "Hospital Ownership and the Practice of Medicine," p. 399.

32. Even under these circumstances, of course, hospitals would still have incentives to encourage physicians to admit patients to their facilities. Although hospitals have engaged in many activities to promote this effect, there is no evidence about differences between for-profit and nonprofit hospitals in encouraging what may be unnecessary use of facilities.

33. Musacchio et al., "Hospital Ownership," p. 398.

34. Roger A. Reynolds and Robert L. Ohsfeldt, eds., *Socioeconomic Characteristics of Medical Practice, 1984* (Chicago: American Medical Association, 1984), p. 34.

35. Alexander M. Capron, "Physicians and Entrepreneurism," speech delivered at conference on For-Profit Enterprise in Health Care, San Francisco, California, June 16, 1986.

36. Evans, *Strained Mercy,* p. 120.

37. Reynolds and Ohsfeldt, *Socioeconomic Characteristics of Medical Practice, 1984,* p. 16.

38. Martin Gonzales and David Emmons, eds., *Socioeconomic Characteristics of Medical Practice, 1988* (Chicago: American Medical Association, 1988), p. 6. Main expenses, as a percentage of revenues, in descending order, were payroll (17 percent), office expenses (12 percent), liability insurance (6 percent), medical supplies (5 percent), and medical equipment (3 percent).

39. Reinforcing the impression of physicians' practices as entrepreneurial enterprises is the rise of the organizational form called the professional corporation. The percentage of physicians (excluding hospital and government employees) who had adopted this legal form for their practice increased from 31 percent to 54 percent between 1975 and 1983. AMA researchers attributed the rise to the tax advantages and to physicians' desire to limit financial liability. Reynolds and Ohsfeldt, *Socioeconomic Characteristics of Medical Practice, 1984*, p. 17.

40. Circumstances under which physicians have a legal obligation to provide uncompensated care are limited. One example arises in the context of an ongoing doctor-patient relationship, in which the physician cannot abandon the patient during a period of care.

41. Eli Ginzberg, "The Monetarization of Medical Care," *New England Journal of Medicine*, May 2, 1984, pp. 1162–65.

42. Robert Wood Johnson Foundation, *Updated Report on Access to Health Care for the American People*, Special Report no. 1 (Princeton, N.J.: Robert Wood Johnson Foundation, 1983), p. 7.

43. Ibid.

44. Robert L. Ohsfeldt, "Uncompensated Medical Services Provided by Physicians and Hospitals," *Medical Care* 23 (December 1985): 1338–44.

45. Frank A. Sloan, Jerry Cromwell, and Janet B. Mitchell, *Private Physicians and Public Programs* (Lexington, Mass.: Lexington Books, 1978), chap. 8; Stephen H. Long, Russell F. Settle, and Bruce C. Stuart, "Reimbursement and Access to Physicians' Services under Medicaid," *Journal of Health Economics* 5 (1986): 235–251.

46. Peter H. Elias, "Physicians Who Limit Their Office Practice to Insured and Paying Patients," *New England Journal of Medicine*, February 6, 1986, p. 391.

47. "For, if such a nostrum be of real efficacy, any concealment regarding it is inconsistent with beneficence and professional liberality; and, if mystery alone give it value and importance, such craft implies either disgraceful ignorance, or fraudulent avarice." *Code of Ethics of the American Medical Association* (Philadelphia: Collins, 1848), p. 16. The code was adopted in May 1847.

48. Veatch, "Ethical Dilemmas of For-Profit Enterprise in Health Care," pp. 125–152.

49. Clark C. Havighurst, *Deregulating the Health Care Industry* (Cambridge, Mass.: Ballinger, 1982), p. 98.

50. Michael R. Pollard, "The Essential Role of Antitrust in a Competitive Market for Health Services," *Milbank Memorial Fund Quarterly/Health and Society* 59 (1981): 35–47.

51. American Medical Association, *Current Opinions of the Council on Ethical and Judicial Affairs of the American Medical Association* (Chicago: American Medical Association, 1986). See also Veatch, "Ethical Dilemmas."

52. A small but symbolically powerful indication of the growing commer-

cialization of medicine is the establishment by the American Medical Association of a mutual fund group called AMA Advisors. Two of the funds specialize in medical technology companies, prompting some criticism about influence on the objectivity with which the AMA renders advice on such issues as government policy regarding the regulation of medical devices. "Just Take 200 Shares and Call Me in the Morning," *Money* (September 1986): 14.

53. Roger A. Reynolds and Jonathan B. Abram, eds., *Socioeconomic Characteristics of Medical Practice, 1983* (Chicago: American Medical Association, 1983), p. 41. The most common measures, in descending order, were demographic studies of the community, surveys of patient satisfaction, satellite clinics or ambulatory care centers, and advertising.

54. Curtis E. Margo, "Selling Surgery," *New England Journal of Medicine,* June 12, 1986, pp. 1575–76.

55. Many questions as to what is misleading will undoubtedly continue to arise as advertising becomes more common. Emerging examples include whether it is misleading to advertise a referral service that refers only to the practitioners who established it; whether it is misleading for practitioners to advertise membership in a group that sounds like a certifying body but is really only a designation that they have given themselves; and what support should underlie assertions of quality using such words as *good, better,* and *best.* John D. Grad, "The Professional Advertiser: How Do We Draw the Line (If There Is a Line)?" *Law, Medicine, and Health Care* 12 (October 1984): 203.

56. The vigilance of competitors is suggested by a case that was described by a legal analyst as typical: a podiatrist's office was brought up on charges of misleading advertising because of having styled itself "The Podiatry Center" in the Yellow Pages. Grad, "Professional Advertiser," p. 203.

57. Michael S. Goldstein, "Abortion as a Medical Career Choice: Entrepreneurs, Community Physicians, and Others," *Journal of Health and Social Behavior* 25 (June 1984): 211–229. See also Michael S. Goldstein, "Creating and Controlling a Medical Market: Abortion in Los Angeles after Liberalization," *Social Problems* 31 (June 1984): 514–529.

58. Goldstein, "Abortion as a Medical Career," p. 226. He describes this process as follows: "[Initially] the law required that abortions be done in licensed hospitals. This meant that each patient had to be admitted to the hospital by a physician who was to perform the abortion and that the hospital's regulations regarding length of stay, operating room procedure, fees, and record-keeping would have to be followed. Quickly, a small number of physicians perceived that the potential demand for abortions was much greater than had been foreseen. They also realized that meeting this demand would involve reducing the cost of abortions, which in turn required that the demands of the hospitals be circumvented. There were a number of small licensed

hospitals in the area that were in very poor financial straits. Some of these came to be dominated and/or owned by the physician entrepreneurs who turned them into what were, essentially, abortion-only facilities run on an assembly line model. To operate efficiently, these facilities required a large number of patients. The necessary quantity was obtained through contracting with referral agencies, family-planning agencies, free clinics, and women's health centers . . . Thus, abortion came to be a commodity that was mass produced along quasi-industrial lines and competitively marketed. Subsequently, legislative and judicial activities that were influenced, in part, by the success, safety, economy, and popularity of the abortions provided by these facilities resulted in the legalization of freestanding outpatient abortion clinics . . . Currently, about 75 percent of all abortions are performed in freestanding abortion clinics, the majority of which are run for profit. While medical costs are rising sharply, the cost of abortions in these competitive facilities has, controlling for inflation, dropped by 28 percent since 1979 . . . The hospitals and clinics that were established by the entrepreneurs we studied currently produce the vast majority of abortions in Los Angeles." Ibid., p. 226.

59. Ibid., p. 225.
60. Goldstein, "Creating and Controlling," p. 520.
61. Incidentally, under these circumstances the interests of third-party payers are not necessarily protected. They may not want to rely on patients' and physicians' determinations of the need for or appropriateness of services in such areas. For example, for many types of outpatient psychiatry the treatment process, with its weekly or biweekly sessions between therapist and patient, may continue as long as the patient finds it useful. So long as the patient wants to continue (a desire shaped in part by ability to pay), the therapist may not be violating any kind of fiduciary responsibility in continuing to provide services. But a third-party payer who is making the service affordable to the patient may decide that some type of utilization control is necessary.
62. Robert J. FitzGibbon, "The Growth of Doctors' Office Testing," *Medical Laboratory Observer* 17 (October 1985): 9.
63. Mark S. Birenbaum, "Where Medicare's Test Work Is Going," *Medical Laboratory Observer* 17 (December 1985): 63.
64. David Mills, "Doctors Bypass Outside Labs for Blood Tests," *Wall Street Journal*, June 4, 1985. According to a trade source physicians can bill $10 to $20 for tests that cost $1 to $2 to perform. FitzGibbon, "Growth of Doctors' Office Testing," p. 9.
65. Patricia M. Johnson, "Government Regulation of In-Office Laboratories: The Debate," *Journal of Medical Technology* 2 (September 1985): 559–562.
66. Shirlyn B. McKenzie et al., "Physician's Office Laboratorians: What Should They Do? How Should They Be Educated?" *Journal of Medical Technology* 2 (September 1985): 570–574.

67. Robert Thomas Grayson, "Effects of Regulatory Controls on the Accuracy of Clinical Laboratory Tests," *Journal of Medical Technology* 1 (August 1984): 632–636.

68. The Institute of Medicine's Committee on For-Profit Enterprise in Health Care summarized these studies as follows: "A study of the use of X-ray by physicians caring for aged persons under a medical assistance program in California in 1965 showed that nonradiologists who provided 'direct X-ray services' to patients (i.e., using their own equipment) used diagnostic X-ray on twice as many patients as did physicians who referred patients to radiologists for X-ray work. A 1983 study by HCFA's Region V offices found that average per-patient reimbursement was 34 percent higher in laboratories in which primary physicians had an ownership interest than in 'non–practice-related laboratories,' because of higher prices (perhaps because it was not necessary to compete for business) and higher utilization levels. The HCFA study also cited a 1981 study by Blue Cross/Blue Shield of Michigan, which found that practice-related laboratories averaged 14–16 services per patient, as compared with 9.94 services per patient in nonpractice-related laboratories. Similarly, a small study of six laboratories by the Michigan Medical Services Administration found that patients referred by physicians who had ownership interest in the laboratories had 41 percent more tests ordered than did patients referred by non-owners.

    "Survey evidence also shows that the rate of laboratory test ordering by physicians was higher for physicians who did tests 'in house' than for physicians who referred their testing out; among those who referred their tests out, rates of testing were higher among physicians who purchased tests and billed patients than among physicians who referred their patients to laboratories that billed patients directly . . . The proliferation of such testing and the level at which it has been reimbursed are a practical explanation of the finding that physicians' incomes have risen faster than fees for their own services. Studies have also shown physicians to change the volume of services provided to patients in response to price controls or changes in payment levels." Gray, *For-Profit Enterprise in Health Care,* pp. 158–159. Citations provided in the original.

69. "The subcommittee found that evidence of improper inducements, kickbacks, and other illegal marketing practices is flagrant and inescapable. Inducements ranged from outright payments of cash to physicians, in the form of $50 deposits in secret Cayman Islands bank accounts for each lens purchased, to free stock in the manufacturer, free lasers and other IOL surgery equipment, the donation of one lens for every one purchased, keys to resort condominiums, yachts, cars and houses, trips to Colorado, Europe, and so on, for medical skiing seminars and large payments for phony consultant work." U.S. Congress, House Select Committee on Aging, Subcommittee on Health and

Long-Term Care, *Cataract Surgery: Fraud, Waste, and Abuse,* 99th Cong., 2d sess., July 19, 1985, pp. 4–5.

70. U.S. Congress, Senate Special Committee on Aging, *Fraud, Waste, and Abuse in the Medicare Pacemaker Industry* (Washington, D.C.: Government Printing Office, 1982), p. 2.

71. Rhonda L. Rundle, "Doctors Stir Controversy by Selling Drugs Directly to Patients," *Wall Street Journal,* September 29, 1986, p. 45.

72. According to trade sources in late 1986, about twenty-five companies that specialize in packaging drugs for sale to and by physicians had sprung up in the previous three years. Howard J. Anderson, "More Physicians Dispensing Commonly Prescribed Drugs," *Modern Healthcare,* November 21, 1986, p. 46.

73. Ibid., p. 46.

74. One report states physicians generally charge $2 to $3 more than their cost per prescription and suggests that a "typical primary care physician who writes 25 prescriptions a day can earn $15,000 per year." Anderson, "More Physicians Dispensing Commonly Prescribed Drugs," p. 46. Another quotes "state medical societies" as estimating that doctors could increase their income by $10,000 to $40,000 by selling the drugs they prescribe. Ronald Sullivan, "Number of Doctors Selling Prescription Drugs Grows," *New York Times,* March 19, 1987, p. B1.

75. Anderson, "More Physicians Dispensing Commonly Prescribed Drugs," p. 46.

76. Ibid., p. 46.

77. American Medical Association, *Current Opinions of the Council on Ethical and Judicial Affairs of the American Medical Association, 1986* (Chicago: American Medical Association, 1986), p. 29.

78. Ronald Sullivan, "Number of Doctors Selling Prescription Drugs Grows." For a variety of views and physician sales of prescription drugs, see Linda Bosy, "MD Drug Dispensing: Patient Convenience or Exploitation?" *American Medical News,* March 27, 1987, pp. 1, 19, 20.

79. Doug Lefton, "Firm Seeks to Market Diet Foods through MDs," *American Medical News,* October 18, 1985, pp. 3, 14. The initial program focused entirely on the overweight, but the company is developing dietary programs for patients with other needs (cholesterol reduction, hypertension, type 2 diabetes).

80. Ibid., p. 3. The company's revenues in its first fourteen months of operation were $27 million, and preparations were under way for a public offering of stock.

81. Arnold Gans, telephone interview, February 26, 1987.

82. Richard P. Kusserow, *Financial Arrangements between Physician's and Health Care Businesses: Report to Congress,* OAI-12-88-01410 (Washington, D.C.: Office of the Inspector General, Department of Health and Human Services, May 1989).

83. See the OIG study cited ibid.; see also note 68.

84. Interestingly, the rise of investor-owned hospital companies substantially reduced the extent of physician ownership of the hospitals to which they referred patients, since such independent proprietary hospitals were the primary source of acquisitions by the companies. Elizabeth Hoy and Bradford H. Gray, "Trends in the Growth of the Major Investor-Owned Hospital Companies," in Gray, *For-Profit Enterprise in Health Care,* pp. 250–259.

85. Michael A. Morrisey and Deal Chandler Brooks, "Hospital-Physician Joint Ventures: Who's Doing What," *Hospitals,* May 1, 1985, p. 74.

86. "Survey Explores Joint Venture Activity," *The Internist* 27 (April 1986): 6.

87. "Integration of the Health Care Sector: Definitions, Trends, and Implications," Report GG (I.85) of the Board of Trustees, referred to Reference Committee G (Chicago: American Medical Association, 1985).

88. "Special Report: Republic Pushes Physician Partnerships as Joint Venture Program Gains Momentum," *FAHS Review* 20 (January–February 1987): 37–38. James Buncher, board chairman and chief executive officer of Republic, was quoted as observing that physicians were looking for opportunities to make investments from which they could receive reasonable returns: "These investments . . . whether they be in surgery joint ventures, equipment joint ventures or a whole facility joint venture are designed to share the success with the physician—if, of course, we are mutually successful. We find that physicians are very receptive to that type of opportunity because if it involves a hospital, they know they can assess the risks and potentials associated with that investment" (p. 37).

89. "Special Report: Republic Pushes Physician Partnerships," p. 38.

90. Form letter dated February 5, 1985, and signed by Philip K. Hensel, M.D. (president), and Jerry B. Silver (senior vice president); emphasis in original.

91. The method of choice for avoiding the risk of losing tax exemptions appears to be corporate restructuring, with the joint venture (and other for-profit activities) located in one subsidiary or set of subsidiaries and the hospital itself in another. See, for example, John J. Gannon and Judith A. Weiland, "Structuring a Successful Joint Venture," *The Internist* 27 (April 1986): 10–12. This issue is largely irrelevant to the physicians' fiduciary responsibilities.

92. Richard A. Blacker and W. Bradley Tully, "Fraud, Abuse Issues in Cooperative Health Care Ventures: An Analysis," *FAHS Review* 20 (January–February 1987): 44.

93. Ibid., p. 44.

94. Ibid., pp. 44–45.

95. Ibid., p. 45. Blacker and Tully note that "although the rationale of Greber might be applicable to arrangements where a purpose of accepting the referring physicians as investors is to give them an incentive to

make referrals, this principle has not yet been embodied in any court decisions." Ibid., p. 45.

96. Ibid., p. 45. Approaches include allowing different investing professionals to buy disproportionate numbers of shares based on their anticipated use of the venture's services, limiting investors to physicians who have an active practice within the service area of the venture, requiring eligible investors to have no ownership interests in similar ventures, limiting investors to physicians who agree to use the venture at a specified level or to use the venture for all work they refer, retaining the venture's right to force redemption of ownership interests where it sees fit, and including prohibitions on transfer of interests to other parties.

97. Ibid., p. 45.

98. Gray, *For-Profit Enterprise in Health Care*, p. 172. It may be argued that the physician's fiduciary responsibilities to the patient extend to determining what facility or hospital can best meet the patient's needs.

99. Office of the Inspector General, "Special Fraud Alert: Joint Venture Arrangements," publication no. OIG-89-04 (Washington, D.C.: U.S. Government Printing Office, 1989).

100. Arnold S. Relman, "The Future of Medical Practice," *Health Affairs* 2 (Summer 1983): 18.

101. Gray, *For-Profit Enterprise in Health Care*, p. 163.

102. Tee L. Guidotti, "Limiting MD Investment in Health Field Ill Advised," *American Medical News*, September 14, 1984, p. 31.

103. For example, the AMA's Council on Ethical and Judicial Affairs holds that "physician ownership interest in a commercial venture with the potential for abuse is not in itself unethical," although in such a situation it would be unethical for the physician to "exploit the patient in any way, as by inappropriate or unnecessary utilization." American Medical Association, *Current Options of the Council on Ethical and Judicial Affairs*, p. 30. In a similar vein, the American Society for Internal Medicine's policy manual for practice management holds that clinical appropriateness, reasonableness of cost, availability and accessibility, and demonstrated quality of service should be the main determinants of utilization of clinical laboratories, and that financial interest in, or ownership of, a clinical laboratory by a referring physician should not in itself prohibit referral of patients to that laboratory.

104. American College of Physicians, *Ethics Manual* (Philadelphia: American College of Physicians, 1984), p. 21.

105. Richard P. Kusserow, *Financial Arrangements between Physicians and Health Care Businesses: State Laws and Regulations: A Management Advisory Report* (Washington, D.C.: Office of the Inspector General, April 1989), p. 4.

106. Ibid., p. 6.

107. Thomas H. Rice, "The Impact of Changing Medicare Reimbursement

Rates on Physician-Induced Demand," *Medical Care* 21 (August 1983): 803–815; Jon R. Gabel and Thomas H. Rice, "Reducing Public Expenditures for Physician Services: The Price of Paying Less," *Journal of Health Politics, Policy, and Law* 9 (1985): 505–609; Michael Schwartz et al., "The Effect of a Thirty Percent Reduction in Physician Fees on Medicaid Surgery Rates in Massachusetts," *American Journal of Public Health* 71:4 (1981): 370–375.

108. American Medical Association, *Current Opinions*, p. 30.
109. Gray, *For-Profit Enterprise in Health Care*, p. 163.
110. Kusserow, *Financial Arrangements: State Laws and Regulations*, p. 5.
111. It should be noted that the Institute of Medicine report, unlike the AMA, calls for disclosure not only to patients and referring physicians but also to third-party payers.

## 9 · *Organizational Dependence and the Fiduciary Ethic*

1. Eliot Freidson, *The Profession of Medicine: An Essay in the Sociology of Applied Knowledge* (New York: Dodd, Mead, 1970).
2. David J. Ottensmeyer and Howard L. Smith, "Patterns of Medical Practice in an Era of Change," *Frontiers of Health Services Management* 3 (August 1986): 5–6.
3. Walter W. Benjamin, "A Reflection on Physician Rights and the Medical Common Good," *Linacre Quarterly* 47 (February 1981): 6–7.
4. James LoGerfo, "The Implications for Quality of Care," in Richard Southby and Warren W. Greenberg, eds., *The For-Profit Hospital* (Columbus: Battelle, 1986), p. 161.
5. Milton I. Roemer, "Proletarianization of Physicians or Organization of Health Services?" *International Journal of Health Services* 16 (1986): 469.
6. Alain C. Enthoven, *Theory and Practice of Managed Competition in Health Care Finance* (Amsterdam: North Holland, 1987); see particularly chap. 2. Enthoven's conceptualization follows C. D. Weller, "'Free Choice' as a Restraint of Trade in American Health Care Delivery and Insurance," *Iowa Law Review* 69 (1984): 1351–91.
7. "Organized medicine has interpreted 'free choice of doctor' to mean that every insurance scheme must leave the patient at all times free in choice of a doctor, and that every doctor must be allowed to participate in every insurance scheme on equal terms. To the extent that the patient is insured, he is unconscious of cost. *'Free choice of provider' means that the third party payor has no bargaining power because it cannot say to the provider 'my insured patients will not go to you if the price isn't right'* . . . Thus, 'free choice of doctor' . . . is not an expression of a basic human right [but] a medical-economic concept designed to insure that there is little or no cost-consciousness on the demand side, therefore, no price competition." Enthoven, *Theory and Practice*, pp. 33–34; emphasis in original.
8. Committee on the Costs of Medical Care, *Medical Care for the Ameri-*

*can People* (Chicago: University of Chicago Press, 1932). To this day, reformers refer to the minority report that called for a national health care system based on prepayment rather than fee-for-service, as well as government integration of levels of care—from physicians to community hospitals to specialized treatment centers.

9. For example, the congressionally created Physician Payment Review Commission found that the number of physician services per Medicare beneficiary doubled between 1975 and 1985 and increased at a rate of 7 percent annually between 1980 and 1987. This was a major reason why expenditures for physician services under Part B of Medicare grew at more than twice the rate of enrollment in the program between 1980 and 1987. See the Physician Payment Review Commission, *Annual Report to Congress* (Washington, D.C.: Physician Payment Review Commission, 1988 and 1989). The growth in the volume of services provided to patients has, of course, not been limited to the Medicare program.

10. It should also be noted that the impetus toward providing a larger number of services was reinforced by the common belief among physicians that leaving something undone creates potential malpractice liability.

11. Mark Pauly, *Doctors and Their Workshops: Economic Models of Physician Behavior* (Chicago: University of Chicago Press, 1980).

12. Physicians might change hospitals for any number of reasons. "I can admit [a patient] to any hospital I want to for any reason I want. I don't have to justify that to anybody. I can admit . . . because I don't like the color of the carpet [at a competing hospital] or I don't like my parking spot." David Spinks, M.D., at a 1986 hospital kickback trial in Texas, quoted in Walt Bogdanich and Michael Waldholz, "Warm Bodies: Hospitals That Need Patients Pay Bounties for Doctors' Referrals," *Wall Street Journal*, February 27, 1989, p. 1.

13. Bogdanich and Waldholz, ibid., describe several arrangements that have been the subject of legal actions or have come to the attention of fraud and abuse authorities in recent years. Bill Stoerkel, a physician and member of a medical group that received $75,000 from an Ohio hospital in 1985 in exchange for patient referrals, is quoted in the article as contending that "most hospitals have arrangements with physicians, one way or another, where they are paying to keep them interested in using their hospital facilities" (ibid., p. A4). Available evidence makes it impossible to evaluate that statement, however, and the hospital in question failed economically after granting similar loan forgiveness to other physicians.

14. Louise B. Russell, *Technology in Hospitals* (Washington, D.C.: Brookings Institution, 1979), p. 161.

15. James C. Robinson and Harold S. Luft, "Competition and the Cost of Hospital Care, 1972 to 1982," *Journal of the American Medical Association* 257 (1987): 3241–45. But see also Glenn A. Melnick and Jack Zwanziger, "Hospital Behavior under Competition and Cost-

Containment Policies: The California Experience, 1980–85," *Journal of the American Medical Association,* November 11, 1988, pp. 2669–75.

16. Susan C. Maerki, Harold S. Luft, and Sandra S. Hunt, "Selecting Categories of Patients for Regionalization: Implications of the Relationship between Volume and Outcome," *Medical Care* 24 (February 1986): 148–158; Harold S. Luft, Sandra S. Hunt, and Susan C. Maerki, "The Volume-Outcome Relationship: Practice-Makes-Perfect or Selective-Referral Patterns?" *Health Services Research* 22 (June 1987): 157–182.

17. Jeff Goldsmith, *Can Hospitals Survive: The New Competitive Health Care Market* (Homewood, Ill.: Dow Jones-Irwin, 1982), pp. 178–180.

18. Bogdanich and Waldholz, "Warm Bodies."

19. Ibid., p. A4.

20. The extent of such joint ventures is unclear. An AMA survey of 1,700 groups found only 6 percent participating in joint ventures, while a survey of 400 groups by a private accounting firm found that 55 percent engaged in joint ventures. Whether the discrepancy is the result of sampling or definitional differences is not known. Dan Richman, "Group Practice Flourishing," *Modern Healthcare,* December 19, 1986, p. 31.

21. Donald L. Holmquest, M.D., J.D., quoted ibid., p. 31.

22. David A. Human and Joel V. Williamson, "Fraud and Abuse: Setting the Limits on Physicians' Entrepreneurship," *New England Journal of Medicine,* May 11, 1989, pp. 1275–78.

23. Freidson, *The Profession of Medicine.*

24. Ibid., p. 107.

25. Ibid.

26. Before the early 1980s it was illegal in most states for insurers or health benefit plans to contract with selected health care providers for alternative rates of payment or to offer beneficiaries economic incentives to use such providers. These are the essential features of preferred provider arrangements. Regarding the law, see Elizabeth S. Rolph et al., *State Laws and Regulations Governing Preferred Provider Organizations* (Santa Monica: Rand Corporation, 1986).

27. Arnold J. Rosoff, "The 'Corporate Practice of Medicine' Doctrine: Has Its Time Passed?" *Supplement to Health Law Digest* 12 (December 1984): 1–7.

28. Alvin R. Tarlov, "HMO Enrollment Growth and Physicians: The Third Compartment," *Health Affairs* 5 (Spring 1986): 27.

29. Milt Freudenheim, "A.M.A. Report Sees Too Many Doctors," *New York Times,* June 14, 1986, p. 15.

30. Not all medical leaders agree that the increase in numbers of physicians will create an oversupply. Joseph Boyle, M.D., executive vice president of the American Society of Internal Medicine and a past president of the American Medical Association, argues that the result will be that patients will have easier access to a physician and that

physicians will work shorter hours. He notes that a decline in physicians' average work week from fifty-five to forty hours would not only create a healthier life-style for physicians but would also create a "need" for 112,000 new physicians. Joseph F. Boyle, "Patient Care Will Still Come First," *The Internist* 27 (May–June 1986): 15–16.

31. The annual rate of decline averaged 1.2 percent during the period 1975–1982 but increased to 3.2 percent annually between 1982 and 1985. Martin L. Gonzalez and David W. Emmons, eds., *Socioeconomic Characteristics of Medical Practice, 1986* (Chicago: American Medical Association, 1986), p. 56.

32. Roger A. Reynolds and Daniel J. Duann, eds., *Socioeconomic Characteristics of Medical Practice, 1985* (Chicago: American Medical Association, 1985), p. 3.

33. Roger A. Reynolds and Robert L. Ohsfeldt, eds., *Socioeconomic Characteristics of Medical Practice, 1984* (Chicago: American Medical Association, 1984), p. 120; U.S. Department of Commerce, *Statistical Abstract of the United States* (Washington, D.C.: U.S. Government Printing Office, 1985), p. 477.

34. This is not to say that misleading advertising does not exist. One issue has been physicians' self-designation of specialty practices in the telephone book Yellow Pages and other places. While some real problems exist, the truthfulness of medical advertising is at least subject to monitoring by competitors, who have a stake in bringing misrepresentations to light.

35. Nonetheless, most hospital admissions still come either through the emergency room or through a physician. The majority of hospital advertising appears aimed at creating a caring, competent image.

36. Kari Super, "For Hospitals, Best Defense Is a Good Campaign," *Modern Healthcare*, April 10, 1987, p. 52.

37. Kari Super, "Produce Developers and Providers View the Benefits of Franchises and Licenses," *Modern Healthcare*, April 10, 1987, p. 60.

38. "Special Report: Republic Pushes Physician Partnerships as Joint Venture Program Gains Momentum," *FAHS Review* 20 (January–February 1987): 37–38.

39. As new cost-containment methods have been adopted by conventional insurers, the relative cost advantages of HMOs have been declining. A 1988 survey by the Health Insurance Assurance of America showed that employers reported that premiums for families under conventional insurance plans ($209 per month) were just slightly higher than premiums for staff and group model HMOs ($203) and were actually lower than premiums in IPA model HMOs ($226). For individual coverage, both types of HMOs' premiums were lower than conventional insurance. *Source Book of Health Insurance Data, 1989* (Washington, D.C.: Health Insurance Association of America, 1989), p. 22.

40. *HMO Industry Profile, 1989* (Washington, D.C.: Group Health Association of America, 1985), reprinted in the GHAA publication *HMO Managers Letter*, October 30, 1989, p. 4.

41. The prepaid group practice model I describe here includes both so-called staff and group models, which are distinguished by the physicians' being employees in the former case and being members of a group that contracts with the HMO in the latter. The so-called network model, in which an HMO contracts with multiple groups of physicians, may be similar either to a prepaid group practice or to an individual practice association, depending on the number of groups involved and the size of the groups.

42. *InterStudy Edge* 4 (1989): 13.

43. It should probably be noted that the origins of IPAs, as with PGPs, go back to the 1930s, but IPAs did not become a significant factor until the 1970s, and then primarily under physician control in response to the growing market share of prepaid group practices, particularly in California and Minneapolis.

44. *InterStudy Edge* 4 (1989): 13.

45. Elizabeth S. Rolph, Paul B. Ginsberg, and Susan D. Hosek, "The Regulation of Preferred Provider Arrangements," unpublished paper, Rand Corporation, 1986.

46. Charles Farkas and Phyllis Yale, "Competition or Regulation: Which Is Most Cost Effective?" presentation at the Group Health Association of America's Tenth Annual HMO Policy Conference, Washington, D.C., January 11–13, 1987.

47. Gonzalez and Emmons, *Socioeconomic Characteristics of Medical Practice, 1986*, pp. 1–3. AMA data show an increase in employed physicians from 23.4 percent in 1983 to 25.7 percent in 1985. (The survey was confined to nonfederal patient-care physicians excluding residents.)

48. Forty percent of physicians below age thirty-seven were employed in 1983. Reynolds and Ohsfeldt, *Socioeconomic Characteristics of Medical Practice, 1984*, p. 16.

49. Ibid.

50. This number is a 1987 estimate by the trade group the National Association of Freestanding Ambulatory Care Centers. Many other ambulatory care centers provide more specialized services (for example, surgery, diagnostic imaging) and receive patients less through self-referral than from physician referrals. From the standpoint of physicians' dependency on organizations for a flow of patients, ambulatory care centers that obtain patients via physician referrals represent only a small change from traditional arrangements. The major change is often the matter of where the work is done, not to whom or by whom the referral is made.

51. American Medical Care and Review Association, *Directory of Preferred Provider Organizations and the Industry Report on PPO Development* (Bethesda, Md.: 1987).

52. Arthur Owen, "What's Prepaid Care Worth to Doctors?" *Medical Economics*, March 2, 1987, pp. 202–219.

53. *InterStudy Edge* (Excelsior, Minn.: InterStudy, 1989); *GHAA National*

*Directory of HMOs* (Washington, D.C.: Group Health Association of America, 1989).

54. American Medical Care and Review Association, *Directory of Preferred Provider Organizations.*

55. Jon Gabel et al., "The Emergence and Future of PPOs," *Journal of Health Politics, Policy, and Law* 11 (Summer 1986): 306.

56. *Report of the Graduate Medical Education National Advisory Committee to the Secretary, Department of Health and Human Services,* vols. 1–7 (Washington, D.C.: Public Health Service, Health Resources Administration, 1980).

57. Tarlov, "HMO Enrollment Growth."

58. Ibid.

59. The major literature review in this area is Harold Luft, *Health Maintenance Organizations: Dimensions of Performance,* 2nd ed. (New Brunswick, N.J.: Transaction Books, 1986).

60. It may also say something about the potential for litigation in such circumstances, a possibility not discussed here. It is noteworthy that an American Bar Association publication on antitrust matters in health care states that "the denial of staff privileges has accounted for the greatest amount of antitrust litigation involving hospitals." Task Force on Antitrust Compliance Program for the Health Care Industry, *The Antitrust Health Care Handbook* (Chicago: American Bar Association, 1988), p. 15. The cases discussed in the ABA book provide no hint that exclusion of physicians on economic grounds has prompted litigation as yet, although such litigation could well arise from grounds other than antitrust (for example, defamation of character).

61. Office of the Inspector General, *National DRG Validation Study: Special Report on Premature Discharges* (Washington, D.C.: Department of Health and Human Services, 1988).

62. This evidence includes a correlation between increased Medicare spending per enrollee and decreased mortality; a shift in the site of death from hospitals to nursing homes (a shift that was largest in states with large declines in hospital lengths of stay and high levels of enrollment in HMOs); and a decline in long-term downward mortality trends in Hennepin County, Minnesota. See, respectively, Jack Hadley, "Medicare Spending and Mortality Rates of the Elderly," *Inquiry* 25 (1988): 485–493; Mark A. Sager, Elaine A. Leventhal, and Douglas Easterling, "The Impact of Medicare's Prospective Payment System on Wisconsin Nursing Homes," *Journal of the American Medical Association* 257 (1987): 1762–66; and Mark A. Sager et al., "Changes in the Location of Death after Passage of Medicare's Prospective Payment System," *New England Journal of Medicine* 320 (1989): 433–443; and Gregory L. Lindberg et al., "Health Care Cost Containment Measures and Mortality in Hennepin County's Medicaid Elderly and All Elderly," *American Journal of Public Health* 79 (November 1989): 1481–85. There is also evidence of increased admissions to nursing homes for hip fractures associated with prospective payment (perhaps

an indicator of premature hospital discharge) and an increase in complication rates in patients undergoing head and neck cancer surgery (perhaps because of shortened presurgical stays for meeting nutritional needs). John F. Fitzgerald et al., "Changing Patterns of Hip Fracture Care before and after Implementation of Prospective Payment System," *Journal of the American Medical Association* 258 (1987): 218–222; Bernard S. Linn and David S. Robinson, "The Possible Impact of DRGs on Nutritional Status of Patients Having Surgery for Cancer of the Head and Neck," *Journal of the American Medical Association* 260 (1989): 510–513.

63. Randall S. Bock, "The Pressure to Keep Prices High at a Walk-In Clinic: A Personal Experience," *New England Journal of Medicine*, September 22, 1988, pp. 785–787.

64. John E. Wennberg, "Dealing with Medical Practice Variations: A Proposal for Action," *Health Affairs* 3 (Summer 1984): 6–32; David M. Eddy and John Billings, "The Quality of Medical Evidence and Medical Practice," paper prepared for the National Leadership Conference on Health Care, Washington, D.C., 1988; Mark Chassin, "Developing Good Medical Standards We All Can Live With," *The Internist* 30 (May–June 1989): 6–9.

65. John M. Eisenberg, *Doctors' Decisions and the Costs of Medical Care* (Ann Arbor: Health Administration Press, 1986).

66. I have in mind here the factors suggested by Freidson's description of the practitioner's way of looking at the world: the aim is action, not knowledge, with action being preferred to inaction; practitioners exhibit a will to believe in the value of their actions even in the face of ambiguity; they are pragmatists who believe in and rely on apparent results rather than theory; they come to trust personal accumulated experience; they emphasize the indeterminacy or uncertainty rather than the regularity or lawful, scientific aspects of medical practice. Eliot Freidson, *The Profession of Medicine*, pp. 168–169.

67. Robert Evans, *Strained Mercy: The Economics of Canadian Health Care* (Toronto: Butterworths, 1984, p. 77).

68. Wennberg's example of mortality from prostatectomy is instructive. Wennberg, "Dealing with Medical Practice Variations," p. 24. The mortality rate generally believed by surgeons to be associated with this common surgical procedure (about 1 percent, according to the literature) turns out to be based on in-hospital experience prior to discharge. Only after patients were followed for months after discharge (which surgeons ordinarily do not do) did it become apparent that mortality from prostatectomy was actually more than 4 percent. Moreover, Wennberg and his colleagues, by linking data on surgery with mortality data from other sources, learned that 40 percent of patients in one subgroup of institutionalized patients in Maine had died within a year after having undergone a prostatectomy. The facts about postdischarge mortality were not known to Maine surgeons before the data were compiled.

69. Ibid., pp. 22–23. Two other leading researchers in this field, Joseph Restuccia and Paul Gertman, have also argued in favor of developing provider-controlled mechanisms to identify inappropriate utilization and to give systematic feedback to physicians and hospital administrators. Failure to do this, they contend, would be likely to lead to systems based on claims denials or even stronger punitive measures of cost and utilization control and thus to a loss of autonomy among providers of health care. See Joseph D. Restuccia et al., "A Comparative Analysis of Appropriateness of Hospital Use," *Health Affairs* 3 (Summer 1984): 138.

70. Eisenberg, *Doctors' Decisions and the Cost of Medical Care*, p. 112.

71. See, for example, the description of an ambulatory utilization reporting system used in the Family Health Plan of Massachusetts, in which each physician is compared to a peer group average on such measures as number of visits, number of procedures, laboratory and radiology utilization, costs, and so on, per "standard patient year." Geoffrey G. Jackson and K. L. Blank, "Utilization Reporting System Facilitates Physician Practice Analysis," *Journal of Ambulatory Care Management* 8 (February 1986): 16–29.

72. Evidence in support of this statement can be found in Chapters 8 and 10.

73. For a description of how such a system works in a successful IPA, see Michael E. Herbert, "Managed Care Systems: A Boon or Bane for Physicians?" *Connecticut Medicine* 49 (January 1985): 26–30.

74. These include a Group Health Association of America Survey of its member organizations in 1986; a Blue Cross and Blue Shield Association Survey of member plans in 1987; a survey of all HMOs by Alan Hillman in 1987; and a 1987 survey by ICF, Inc., under contract with the U.S. Department of Health and Human Services. The General Accounting Office has also made reports on this topic. For references, see Joan B. Trauner and Sibyl Tilson, "Utilization Management and Quality Assurance in Health Maintenance Organizations: An Operational Assessment," pp. 205–245 in Bradford H. Gray and Marilyn Field, eds., *Controlling Costs and Changing Patient Care? The Role of Utilization Management* (Washington, D.C.: National Academy Press, 1989).

75. Ibid., p. 226.

76. Alan L. Hillman, Mark V. Pauly, and Joseph J. Kerstein, "How Do Financial Incentives Affect Physicians' Clinical Decisions and the Financial Performance of Health Maintenance Organizations?" *New England Journal of Medicine,* July 13, 1989, pp. 86–92; see also Mathematica Policy Research, Inc., *National Medicare Competition Evaluation, Final Analysis Report: The Structure of Quality Assurance Programs in HMOs and CMPs Enrolling Medicare Beneficiaries* (Washington, D.C.: Mathematica, 1987).

77. David J. Ottensmeyer and Howard L. Smith, "Patterns of Medical Practice in an Era of Change," *Frontiers of Health Services Management* 3 (August 1986): 11.

78. This point was made in a draft of the paper that was eventually published as Donald L. Madison and Thomas R. Konrad, "Large Medical Group-Practice Organizations and Employed Physicians: A Relationship in Transition," *Milbank Quarterly* 66 (1988): 240–282.

79. Robert A. Berenson, "Capitation and Conflict of Interest," *Health Affairs* 5 (Spring 1986): 141–146.

80. The HMO was to be paid a capitation rate equivalent to 95 percent of the average adjusted per capita cost (AAPCC) that Medicare spends for patients in the fee-for-service system in that geographic area.

81. Ira Burney et al., "Medicare Physician Payment, Participation, and Reform," *Health Affairs* 3 (Winter 1984): 9.

82. Berenson, "Capitation and Conflict of Interest."

83. For a detailed empirical demonstration of the truth of this observation, see Eliot Freidson, *Doctoring Together: A Study of Professional Social Control* (New York: Elsevier, 1975).

84. *The Antitrust Health Care Handbook* (Chicago: American Bar Association, 1988), p. 33.

85. It should not be surprising that trade sources report that networks are seeking ways to increase selectivity in providers. Judith A. Hale and Mary Hunter, *From HMO Movement to Managed Care Industry: The Future of HMOs in a Volatile Healthcare Market* (Excelsior, Minn.: InterStudy, 1988), pp. 28–29.

86. Sanford Marcus, "Trade Unionism for Doctors: An Idea Whose Time Has Come," *New England Journal of Medicine,* December 6, 1984, pp. 1508–11. See also Eliot Freidson, *Professional Powers: A Study of the Institutionalization of Formal Knowledge* (Chicago: University of Chicago Press, 1986), chap. 7.

87. Freidson notes that professional employees are not eligible for protection under the act if they work as supervisors, which is defined as spending 50 percent or more of working time supervising nonprofessionals. Freidson, *Professional Powers,* pp. 141–142.

88. For example, the major issues in the 1986 strike by the Capital Alliance of Physicians against the Group Health Association (GHA), the largest HMO in Washington, D.C., were (1) the minimum number of hours per week that physicians had to spend seeing patients and (2) the creation of an incentive system tied to productivity whereby physicians who saw more patients than an "average goal" would receive financial rewards. The physicians argued that these issues would negatively affect the quality of care by turning doctors into "electronic robots" and GHA members into "machines." "D.C. Physicians' Strike against HMO Ends," *Labor Law in the Health Care Industry,* July 1986. This publication is a quarterly for clients of Epstein Becker Borsody & Green, P.C., New York.

89. Reynolds and Ohsfeldt, *Socioeconomic Characteristics of Medical Practice, 1984,* p. 15.

90. American Medical Association, *Medical Groups in the United States* (Chicago: American Medical Association, 1986).

91. Madison and Konrad, "Large Medical Group-Practice Organizations," p. 245.
92. Dan Richman, "Group Practice Flourishing," *Modern Healthcare,* December 19, 1986, p. 31. The Wichita Clinic, for example, with one hundred physicians, had a day-surgery facility, a large home health care department, and a durable medical equipment business, and was planning to provide magnetic resonance imaging services.
93. "The Trend Is toward Group Practice," *The Internist* 27 (May–June 1986): 9.
94. Madison and Konrad, "Large Medical Group-Practice Organizations."
95. Ibid., p. 250.
96. Ibid., p. 252.
97. Ibid., p. 268.
98. Mark Schlesinger, Paul D. Cleary, and David Blumenthal, "The Ownership of Health Facilities and Clinical Decisionmaking: The Case of the ESRD Industry," *Medical Care* 27 (March 1989): 244–257.

## 10 · Payers and Physicians' Patient Care Decisions

1. Indeed, third-party payers came to be criticized for being passive financiers for providers rather than organizations "primarily responsive and accountable to the public interest." See Sylvia A. Law, *Blue Cross: What Went Wrong* (New Haven: Yale University Press, 1974), p. 2. Today, although it can still be debated how well they serve the public interest—changes in the federal tax exemptions of Blue Cross in 1986 convey the view of the 99th Congress—insurance companies have had to become much more aggressive in serving the interests of their customers, particularly large employers.
2. Andrew Webber and Willis B. Goldbeck, "Utilization Review," pp. IV: 1–31 in Lewin and Associates, *Synthesis of Private Sector Health Care Initiatives* (Washington, D.C.: Assistant Secretary for Health, Department of Health and Human Services, 1984), pp. IV: 20–26.
3. Some analogies come to mind. The reviews of hospitals and HMOs in consumer-oriented publications in a few cities suggest a similarity to critiques of movies and restaurants. The publication of hospitals' mortality rates by the Health Care Financing Administration and the California PRO (California Medical Review of San Francisco) suggests a parallel with professional sports; indeed, the procompetition theorist and activist Walter McClure, in speaking of the uses of data systems about hospitals, refers to comparisons of hospitals' and physicians' batting averages. See Walter McClure, "Buying Right: The Consequences of Glut," *Business and Health* 2 (September 1985): 43.
4. Terminology in this area is far from precise and is not used in consistent ways in the field. *Managed care* often refers to alternative delivery systems, such as HMOs, which have contracted to provide a defined package of services at a fixed cost for enrollees and which, therefore, must control their costs or lose money. Yet, the extent to which HMOs

actually seek to manage the care that is provided to patients as a way of controlling costs is not well documented, and recent case studies show it to be quite variable. See Peter D. Fox, LuAnn Heinen, and Richard J. Steele, *Determinants of* HMO *Success* (Washington, D.C.: Lewin and Associates, 1986). Furthermore, neither the cost-control imperative nor active efforts to manage care are limited to HMOs. *Managed fee-for-service* generally refers to standard fee-for-service payment systems to which various types of utilization review and utilization management requirements are attached. The term *utilization management* can be used broadly to refer to the family of methods by which purchasers of service can seek to influence the behavior of providers of health care. Thus, the term would include benefit design and incentive arrangements meant to encourage cost containment, as well as the methods that are included within the narrower definition of utilization management. This definition was used in the 1989 Institute of Medicine (IOM) study on this topic, which limited utilization management to methods by which a party concerned with costs becomes involved in patient care decisions prior to the provision of services. It is this definition that I will use in this chapter and Chapter 11.

5. For example, here is a description of a problem that one utilization review company brought before its medical advisory committee for assistance in developing utilization standards.

"Problem: Freestanding centers are being established which offer multiple modality screening for vascular disease. Physicians are referring patients to the centers on a "rule out" basis, often with the most minimal clinical indications. The entrepreneurs circulate material through the medical community which at least implies that should a patient subsequently develop one of the conditions for which screening can be done, the primary physician would be at risk for a malpractice action if the patient had not been sent for screening. There is often the very clear implication that third party payments will cover all of the costs. The centers offer intravenous digital substraction angiography, intra-arterial digital substractional angiography (DSA), and CT head scans to rule out intracranial and carotid artery disease. A typical charge for intravenous DSA is $735 plus $35 for each extra run. Intra-arterial DSA begins at $1,000 and progresses upward, depending upon the number of runs. CT head scans in these centers range from $500 to $800. The total cost for screening for intracranial disease can, therefore, approach $3,000.

"Other centers offer [other screening procedures] for carotid artery disease . . . and peripheral vascular disease . . . A typical charge for these non-invasive procedures is $375.

"The literature provides no basis for patient selection, and the promotional material of the centers suggests that the entire population should be screened, implying that such screening will prevent strokes,

pulmonary emboli, and other complications of vascular disease."
(Taken from slide used in presentation by Marvin J. Shapiro, M.D.,
vice president for medical affairs, U.S. Administrators, at National
Health Policy Forum, Washington, D.C., 1986.)

6. PSROs were private organizations, often created by medical societies,
whose funding, at least initially, was from federal contracts; most
PSROs delegated many review activities to the hospitals themselves.
Hence, my use of the term *quasi-independent.*

7. For example, among the challenges in the development of valid and
useful taxonomies and criteria were the following: the extraordinary
variety that is represented by clinical medicine; the imprecision of
diagnostic labeling; various inadequacies of medical records and the
difficulty of achieving reliable results when diagnostic information is
abstracted from such records; discrepancies between diagnoses upon
admission and upon discharge; the error rate in discharge diagnoses
shown in billing information; the complexity of the factors going into
medical decision making; the paucity of the research base for much of
medical practice and the accompanying variability in how different
physicians respond to similar cases. The development of taxonomies
and criteria was clearly a formidable undertaking.

8. Health benefits are part of the total compensation for employees, and
their magnitude may affect the level of wages. From the standpoint of
international competition, total employee compensation cost is a
more significant factor than is the cost of health benefits. See Uwe E.
Reinhardt, "Health Care Spending and American Competitiveness,"
*Health Affairs* 8 (Winter 1989): 5–21.

9. J. Sanford Schwartz, "The Role of Professional Medical Societies in
Reducing Practice Variations," *Health Affairs* 3 (Summer 1984): 94.

10. Sean Sullivan, *Managing Health Care Costs: Private Sector Initiatives*
(Washington, D.C.: American Enterprise Institute, 1984), p. 16.

11. Wyatt Company, *1986 Group Benefits Survey* (n.p., n.d.), p. 18; Andrew
Webber and Willis B. Goldbeck, "Utilization Review," in *Health Care
Cost Management: Private Sector Initiatives*, ed. Peter B. Fox, Willis
B. Goldbeck, and J. J. Spies (Ann Arbor: Health Administration Press,
1984). For example, in a pilot program at Ford Motor Company in 1985,
bills were audited for 476 cases at ten hospitals where Ford's payment
had exceeded $10,000. For each billed service, registered nurse-
auditors sought documentation in patients' medical records and other
hospital records to verify that the services had been ordered, provided,
and charged properly. Errors were found in all hospitals and in 465 of
the 476 cases, and included the absence of written physician orders,
absence in patients' medical records of any documentation that the
service had been provided, and absence of charge breakdowns, as well
as billing errors and services not billed. See David J. Chinsky, "Making
More Informed Choices: Responsibilities and Opportunities for Purchasers," speech delivered at conference of Hospital Patient Account-

ing Association, February 19, 1986. Chinsky was in the Employee Insurance Department of Ford Motor Company.

12. Under the courts' interpretation of provisions of the 1973 Employee Retirement Income Security Act (ERISA), employers who created benefit plans under ERISA terms were exempted from state regulations that applied to health insurance. See Daniel M. Fox and Daniel C. Schaffer, "Health Policy and ERISA: Interest Groups and Semipreemption," *Journal of Health Politics, Policy, and Law* 14 (Summer 1989): 239–260.

13. Wyatt Company, *1986 Group Benefits Survey,* p. 18; *Employee Health Care Cost Containment,* Factpack Series no. 10 (Philadelphia: Leonard Davis Institute of Health Economics, 1986), p. 15.

14. John P. Bunker, "Surgical Manpower: A Comparison of Operations and Surgeons in the United States and in England and Wales," *New England Journal of Medicine,* January 15, 1970, pp. 135–144. A study of surgery rates in Canada and England found similar differences and strengthened the conclusion that it was numbers of surgeons, not payment systems, that accounted for the result. Eugene Vayda, "A Comparison of Surgical Rates in Canada and in England and Wales," *New England Journal of Medicine,* 1973, pp. 1224–29; see also Charles Lewis, "Variations in the Incidence of Surgery," *New England Journal of Medicine,* October 16, 1969, pp. 880–884.

15. These and other variations are documented in National Center for Health Statistics, *Utilization of Short-Stay Hospitals, United States, 1982, Annual Summary,* ser. 13, no. 78 (Hyattsville, Md.: Department of Health and Human Services, 1984); John E. Wennberg, "Dealing with Medical Practice Variations: A Proposal for Action," *Health Affairs,* Special Issue, *Variations in Medical Practice* 3 (Summer 1984): 9. See also Kathleen N. Lohr, William R. Lohr, and Robert H. Brook, *Geographic Variations in the Use of Medical Services and Surgical Procedures: A Chartbook* (Washington, D.C.: George Washington University National Health Policy Forum, 1985); John M. Eisenberg, *Doctors' Decisions and the Cost of Medical Care* (Ann Arbor: Health Administration Press, 1986); Karen M. Sandrick, "Blue Cross and Blue Shield of Michigan's Efforts to Change Practice Patterns," *Quality Review Bulletin* 10 (November 1984): 349–352.

16. A study of hospital discharges in Maine between 1980 and 1982 found that 85 percent were in diagnostic categories for which utilization rates varied across hospital service areas even more than did hysterectomy rates, "which had heretofore been considered to be a high-variation procedure (about fourfold)." Philip Caper, "Variations in Medical Practice: Implications for Health Policy," *Health Affairs* 3 (Summer 1984): 114.

17. Ibid., p. 115.

18. Robert H. Brook and Kathleen N. Lohr, "Will We Need to Ration Effective Medical Care?" *Issues in Science and Technology* 2 (Fall 1985): 68–77. Notwithstanding the obvious possibility that inap-

propriate services account for much of the variation, this has not been documented. In fact, a study of three highly variable procedures— coronary angiography, carotid endarterectomy, and upper gastrointestinal tract endoscopy—concluded that inappropriate use explained a significant share of county-to-county variation only for coronary angiography, and the authors reached the overall conclusion that little of the variation was explained by this factor. Lucian L. Leape et al., "Does Inappropriate Use Explain Small-Area Variations in the Use of Health Care Services?" *Journal of the American Medical Association* 263 (February 2, 1990): 669–672. The same group of researchers reached a similar conclusion in another study of the same three procedures. See Mark R. Chassin et al., "Does Inappropriate Use Explain Geographic Variations in the Use of Health Care Services? A Study of Three Procedures," *Journal of the American Medical Association* 258 (1987): 2533–37.

19. Brook and Lohr, "Will We Need to Ration Effective Medical Care?"
20. J. F. Sparling, "Measuring Medical Care Quality: A Comparative Study," *Hospitals* 36 (March 1962): 67; data reprinted in Avedis Donabedian et al., *Medical Care Chartbook,* 8th ed. (Ann Arbor: Health Administration Press, 1986), p. 315.
21. J. J. White, M. Satillana, and J. A. Haller, Jr., "Intensive In-Hospital Observation: A Safe Way to Decrease Unnecessary Appendectomy," *American Surgeon* 41 (December 1975): 794.
22. A full report of McCarthy's initial studies of second surgical opinions in New York City showed even higher rates: approximately 24 percent of recommended procedures were not confirmed and another 2 percent were found not to require hospitalization. E. G. McCarthy and G. Widmer, "Effects of Screening by Consultants on Recommended Elective Surgical Procedures," *New England Journal of Medicine* 291 (1974): 1331–35.
23. American College of Surgeons, *Second Surgical Opinion Programs: A Review and Progress Report* (Chicago: American College of Surgeons, 1982), p. 3.
24. For example, a study of teamster family members in New York City in 1962 found 15 percent of hospital admissions (and 40 percent of pediatric admissions) to have been unnecessary. Unnecessary admissions were notably low in teaching hospitals and high in proprietary hospitals. These data, from M. A. Morehead et al., *A Study of the Quality of Hospital Care Secured by a Sample of Teamster Family Members in New York City* (New York: Columbia University School of Public Health, 1964), pp. 52–54, are reprinted in Donabedian et al., *Medical Care Chartbook,* p. 338, which also reprints a table showing that both admission and length of stay were "appropriate" for only 74 percent of patients hospitalized in Hawaii in 1968. Beverly C. Payne et al., *The Quality of Medical Care: Evaluation and Improvement* (Chicago: Hospital Research and Educational Trust, 1976), p. 14.

25. John M. Eisenberg et al., "Computer-Based Audit to Detect and Correct Overutilization of Laboratory Tests," *Medical Care* 15 (1977): 915–921; Steven A. Schroeder, L. P. Myers, and S. J. McPhee, "The Failure of Physician Education as a Cost Containment Strategy: Report of a Prospective Controlled Trial at University Hospital," *Journal of the American Medical Association* 252 (1984): 225–230; Robert A. Hughes et al., "The Ancillary Services Review Program in Massachusetts: Experience of the 1982 Pilot Project," *New England Journal of Medicine*, October 5, 1984, pp. 1727–32.

26. D. E. Knapp et al., "Relationship of Inappropriate Drug Prescribing to Increased Length of Hospital Stay," *American Journal of Hospital Pharmacy* 36 (1979): 1333–37.

27. Constance M. Winslow et al., "The Appropriateness of Use of Coronary Angiography and Coronary Artery Bypass Surgery," *Clinical Research* 34 (April 1986): 635A. See also Mark Chassin et al., "How Coronary Angiography Is Used," *Journal of the American Medical Association*, November 13, 1988, pp. 2543–47.

28. Constance Winslow et al., "The Appropriateness of Carotid Endarterectomy," *New England Journal of Medicine*, March 24, 1988, pp. 721–727.

29. For example, a study of six hospitals by a Maryland PSRO found 25 percent of hospital days to be for "non-acute" care (that is, the patient did not need the services of an acute-care inpatient facility). Peter Borchardt, "Non-Acute Profiles," *Quality Review Bulletin* 7 (November 1981): 21. A study of 1,232 patient days at each of twenty-five sample U.S. hospitals in 1980 found that 19.1 percent of admissions were inappropriate; for patients who had been admitted appropriately, 20 percent of their days in the hospital were inappropriate. Joseph D. Restuccia et al., "A Comparative Analysis of Appropriateness of Hospital Use," *Health Affairs* 3 (Summer 1984): 130–138. Overall, the percentage of unnecessary patient days ranged from 20.5 in the rural West to 36.6 in the urban East. An analysis of data on 1,132 adults who were hospitalized during the Rand Health Insurance Experiment between 1972 and 1982 found that 23 percent of admissions were inappropriate, and another 17 percent could have been avoided through the use of ambulatory surgery. Albert L. Siu et al., "Inappropriate Use of Hospitals in a Randomized Trial of Health Insurance Plans," *New England Journal of Medicine*, November 13, 1986, pp. 1259–66. In the first study to adjust the AEP criteria to include corroboration by physician-reviewers, a sample of records of patients hospitalized in southeastern Michigan in 1983 was evaluated. For medical admissions, 12 percent of admissions and 22 percent of days of stay were found to be for "non-acute care" (care for which hospitalization was not necessary); rates for surgery were much lower—5 percent and 7 percent, respectively. Ira Strumwasser et al., "Determining Non-Acute Hospital Stays," *Business and Health* 4 (February 1987): 19.

30. Health Data Institute, *The Appropriateness Evaluation Protocol, January 1985: Lahey Clinic* (Newton, Mass.: Health Data Institute, 1985), p. 2. HDI also suggests that discretionary admissions for ambulatory procedures should be less than five percent of all admissions. These suggested levels to which inappropriate utilization might be reduced, it should be noted, come from a company that sells tools for reducing inappropriate utilization.

31. The norms against which physicians' patterns are compared have most commonly been statistical rather than professionally developed standards. For a sampling of the literature on this topic, see John E. Wennberg et al., "Changes in Tonsillectomy Rates Associated with Feedback and Review," *Pediatrics* 59 (June 1977): 824; Health Care Financing Administration, *Professional Standards Review Organizations: 1978 Program Evaluation* (Washington, D.C.: Department of Health, Education and Welfare, 1979), pp. 34–37; Peter Borchardt, "Non-Acute Profiles," *Quality Review Bulletin* 7 (November 1981): 21; Joseph D. Restuccia, "The Effect of Concurrent Feedback in Reducing Inappropriate Hospital Utilization," *Medical Care* 20 (January 1982): 46; Geoffrey G. Jackson and K. L. Blank, "Utilization Reporting System Facilitates Physician Practice Analysis," *Journal of Ambulatory Care Management* 8 (February 1986): 16–29. For a summary of studies on the efficacy of education and feedback in modifying physicians' decisions, see John M. Eisenberg, *Doctors' Decisions and the Cost of Medical Care* (Ann Arbor: Health Administration Press, 1986), chap. 6.

32. Frank J. Dyck et al., "Effect of Surveillance on the Number of Hysterectomies in the Province of Saskatchewan," *New England Journal of Medicine* 296 (1977): 1326–28.

33. Arnold M. Epstein, Colin B. Begg, and Barbara J. McNeil, "The Use of Ambulatory Testing in Prepaid and Fee-for-Service Group Practices," *New England Journal of Medicine*, April 24, 1986, pp. 1089–94.

34. Louis F. Rossiter and Gail R. Wilensky, "A Reexamination of the Use of Physician Services: The Role of Physician-Initiated Demand," *Inquiry* 20 (1983): 162–172.

35. Thomas H. Rice, "The Impact of Changing Medicare Reimbursement Rates on Physician-Induced Demand," *Medical Care* 21 (August 1983): 803–815.

36. Jon R. Gabel and Thomas H. Rice, "Reducing Public Expenditures for Physician Services: The Price of Paying Less," *Journal of Health Politics, Policy, and Law* 9 (1985): 505–609.

37. Michael Schwartz et al., "The Effect of a Thirty Percent Reduction in Physician Fees on Medicaid Surgery Rates in Massachusetts," *American Journal of Public Health* 71, no. 4 (1981): 370–375. For an excellent discussion of evidence regarding "the physician as a self-fulfilling practitioner," see Eisenberg, *Doctors' Decisions and the Costs of Medical Care*, chap. 2.

38. Harold S. Luft, *Health Maintenance Organizations: Dimensions of Performance* (New York: John Wiley & Sons, 1981), pp. 114, 250. It is important to bear in mind that most available evidence about HMOs comes from nonprofit HMOs operating in a less competitive and commercial environment than now exists.

39. Ibid., p. 114.

40. Ibid., p. 200.

41. Willard G. Manning et al., "A Controlled Trial of the Effect of a Prepaid Group Practice on Use of Services," *New England Journal of Medicine* 310 (1984): 1505–10. Regarding health outcomes, high-income people did as well (or better) in the HMO as in the fee-for-service system. This was not true for poor people, however. John E. Ware, Jr., et al., "Comparison of Health Outcomes at a Health Maintenance Organization with Those of Fee-for-Service Care," *Lancet*, May 31, 1986, pp. 1017–22.

42. Chinsky, "Making More Informed Choices."

43. Lee Iacocca, *Iacocca: An Autobiography* (New York: Bantam Books, 1984), p. 236.

44. Patricia M. Nazemetz, "Health Care Management Directions at Xerox," speech delivered at Government Research Health Leadership Conference, Washington, D.C., April 1986.

45. Glenn Richards, "Business Spurs UR Growth," *Hospitals*, March 1, 1984, p. 96.

46. For example: "At the Midwest Business Group, [Steve] King says that a lot of talking and a willingness to accommodate provider concerns usually lift resistance. 'We think there need not be coercion,' he says. However, the 'rough boys' among large companies trying to start UR programs sometimes behaved differently, he points out. Says King: 'Some companies have said to providers, "Either you do things the way we want, or we will begin retrospectively reviewing and denying claims. We will hold our employees harmless [for reimbursement], and if you want to pursue payment, you'll have to sue." Not every company has a personality to stand up like that to the hospital community.'" Ibid., p. 98.

47. Some did this by developing their own products (Blue Cross's HMOs, Humana's HumanaCare insurance products, Maxicare's acquisition of an insurance company); and some did it through joint ventures between insurers and hospital chains—Aetna and Voluntary Hospitals of America (VHA), Occidental/Provident and American Healthcare Systems (AHS), Equitable and Hospital Corporation of America (HCA).

48. A striking feature of these developments is that each type of organization apparently saw the move into the other's sector as a way to increase profit margins. The hospital companies' interest in moving into insurance developed when economic conditions for hospitals became more difficult as a result of declining admissions and tougher utilization review in the 1980s. Insurance companies, faced with small

profit margins, found the larger margins of the HMOs attractive. See Robert Patricelli, "Musings of a Blind Man: Reflections on the Health Care Industry," *Health Affairs* 5 (Summer 1986): 128–134. Obviously, when everyone thinks everyone else's grass is greener, the risk of disappointment is high.

49. Both American Medical International and National Medical Enterprises moved out of the insurance-HMO side of health care in 1986 and 1987.

50. *Review Resources: Sourcebook of Private Independent UR Companies* (Washington, D.C.: McGraw-Hill, 1987).

51. Richard M. Scheffler, James O. Gibbs, and Deborah Gurnick, *The Impact of Medicare's Prospective Payment System and Private Sector Initiatives: Blue Cross Experience, 1980–1986* (Berkeley: Research Program in Health Economics, University of California, 1988).

52. Mayo Clinic, "The Cost of Effective Utilization Review Programs," paper prepared for the Institute of Medicine Committee on Utilization Management by Third Parties, Washington, D.C., May 20, 1988.

53. American Hospital Association, *Private Utilization Review*, State Issues Monograph Series (Chicago: American Hospital Association, 1989).

54. A 1983 survey by the American Medical Peer Review Association showed that 81 PSROs had contracts to carry out utilization review activities for private organizations, in addition to their review activities for Medicare, and 192 contracts were under negotiation. Richards, "Business Spurs UR Growth," p. 98.

55. In Washington, D.C., for example, the major firms offering utilization management services in 1986 were Health Management Strategies (a Blue Cross subsidiary), Aetna, Equitable, John Hancock, Metropolitan, Prudential, Travelers, and Intracorp (which administers a psychiatric utilization review program for the American Psychiatric Association).

56. Notable in this regard are Interqual, SysteMetrics, and the Health Data Institute. HDI, for example, developed and leases utilization management software, which it estimated in 1986 was being applied to as many as 2 million beneficiaries of employee benefit packages and insurance companies. (Although this figure conveys something of the impact that the criteria and standards developed by particular companies can have, it is not particularly large by industry standards. Some of the major insurance companies that have developed utilization management programs, such as Prudential, have at least the potential to apply their programs to as many as 25 million or more people.) HDI also offers claims analysis services to enable clients to review utilization patterns and trends so as to identify possible quality problems or opportunities to reduce costs; evaluation services for possible changes in benefit plans; selective contracting services to assist insurers, employers, and health care coalitions in establishing or evaluating proposed preferred provider and selective contracting arrange-

ments; chart auditing services to evaluate appropriateness of care being provided to beneficiaries; claims monitoring software to help insurers and third-party administrators evaluate the accuracy of claims and the necessity of services prior to payment; hospital discharge data analysis services; and case management services.

57. I refer here to criteria sets such as the Appropriateness Evaluation Protocol and the Intensity of Service, Severity of Illness, and Discharge Appropriateness Screening Criteria that were developed and published by health services researchers who were involved in the PSRO program in the late 1970s (these criteria are discussed further elsewhere in this chapter) and to average length-of-stay data that are published by the Commission on Professional and Hospital Activities.

58. For a description of such a system in operation, see Michael E. Herbert, "Managed Health Systems: A Boon or Bane for Physicians," *Connecticut Medicine* 49 (January 1985): 26–30. For data on incentive arrangements in HMOs, see Alan L. Hillman, "Financial Incentives for Physicians in HMOs: Is There a Conflict of Interest?" *New England Journal of Medicine,* December 31, 1987, pp. 1743–48.

59. An advantage of fee-for-service is that it gives the payer—who is distinct and has an interest different from that of the provider—a stream of data that can be used to monitor patterns of care. A disadvantage of approaches that shift the risk to a provider organization is that the utilization management activities can all be internal to the provider organization, reaching the payer or purchaser in the form of a price. It is interesting, therefore, that employers seem to be making increased demands for utilization and cost data from HMOs, although to date this demand seems not to be motivated by the desire to monitor quality but by the belief that the HMO (not the purchaser) is reaping the benefits of good utilization control by shadow pricing (that is, setting prices just below those in the fee-for-service system) rather than passing the savings on to the purchaser.

60. An example of this last purpose is the requirement that Medicare's PROs monitor and calculate hospital-specific adverse outcome rates for each of the following six generic quality screens: adequacy of discharge planning, medical stability at discharge, deaths, nosocomial infections, unscheduled return to surgery, and trauma suffered in the hospital. PROs are required to set goals for improvement and follow hospitals' performance over time.

61. In the private sector the patient is generally responsible for the bill, so payment denials by payers are ineffective regarding providers.

62. This information is based on an interview with Michael Spinharney of Utilization Management Systems and is reported by Arnold Milstein, Linda Bergthold, and Leslie Selbovitz, "In Pursuit of Value: American Utilization Management at the Fifteen Year Mark," in *Managed Healthcare* (New York: McGraw-Hill, in press).

63. Obviously such information is most useful when it is acted on, which does not always happen. For example, a 1986 General Accounting

Office study of PROs in California, Georgia, and Florida found that although they were developing data about *instances* of substandard care, they were not using these data to develop profiles identifying providers with *patterns* of quality problems that warranted further review and action. General Accounting Office, *Medicare: Review of Quality of Care at Participating Hospitals* (Washington, D.C.: General Accounting Office, 1986). When the GAO did its own profiles of the Florida and Georgia data, it found that quality problems were heavily concentrated in a handful of institutions and physicians.

64. This approach was developed by Donald Harrington, M.D.

65. This information, like much else in this area, comes from rather occult sources. In this case my source is a paper by the leaders of National Medical Audit, a company that evaluates utilization management services for corporations. They cite a 1989 internal memo from Anthony Treni, vice president, Metropolitan Life, to "Group Field Personnel." Milstein, Bergthold, and Selbovitz, "In Pursuit of Value."

66. According to Milstein, Bergthold, and Selbovitz, "In Pursuit of Value," as of October 1989 Metropolitan had not made public any detailed information about the magnitude of savings as a percentage of total outpatient claims, or about the basis of the savings calculation. This is not unusual for claims of savings via utilization review and management.

67. Interview with Ed Zalta, president of CAPP CARE, December 1988, reported ibid.

68. Linda E. Demkovich, "Controlling Health Care Costs at General Motors," *Health Affairs* 5 (Fall 1986): 62.

69. Chinsky, "Making More Informed Choices."

70. *Business and Health* 4 (December 1986): 53.

71. A survey in early 1986 showed that 37 percent of PPOs founded after June 1984 were hospital sponsored, compared with 49 percent of PPOs founded earlier. See Jon Gabel et al., "The Emergence and Future of PPOs," *Journal of Health Politics, Policy, and Law* 11 (Summer 1986): 310. Another 1986 survey found most enrollees (59 percent) were in PPOs that were sponsored by purchasers or payers rather than providers. Gregory de Lissovoy, Thomas Rice, Jon Gabel, and Heidi J. Gelzer, "Preferred Provider Organizations One Year Later," *Inquiry* (Summer 1987): 127–135.

72. Gabel et al., "Emergence and Future of PPOs," p. 308, citing Peter Boland.

73. The discussion of disincentives is based on Walter McClure's remarks at a seminar, "Buying Right: A Case Study of Pennsylvania's Health Data Collection Legislation" sponsored by the National Health Policy Forum in Washington, D.C., November 13, 1986.

74. Although McClure (see note 73) suggests that an adequate program for ensuring and documenting the quality of care within a hospital would cost 1.2 percent of revenues, it is difficult to estimate the costs that

might result if providers knew that future business depended on their ability to maintain and document quality. Donald Berwick, M.D., a leading expert on health care quality assurance, notes that quality control activities account for 5 to 30 percent of revenues in other industries. Donald Berwick, "In Search of Practical Quality Measurement in Health Care," presentation to the National Health Policy Forum, Washington, D.C., December 12, 1986.

75. For example, in talking about his experience with cost containment and HMO development efforts in Des Moines in the late 1970s, Robert Burnett, CEO of Meridith Publishing Company, noted: "Health-care cost containment is a dirty project—it's filled with personal and sensitive relationships and interrelationships that cause any thinking person, if at all possible, to want to avoid it. Any CEO who tells you he relishes getting into the middle of that can of worms, I think, is suspect. I don't feel that way. I've been in the middle of it, and my family and I would have to leave town to get medical care in the next two or three years. I don't think it's fun and I don't like it and I wouldn't want to do it again . . . [Nonetheless] I can make more money for this corporation in the next three or four or five years . . . by doing something effective in the way of cost control than I can by selling . . . Every dollar of health care cost that's saved goes straight to the bottom line." Quoted in John K. Iglehart, "Health Care and American Business," *New England Journal of Medicine,* January 14, 1982, p. 124.

76. As one executive noted, why should an executive take risks and devote serious time to health care cost containment "when his own compensation committee review and his performance standard review don't say a damn thing about health care costs [or] health care standards? The whole arena to most CEOs is a bit on the esoteric side." Ibid., p. 124.

77. Although Pennsylvania's law is both new and notably ambitious, at least twenty-four states have programs under which statewide patient utilization data are collected. *Business and Health* 3 (April 1986): 49–50; 4 (December 1986): 48.

78. Harold S. Luft and Sandra S. Hunt, "Evaluating Individual Hospital Quality through Outcome Statistics," *Journal of the American Medical Association* 255 (May 23–30, 1986): 2780–84.

79. Douglas P. Wagner, William A. Knause, and Elizabeth A. Draper, "The Case for Adjusting Hospital Death Rates for Severity of Illness," *Health Affairs* 5 (Summer 1986): 148–153.

80. For a more extensive discussion of the arguments regarding the disclosure of utilization review data, see Institute of Medicine, *Access to Medical Review Data* (Washington, D.C.: National Academy Press, 1981).

81. See, for example, the release of mortality statistics for cardiac surgery, *Washington Post,* August 13, 1982, p. 1; *Los Angeles Times,* March 12, 1982, p. 1.

82. Press release, January 10, 1986.
83. Mark F. Baldwin, "Hospital Industry Leaders Criticize Publication of Hospital Death Rates," *Hospitals*, March 28, 1986, p. 26.
84. In addition, a growing number of states, including Florida and California, now collect and routinely publish data on utilization and costs in health facilities. The possibility of integrating such data with mortality and other outcome data is obvious.
85. Health Care Financing Administration, *Medicare Hospital Mortality Information: 1986*, 7 vols. (Washington, D.C.: Government Printing Office, 1987).
86. *Medicare Hospital Mortality Information: 1986, 1987, 1988* (Washington, D.C.: U.S. Department of Health and Human Services, n.d.).
87. "HCFA Issues Nursing Home Report Card," *Medicine & Health*, May 28, 1990, p. 1.

## 11 · Utilization Management by Third Parties

1. A California Supreme Court decision, *Sarchett v. Blue Shield of California*, 43 Cal. 3d 1, 233 Cal. Rptr. 76, 729 P. 2d 267 (1987), has upheld an insurer's right to disagree with a treating physician's determination of medical necessity and to deny payment accordingly. Yet the court also noted that any doubts should be construed in favor of coverage for the insured. See William Helvestine, "Legal Implications of Utilization Review," pp. 169–204 in Bradford H. Gray and Marilyn Field, eds., *Controlling Costs and Changing Patient Care? The Role of Utilization Management* (Washington, D.C.: National Academy Press, 1989). My reference to liability stems from another set of cases in the insurance world that pertain to good faith and fair dealing. As Helvestine (p. 180) describes it: "Many states recognize tort liability against an insurance company for breach of implied covenant of good faith and fair dealing. This cause of action exposes the defendant to punitive damages that ordinarily would not be available in a simple negligence or breach of contract case. Insurance bad faith theories are also useful to the plaintiff because they inquire directly into the process used to reach a coverage decision, and not merely the correctness of the decision itself. Similarly, the failure to provide adequate appeal rights may itself be the basis for bad faith liability."
2. Some attempts have been made in the literature to draw distinctions between unnecessary and inappropriate services, with *unnecessary* referring to services that will not help prevent, correct, or ameliorate a patient's problem, and *inappropriate* referring to a poor fit between the patient, the service needed, and the *setting* in which the service is provided. One can refer to whether a surgical procedure is *necessary* or whether the use of the hospital for a particular patient undergoing the procedure is *appropriate*. In many practical situations the distinction is difficult to adhere to. Because many third-party payment programs

limit coverage to medically necessary and/or appropriate services, these matters have been the subject of numerous lawsuits between payers that try to deny payment on those grounds and patients or providers who seek payment. For example, see Anita F. Sarro, "Determining Medical Necessity within Medicaid: A Proposal for Statutory Reform," *Nebraska Law Review* 63 (1984): 835.

3. Terminology is not standardized in this area, but I am limiting the term *utilization management* to cost-containment methods in which a party other than doctor and patient becomes involved in patient care decisions prior to the provision of services. The term *utilization review* is often used in the field in a way that encompasses both UM and retrospective review, but I am trying to maintain a distinction.

4. Gray and Field, *Controlling Costs and Changing Patient Care.* This chapter (as well as Chapter 10) has a complex relationship to the Institute of Medicine study; see footnote on first page of Chapter 10.

5. The information obtained in those site visits can be found in Chapter 3 and Appendix E of Gray and Field, *Controlling Costs and Changing Patient Care.*

6. Blue Cross and Blue Shield Association, *Second Surgical Opinion Programs: Status and Development* (Chicago: Blue Cross and Blue Shield, 1984), p. 16.

7. Among voluntary participants in the first eight years of the Cornell–New York Hospital program, nonconfirming opinions were notably high for knee surgery (51 percent), bunionectomy (47 percent), hysterectomy (41 percent), and prostatectomy (41 percent). These data come from a 1982 American College of Surgeons report on second-opinion surgery programs, which cites a contract report to the Health Care Financing Administration as the source. The most detailed presentation of results from the Cornell–New York Hospital program can be found in Eugene McCarthy, Madelon L. Finkel, and Hirsch Ruchlin, *Second Opinion Elective Surgery* (Boston: Auburn House, 1981). For a useful literature review that was published after my discussion of second opinions was written, see Ira M. Rutkow and Steven Sieverts, "Second Surgical Opinion Programs," pp. 200–214 in Ira M. Rutkow, ed., *Socioeconomics of Surgery* (St. Louis: C. V. Mosby, 1988).

8. Linda K. Demlo, "Assuring Quality of Health Care: An Overview," *Evaluation and the Health Professions* 6 (June 1983): 185; Blue Cross and Blue Shield Association, *Second Surgical Opinion Programs,* p. 17.

9. During that period, however, almost half of the patients who did not have surgery had received a *confirming* second opinion.

10. American College of Surgeons, *Second Surgical Opinion Programs: A Review and Progress Report* (Chicago: American College of Surgeons, 1982), pp. 7–8.

11. Eugene G. McCarthy, "Second Opinions in Perspective," *Business and Health* 1 (December 1983): 7.

12. Steven Sieverts, "The Effects of Surgical Second Opinions," *Bulletin of the American College of Surgeons* 66 (April 1981): 9.

13. Some studies of such case management in Medicaid programs have found that it increases costs, probably because it provides a point of entry into the health care system for beneficiaries who otherwise face difficulties in finding providers. Stephen H. Long and Russell F. Settle, "An Evaluation of Utah's Primary Care Case Management Program for Medicaid Recipients," *Medical Care* 26 (November 1988): 1021–32.

14. In Gray and Field, *Controlling Costs and Changing Patient Care,* studies are cited (p. 120) that show that in different groups 1 percent of patients account for 29 percent of expenditures, that 2 percent of patients account for 38 percent of expenses, and that 6 percent of patients account for 55 percent of expenses.

15. Foster Higgins Health Care Benefits Survey, *Report of Survey Findings* (New York: A. Foster Higgins & Co., 1987).

16. This quote comes from descriptive information about the Health Data Institute (HDI), enclosed with a letter from Howard Birnbaum, assistant vice president, July 14, 1986. Elsewhere, HDI officials observe that "any sense that the [case management consultant] is just trying to save an employer or insurance company money would cause the effort to fail." David L. Rosenbloom and Paul M. Gertman, "An Intervention Strategy for Controlling Costly Care," *Business and Health* 2 (July–August 1984): 18.

17. Some probably rare actions by case managers are so frequently mentioned that they take on a mythical quality—for example, getting the employer to pay for having ramps built and doors widened so that a patient who requires a wheelchair can return home.

18. Mary G. Henderson and Stanley S. Wallach, "Evaluating Case Management for Catastrophic Illness," *Business and Health* 4 (January 1987): 7.

19. Gray and Field, *Controlling Costs and Changing Patient Care,* p. 131.

20. Ibid., p. 131.

21. Anecdotes are available of dramatic success stories, such as the following example from the General Motors Informed Choice Plan: "GM and the union have now instituted separate coverage for substance abuse for all its employees. The benefit will use a 'gatekeeper' approach to monitor a person's progress and avoid the 'revolving door' syndrome. Records on one employee, for instance, showed an average of 106 days of absence a year for ten years, most related to alcoholism. The cost to the company's health plan: more than $6,200 a year. After enrolling in the program, the employee had no sickness or accident days in 1982, 1983, or 1984." Linda Demkovich, "Controlling Health Care Costs at General Motors," *Health Affairs* 5 (Fall 1986): 66.

22. Estimates suggest that from 20 to 40 percent of the 18 million surgical procedures performed in hospitals each year could be done in outpatient settings. Comptroller General, *Constraining National Health*

*Care Expenditures*, GAO/HRD 85.105 (Washington, D.C.: General Accounting Office, 1985), pp. 15–16. Many employers and third-party payers encourage outpatient surgery through incentives and preadmission certification requirements.

23. Foster Higgins, *Report of Survey Findings.*

24. Gabel et al., "The Emergence and Future of PPOs," *Journal of Health Politics, Policy, and Law* 11 (Summer 1986): 312.

25. The "direct controls" used by the eight HMOs studied include preauthorization for elective inpatient admissions and certain costly ambulatory services, for example, CT scans, home health care, expensive drug therapies; mandatory second opinions for certain surgical procedures (such as hysterectomies for women under age thirty-five); rules regarding procedures that must be done on an outpatient basis; rules requiring that certain presurgical testing be done either on an outpatient basis or on the day of surgery; rules prohibiting weekend admissions in nonemergency situations; and continued-stay reviews for hospital inpatients. Peter D. Fox, LuAnn Heinen, and Richard J. Steele, *Determinants of HMO Success* (Washington, D.C.: Lewin and Associates, 1986), pp. 46–47.

26. The continued-stay review process is not described separately here because it works similarly, although it is triggered differently—most commonly by the patient's approach to a length-of-stay screen.

27. Activation of the precertification process is thus usually the responsibility of the insured persons, whose health insurance benefits are structured to depend in part on their complying with the requirements. For example, requirements to pay copayments or deductibles may come into play if proper authorization is not obtained before services are provided. Such programs may also in effect increase the provider's financial risk and give an incentive to make sure that preadmission requirements have been met. For example, if a required preadmission certification is not obtained and a later determination is made by the payer's utilization management organization that the admission was not medically necessary, the provider may have little recourse against the third-party payer and may have to seek payment from a patient who had assumed that he was insured and who has learned that the services have been deemed to be medically unnecessary. For an example of such a case and an analysis of the legal issues involved, see Nathan Hershey, "Fourth-Party Audit Organizations: Practical and Legal Considerations," *Law, Medicine, and Health Care* 14 (1986): 54–65.

28. See note 4.

29. As a practical matter, initial calls are often made by hospitals because they stand to lose financially from an unauthorized admission.

30. With emergency admissions a common practice is to review the admission within forty-eight hours to certify its necessity and to assign an approved length of stay.

31. Beverly Spadotto, U.S. Administrators, telephone communication, December 11, 1986.
32. Gray and Field, *Controlling Costs and Changing Patient Care,* pp. 276–277.
33. Ibid., p. 276. Precision in reporting such figures is not warranted because most organizations provided only estimates to site visitors and because organizations differ to some extent in the amount of authority that they give to review nurses. Some organizations limit the nurse's role to obtaining information and conveying approval if the screens are passed, while other organizations allow the nurses to engage in some negotiation with providers. (One organization reported that the nurse's role was limited to obtaining information, and another used "medical secretaries" rather than nurses in this role.)
34. Hershey, "Fourth-Party Audit Organizations."
35. Arnold Milstein, Linda Bergthold, and Leslie Selbovitz, "In Pursuit of Value: American Utilization Management at the Fifteen Year Mark," in *Managed Healthcare* (New York: McGraw-Hill, forthcoming).
36. Helvestine, "Legal Implications," p. 172. The leading case is *Wickline v. California,* 192 Cal. App. 3d 1630, 239 Cal. Rptr. 810 (1986). Helvestine's article includes a summary of the facts of this case.
37. The logic of some purpose-oriented approaches is to try to list, parsimoniously yet exhaustively, all of the reasons for which the provision of the service in question (such as hospitalization) is appropriate and to do so in a way that would not also result in the inclusion of cases for which that service is not appropriate. Such lists are not made up of diagnoses, for a person with a given diagnosis might or might not need a particular service. Instead, the lists generally are composed of three categories of information: intensity of services required, severity of illness, and need for nursing and/or life-support services.
38. An example is the criteria used by at least one PRO (in Minnesota) for certifying the necessity for elective coronary artery bypass surgery: the patient must be experiencing angina pain that limits life-style; there must be evidence from a coronary angiogram that demonstrates 50 percent or more narrowing of a vessel (the angiogram must be provided to the PRO by the physician); and there must be positive evidence from a treadmill test (with exceptions for unstable angina) or status post-MI pain after MI (myocardial infarction).
39. A variant on the algorithm approach is the Model Treatment Plan (MTP) developed and used by U.S. Administrators (USA), a very large third-party administrator, with more than sixty self-insured clients and $780 million in claims in the mid-1980s. *Business Insurance,* January 27, 1986. USA describes its use in the claims-control–administration process as follows:

"MTP tracks physician practice patterns and is instrumental in screening for medical necessity. USA routinely tracks over 14,000 ICD9-CM diagnoses and all CPT-4 procedures to assist in evaluating

whether treatment rendered is appropriate and necessary for the diagnosis. Each diagnosis has been grouped into related diagnostic categories called screens. For each diagnostic screen, the type and frequency
of allowable procedures is encoded. The most common range of physician, laboratory and radiological services are specified, along with special tests that would frequently be required . . . For each procedure
listed, the frequency limitations are delineated in terms of allowable
visits per month, per quarter, and per year. The system checks the
diagnosis and procedures on each claim, comparing it against the
patient's history to determine if the MTP parameters have been exceeded. If so, the claim pends for review by the Registered Nurse
Health Care Coordinators. "The nurses review the claim, taking into
consideration other factors, such as the patient's age and general
health, and any other illnesses or conditions. The nurses may make
the decision to pay the charges. They may determine that the services
should be denied; they refer such recommendations to the Physician
Advisor for final determination." U.S. Administrators, promotional
brochure, "Health Benefits Administration Program."

40. The Appropriateness Evaluation Protocol (AEP), developed at Boston
University in the early 1970s, consists of two related lists. See Paul M.
Gertman and Joseph D. Restuccia, "The Appropriateness Evaluation
Protocol: A Technique for Assessing Unnecessary Days of Hospital
Care," *Medical Care* 19 (1981): 855–871. One is a set of eighteen
criteria (shown in Table 11.1), any one of which justifies a medical
admission to the hospital. The original version applied only to medical
admissions; before the rise of ambulatory surgery, admission for the
purpose of surgery was simply treated as appropriate. The second was a
set of twenty-seven criteria, any one of which justifies any given day of
hospitalization (medical or surgical).

41. The Intensity of Service, Severity of Illness, Discharge, and Appropriateness Screening Criteria (ISD-A), developed by Charles Jacobs, Alan
Brewster, and their colleagues at InterQual, is not easy to summarize.
It has been revised five times since its original publication in 1978 and
is now accompanied by a third edition of a set of criteria for surgery
(surgical indications monitoring, or SIM), for special care units (for
example, coronary care and intensive care), rehabilitation units, and
pediatric care. The basic ISD (now called the ISD-A since appropriateness criteria have been added) includes both a set of generic criteria
and thirteen sets of system-specific criteria (such as cardiovascular and
blood, central nervous system and head, male reproductive, psychiatric). InterQual, *The ISD-A Review System with Adult Criteria*
(Chicago: InterQual, 1986). Each set of criteria contains three subsets:
severity of illness criteria (physical findings, sudden onset of functional impairments, vital sign and blood pressure readings, laboratory
evidence), intensity of service criteria (the monitoring, medications,
treatments, and procedures being used with the patient), and discharge
screens. The generic set includes forty-one severity and seventeen ser-

vice criteria; additional criteria are built into each system-specific set. In general (and there are exceptions), an admission is deemed appropriate if the patient meets either one severity of illness criterion (for example, respiratory rate above 28 per minute) or one intensity of service criterion (such as receiving parenteral analgesics three or more times daily); after the first day both severity and intensity criteria must be met. When, during the course of a hospitalization, the intensity criteria are no longer met, the discharge screens are applied. By design, insofar as is possible, the criteria are based on objective findings, not on the physician's interpretation.

42. The Standardized Medreview Instrument (SMI) is more recent than AEP or ISD-A (having been completed in 1983) and was designed to synthesize the earlier approaches. SysteMetrics, *Standardized Medreview Instrument Reviewer's Training Manual* (Santa Barbara, Calif.: SysteMetrics, n.d.), p. 3. Like the AEP, the SMI contains separate criteria for review of appropriateness of admissions and appropriateness of days of care. The criteria are designed to determine whether the patient's condition warrants hospital-level services or whether the services that the patient is being admitted to receive can best be provided on an inpatient basis. There are 117 admission criteria in the SMI, divided into four sets: laboratory abnormalities (28 criteria, such as hemoglobin below 6 or above 18); medical problems/diseases/complications of medical or surgical care (47 criteria, such as infarction, whether bowel, brain, cerebrovascular, myocardial, or pulmonary); abnormal signs (16 criteria, including bowel distention evidenced by air fluid levels on radiology); and symptoms (24 criteria, including bleeding or hemorrhage, gross or uncontrolled). There are 56 day-of-care criteria in the SMI, 30 of which refer to acute care services being received by the patient and 26 of which refer to the patient's condition. As with the other systems, unnecessary utilization is deemed to be indicated when none of the criteria are met.

43. Milstein, Bergthold, and Selbovitz, "Pursuit of Value," pp. 28, 29.
44. Ibid.
45. See Peter S. O'Donnell, "Controlling Costs under a Fee-for-Service Plan," *Business and Health* (March 1987): 38–41; and Paul J. Feldstein, Thomas M. Wickizer, and John R. C. Wheeler, "Private Cost Containment: The Effects of Utilization Review Programs on Health Care Use and Expenditures," *New England Journal of Medicine*, May 19, 1988, pp. 1310–14. This study, based on an analysis of groups covered by one insurance company, found lower levels of hospital admissions, inpatient days, and medical expenditures among groups covered by a Health Care COMPARE utilization management program than in groups that were not covered; the possibility that the groups were different at the outset, however, was not ruled out, and a comparison of trends over a one-year period (1984–85) showed no difference between groups. For a further analysis, see Thomas M. Wickizer, John R. C. Wheeler, and Paul J. Feldstein, "Does Utilization Review Reduce

Unnecessary Hospital Care and Contain Costs?" *Medical Care* 27 (June 1989): 632–647.

46. For a more detailed discussion of the methodological issues in assessing the effects of UM programs, see Gray and Field, *Controlling Costs and Changing Patient Care*, pp. 99–116.

47. Ibid., pp. 3–4.

48. Thomas Imperiale et al., "Preadmission Screening of Medicare Patients," *Journal of the American Medical Association*, June 17, 1988, pp. 3418–21; Project HOPE, "A Study of the Preadmission Review Process," report prepared for the Prospective Payment Review Commission, Washington, D.C., 1987.

49. Even in the well-known *Wickline* case, the facts did not suggest that the utilization process had anything to do with the patient's complications. See Helvestine, "Legal Implications."

50. American Medical Association, *Guidelines for the Conduct of Prior Authorization Programs* (Chicago: American Medical Association, 1989).

51. Randall D. Cebul and Roy M. Poses, "The Comparative Cost-Effectiveness of Statistical Decision Rules and Experienced Physicians in Pharyngitis Management," *Journal of the American Medical Association* 256 (December 26, 1986): 3353–57.

52. Philip Caper, "Cost Containment Policy: Implications for the Future," *The Internist* 27 (May–June 1986): 27.

53. James B. Holloway, Jr., quoted in "Preadmission Review Angers KY Physicians," *Hospitals*, November 16, 1983, p. 52.

54. See, for example, A. E. Miller, Jr., "Thou Shalt Not Do Routine Tests," *American Medical News*, August 15, 1986, pp. 21–22.

55. Harold P. Lazar, "Doctor, Patient, Bureaucrat," *New York Times*, December 20, 1986, op. ed. page.

56. I am grateful to Stanley B. Jones for this point.

57. Harry Schwartz, "The Veterinarian Ethic," *Wall Street Journal*, July 9, 1986, p. 22.

58. Jennifer Fine, "Physicians' Group Plans to Expand National Campaign against HMOs," *Modern Healthcare*, October 24, 1986, p. 92. Examples include Physicians Who Care, of San Antonio; Traditional Health Care, in Detroit; Physicians Who Care of Southern California; and Independent Physicians of Hawaii. Even the names of these groups create ambiguity over whether the greatest concern is quality of care or physician autonomy. Among the methods used by Physicians Who Care (San Antonio) are advertising expressing their point of view, a second-opinion service for HMO enrollees, and a physician referral service. The organization was also the subject of a Federal Trade Commission investigation for an alleged boycott against three Humana-owned hospitals in San Antonio. Physician opposition to HMOs is, of course, as old as HMOs themselves. Yet the fact that so many of today's changes in health care have an explicit goal of reducing costs by cur-

tailing services lends plausibility to doctors' groups' claims that quality of care is a true concern, even though issues of self-interest are also apparent.

59. *Wickline v. State of California* (see note 36).

60. John Horty, "Payers May Be Sued for Harm Caused by Early Discharge," *Modern Healthcare*, December 5, 1986, pp. 60–61.

61. Quoted in Joseph A. Carabillo, "Liability for Treatment Decisions: How Far Does It Extend?" in *Managed Health Care: Legal and Operational Issues Facing Providers, Insurers, and Employers,* Commercial Law and Practice Course Handbook Series no. 393 (New York: Practicing Law Institute, 1986), pp. 347–348.

62. Ibid., p. 349.

63. Glen Richards, "Business Spurs UR Growth," *Hospitals,* March 1, 1984, p. 99.

64. Referring to the leading case in this area, Helvestine, "Legal Implications," p. 191, writes: "*Wickline* held that the responsibility for the hospital discharge was solely that of the physicians . . . But *Wickline* did not say how far a physician must go in appealing a denial decision . . . The hard case will arise where the physician vigorously appeals a denial, to no avail . . . At some point, if the physician's appeal is strong enough, a court is likely to hold the review entity responsible for causing at least part of the harm. But the possibility of sharing liability with another defendant is little solace to the treating physician who still remains a clear potential defendant if he withholds treatment."

65. Ibid., p. 192.

66. See *Edelman v. John F. Kennedy Hospital,* 96 N.J. 289, 475 A. 2d 585 (1984). By contrast, many hospitals provide services that physicians order but payers deem unnecessary. According to its director, Jerome Grossman (personal communication, 1988), the New England Medical Center estimates such costs at $8 million to $10 million per year, although it is not clear how much of this amount results from services that were deemed *prospectively* to be ineligible for payment.

67. This language comes from the *Wickline* case, cited in note 36. For citation and full discussion, see Helvestine, "Legal Implications."

68. See also Marilyn J. Field and Bradford H. Gray, "Should We Regulate 'Utilization Management'?" *Health Affairs* 8 (Winter 1989): 103–112.

69. There are exceptions. Among the published criteria used by some UMOs are the Appropriateness Evaluation Protocol (which is widely used although most UMOs say that they have made adaptations) and the length-of-stay norms published by the Commission on Professional and Hospital Activities. The equally widely used InterQual criteria are available for the price of a publication. The Pittsburgh Program for Affordable Health has developed and published criteria of appropriateness. Notwithstanding these examples, the basic point is true that the criteria used by UMOs are generally not open to outside review.

70. Gertman and Restuccia, "Appropriateness Evaluation Protocol."
71. Alan Brewster, M.D., president of InterQual, telephone conversation, December 2, 1986.
72. Ira Strumwasser et al., "Non-Acute Hospitalization, Cost Containment, and Resource Management," unpublished paper, March 1981.
73. Ibid.
74. The decision is also influenced by whether the validating physicians are from fee-for-service practices or from an HMO. Ira Strumwasser, personal communication.
75. Gray and Field, *Controlling Costs and Changing Patient Care*, p. 154.
76. See Helvestine, "Legal Implications," pp. 190–191.
77. Gray and Field, *Controlling Costs and Changing Patient Care*, pp. 276–279.

### 12 · The Profit Motive and Accountability in the Future

1. Other factors that underlie the accountability structure of American health care include the oft-noted American distrust of too much power centralized in government, the energetic political activities of professional and trade associations in health care, and the private nature of the doctor-patient relationship.
2. See Theodore N. McDowell, "The Medicare-Medicaid Anti-Fraud and Abuse Amendments: Their Impact on the Present Health Care System," *Emory Law Journal* 36 (1987): 691–754. The National Association of Attorneys General now has a regular publication called the *Medicaid Fraud Report*. Among private insurers an organization (the Health Care Anti-Fraud Association) has been formed to communicate about fraudulent activities among health care providers.
3. Edmund D. Pellegrino and David Thomasma, *For the Patient's Good: The Restoration of Beneficence in Health Care* (New York: Oxford University Press, 1988).
4. An American Medical Association survey in the fall of 1988 asked physicians about their experience in appealing prior-authorization decisions in the previous six months. Fewer than 25 percent said that they had "always" been able to explain medical necessity to a utilization management physician before the decision was finalized, and 27 percent said that they were "never" able to do so. *Summary Report: 1988 Payor Accountability Monitoring Survey* (Chicago: American Medical Association, May 1989). Just what these numbers mean is not altogether clear because of limitations of the survey. (For example, no data were collected on the number of cases in which appeals were actually made, and respondents were asked to report experiences in percentage terms for each of five types of third-party payers.)
5. *Wickline v. State of California* 192 Cal. App. 3d 1630, 239 Cal. Rptr. 810 (1986).
6. Eliot Freidson, *Doctoring Together* (New York: Elsevier, 1975).

7. This phrasing is borrowed from David Braybrooke, *Ethics in the World of Business* (Totowa, N.J.: Rowman and Littlefield, 1983), p. 23.

8. Darrel W. Amundsen and Gary B. Ferngren, "Philanthropy in Medicine: Some Historical Perspectives," pp. 1–31 in Earl E. Shelp, ed., *Beneficence and Health Care* (Dordrecht, Holland: D. Reidel, 1982), p. 1.

9. U.S. Congress, Senate Finance Committee, Subcommittee on Health, testimony of Carol M. McCarthy of American Hospital Association, 100th Cong., 2d sess., July 25, 1988. See also U.S. General Accounting Office, *Health Insurance: An Overview of the Working Uninsured* (Washington, D.C.: General Accounting Office, 1989).

10. Data supplied in February 1990 by Mike O'Grady of the Congressional Research Service. The number of uninsured remained quite stable in 1985 and 1986. Unofficial preliminary reports on 1987 put the figure at 31.3 million. Though not yet fully understood, this reduction appears to be due to changes in the questions used in the survey, not to an actual decline in the number of uninsured. The changes in the survey may have improved the count of the insured, particularly among college students living away from home and early retirees who were still covered by their employment-based insurance. The large *increase* in uninsured in the early 1980s, however, appears to have been real, but the *number* of uninsured may have been overestimated by several million in the years prior to 1987.

11. Depending on local circumstances, examples might include obstetrical care or neonatal intensive care units, emergency services offered in early morning hours, burn units, AIDS treatment units, units that offer experimental therapies for which third-party payers refuse to pay, and community-oriented services (such as educational programs and counseling) that are often associated with hospitals.

12. Moreover, because the nonprofits need not generate revenues to cover tax payments, and because they can raise charitable contributions as a way to defray some expenses, certain cost advantages accompany that organizational form.

13. I have in mind the adoption of such money-saving steps as Medicare's directing fiscal intermediaries and carriers to introduce unnecessary delays into the claims payment process. The federal government's methods in dealing with payment disputes have also been strongly criticized, including in the courts. See David Burda, "HHS Antics Trying Courts' Patience," *Modern Healthcare* 18 (September 2, 1988): 65–66.

14. I refer here to Internal Revenue Ruling 69-545 (issued in 1969 and still in effect) that changed IRS's criterion for tax exemptions for hospitals. In 1956 the IRS had stated (in Revenue Ruling 56-185) that for a hospital to be considered charitable under section 501(c)(3) of the Internal Revenue Code, "it must be operated to the extent of its financial ability for those not able to pay for the services rendered and not

exclusively for those who are able and expected to pay." By contrast, the 1969 ruling held that "the promotion of health is considered to be a charitable purpose," a position that was later supported in an appellate court ruling that the term *charitable* was not intended by Congress to be restricted to serving the poor. For a recent summary of the law on this point, see Elizabeth Miller Guggenheimer, "Making the Case for Voluntary Health Care Institutions: Policy Theories and Legal Approaches," pp. 35–64 in J. David Seay and Bruce C. Vladeck, eds., *In Sickness and in Health: The Mission of Voluntary Health Care Institutions* (New York: McGraw-Hill, 1988).

15. For historical data, see Herbert E. Klarman, "The Role of Philanthropy in Hospitals," *Journal of Public Health* 52 (August 1962): 1227–37. American Hospital Association data show that the average nonprofit community hospital in the United States receives 0.4 percent of its revenues via "contributions." Bradford H. Gray, ed., *For-Profit Enterprise in Health Care* (Washington, D.C.: National Academy Press, 1986), p. 100.

16. Most notable were five days of hearings by the Subcommittee on Oversight of the House Committee on Ways and Means from June 22 to June 30, 1987. These hearings, entitled "Unrelated Business Income Tax," were published in three volumes by the Ways and Means Committee.

17. Manifestations include the United Hospital Fund Project that led to the publication of *Mission Matters: A Report on the Future of Voluntary Health Care Institutions* (New York: United Hospital Fund, 1988), and J. David Seay and Bruce C. Vladeck, eds., *In Sickness and in Health* (New York: McGraw-Hill, 1988); the development by the Catholic Health Association of a model process by which member hospitals could define and document a "social accountability budget"; and a New York University project funded by the Kellogg Foundation to work with a number of hospitals to demonstrate the feasibility of a new "community benefit standard" for nonprofit hospitals. The elements of such a standard are set forth in J. David Seay and Robert M. Sigmond, "Community Benefit Standards for Hospitals: Perceptions and Performance," *Frontiers of Health Services Management* 5 (Spring 1989): 3–39.

18. This problem could also be considered from the standpoint of professional education, but that is outside the scope of this discussion.

19. Douglas F. Levinson, "Toward Full Disclosure of Referral Restrictions and Financial Incentives by Prepaid Health Plans," *New England Journal of Medicine*, December 31, 1987, pp. 1729, 1731.

20. For two recent examples, see Randall S. Bock, "The Pressure to Keep Prices High at a Walk-In Clinic: A Personal Experience," *New England Journal of Medicine*, September 22, 1988, pp. 785–787; and Henry Scovern, "A Physician's Experiences in a For-Profit Staff-Model HMO," *New England Journal of Medicine*, September 22, 1988, pp. 787–790.

21. Arnold S. Relman, "Salaried Physicians and Economic Incentives," *New England Journal of Medicine,* September 22, 1988, p. 784.

22. For example, many centers are subsidiaries of other organizations (such as hospitals) and operate under those organizations' licenses. In a similar vein, the National Association for Ambulatory Care has vigorously argued that primary care or urgent care centers are simply augmented physicians' offices and, as such, are adequately covered by the licensure requirements that apply to physicians. This argument ignores the role of organizational auspices and arrangements in influencing the behavior of physicians. Few states have licensure requirements for such centers. The development of separate accountability mechanisms may also have been retarded by the suspicion that at least some calls for licensure, accreditation, or certificate-of-need requirements are only thinly veiled attempts to protect existing institutions from competition.

23. Telephone interview with Elizabeth Flanagan, director of ambulatory care, Joint Commission for Accreditation of Healthcare Organizations, Chicago, August 22, 1985.

24. Institute of Medicine, *Improving the Quality of Care in Nursing Homes* (Washington, D.C.: National Academy Press, 1986); American Bar Association, *The "Black Box" of Home Care* (Chicago: American Bar Association, 1986). See also U.S. Congress, Senate Special Committee on Aging, "Home Care: The Agony of Indifference," 100th Cong., 1st sess., April 27, 1987.

25. U.S. General Accounting Office, *Health Care: Limited State Efforts to Assure Quality of Care outside Hospitals,* GAO HRD 90.53 (Washington, D.C.: General Accounting Office, 1990), pp. 2–3.

26. See "Summary Report: 1988 Payor Accountability Monitoring Survey" (Chicago: American Medical Association, 1989).

27. The final product of an organizing meeting that was held in Washington, D.C., in December 1989 was a document entitled "National Utilization Review Standards," American Managed Care and Review Association, January 22, 1990.

28. This was a strong theme in the Institute of Medicine report on utilization management. Bradford H. Gray and Marilyn Field, eds., *Controlling Costs and Changing Patient Care? The Role of Utilization Management* (Washington, D.C.: National Academy Press, 1989).

29. Elise Gemeinhardt, "Employer Liability in Managed Care Settings: A Discussion Paper" (Washington, D.C.: Washington Business Group on Health, 1990).

30. Notably, in his pathbreaking work on creating a health care system that has all the right internal incentives regarding cost, quality, access, and innovation, Alain Enthoven stresses the role of "plan sponsors"— the purchasers of health benefit plans whose work is essential to ensuring that quality does not suffer in the face of the competitive conditions that Enthoven favors. For a discussion of his approach, see

Alain Enthoven and Richard Kronick, "A Consumer-Choice Health Plan for the 1990s: Universal Health Insurance in a System Designed to Promote Quality and Economy," *New England Journal of Medicine,* January 5, 1989, pp. 29–37.

31. The 1989 version, entitled *Medicare Hospital Mortality Information: 1986, 1987, 1988* (Washington, D.C.: U.S. Department of Health and Human Services, n.d.), consisted of at least thirteen volumes. The volume at hand as I wrote this section was just for California and was approximately seven hundred pages long.

32. An exceptionally current, clear, and comprehensive survey of the state of the art in quality assessment can be found in Kathleen N. Lohr, ed., *Medicare: A Strategy for Quality Assurance* (Washington, D.C.: National Academy Press, 1990).

33. State of New York, Department of Health, "A Critique of the 1987 HCFA Mortality Study Based on N.Y. State Data," July 1988. Quoted in *Medical Benefits,* September 15, 1988, p. 4.

34. See Gray and Field, *Controlling Costs and Changing Patient Care,* esp. Chap. 3 and Appendix E.

# Index